COMPLICATIONS IN CUTANEOUS LASER SURGERY

[redacted]

This book is dedicated to my Research Assistant, Mussarrat Hussain MD.
He worked tirelessly in helping me organize and write this book.
Without his gallant efforts this book would never have become a reality.

COMPLICATIONS IN CUTANEOUS LASER SURGERY

DAVID J GOLDBERG MD

Clinical Professor of Dermatology
Director of Laser Research and Mohs Surgery
Mount Sinai School of Medicine, New York

Clinical Professor of Dermatology
Director of Dermatologic Surgery
UMDNJ – New Jersey Medical School

Adjunct Professor of Law
Fordham Law School, New York

Director of Skin Laser & Surgery Specialists of New York and New Jersey
Hackensack, New Jersey
USA

Taylor & Francis
Taylor & Francis Group
LONDON AND NEW YORK
A MARTIN DUNITZ BOOK

First published in the United Kingdom in 2004
by Taylor & Francis, an imprint of the Taylor & Francis Group, 2 Park Square, Milton Park, Abingdon, Oxfordshire, OX14 4RN

Tel: +44 (0) 1235 828600
Fax: +44 (0) 1235 829000
E-mail: info@dunitz.co.uk
Website: http://www.dunitz.co.uk

A CIP record for this book is available from the British Library.

Library of Congress Cataloging-in-Publication Data

Data available on application

ISBN 1 84184 245 1

Distributed in North and South America by

Taylor & Francis
2000 NW Corporate Blvd
Boca Raton, FL 33431, USA

Within Continental USA
Tel.: 800 272 7737; Fax.: 800 374 3401
Outside Continental USA
Tel.: 561 994 0555; Fax.; 561 361 6018
E-mail: orders@crcpress.com

Distributed in the rest of the world by
Thomson Publishing Services, Cheriton House
North Way, Andover
Hampshire SP10 5BE, UK
Tel.: +44 (0) 1264 332424
E-mail: salesorder.tandf@thomsonpublishingservices.co.uk

Composition by Tek-Art, Croydon, Surrey

Printed and bound in Spain by Grafos SA Arte Sobre Papel

CONTENTS

PREFACE

The concept of selective photothermolysis, conceived in 1983, revolutionized cutaneous laser therapy. A new generation of highly selective pulsed lasers that conformed to these principles was developed in the late 1980s and early 1990s. Newer systems are still evolving with each year. These lasers have been successfully employed in clinical practice for the treatment of various disorders. Selective photothermolysis remains the basis of low-risk laser treatment of photoaging skin, benign pigmented lesions and tattoos, unwanted hair, and the cutaneous vascular lesions seen within both medical and cosmetic laser dermatology. The American Society for Dermatologic Surgery estimated that, among its members, 100 million skin laser and light procedures were performed in 2003. These numbers continue to increase. With the increasing worldwide availability of more powerful lasers and light sources, complications are going to be seen with these technologies.

A basic understanding of laser–tissue interaction, as described in Chapter 1 of this book, will lessen the incidence of such complications. However, complications can and do happen. Chapter 2 describes complications seen with laser resurfacing. Chapter 3 describes complications seen after laser treatment of pigmented lesions and tattoos. Chapter 4 describes complications seen after laser treatment of unwanted hair. Finally, Chapter 5 describes complications seen after laser treatment of vascular lesions. Each chapter begins with several key points. These are followed by a discussion of the lasers used to treat the entity described in each chapter. The core of each chapter describes and illustrates the complications that can be seen with today's cutaneous lasers.

1 LASER COMPLICATIONS: LASER–TISSUE INTERACTION

KEY POINTS

(1) An understanding of basic laser–tissue interaction will lead to a lessened incidence of laser complications
(2) Complications are more common after ablative laser resurfacing as compared to non-ablative techniques. However, no dermal remodeling technique will have a zero incidence of complications
(3) Complications from pigment-specific lasers are usually related to collateral tissue damage occurring during treatment. This will be more common from millisecond, as compared to nanosecond pigmented lesion and light sources
(4) Complications from laser hair removal systems occur because of either too much heat delivered into the dermis or alternatively not enough epidermal cooling
(5) Complications from vascular lasers are generally related to excess heat or insufficient cooling. This is more common with longer wavelength systems

INTRODUCTION

Lasers represent the most precise and selective surgical tools ever made. For years electromagnetic radiation (EMR) from lasers, lamps, and other EMR sources has been used to treat a variety of medical conditions in ophthalmology, dermatology, urology, otolaryngology, and other specialties.

Dermatologic EMR sources have been used to perform a wide variety of procedures including hair removal, treatment of pigmented lesions, removal of unwanted vascular lesions, tattoo removal, and skin resurfacing (Figure 1.1). For all these treatments, a natural or artificial chromophore present in the body is heated by absorption of either monochromatic or broadband EMR. Typical natural

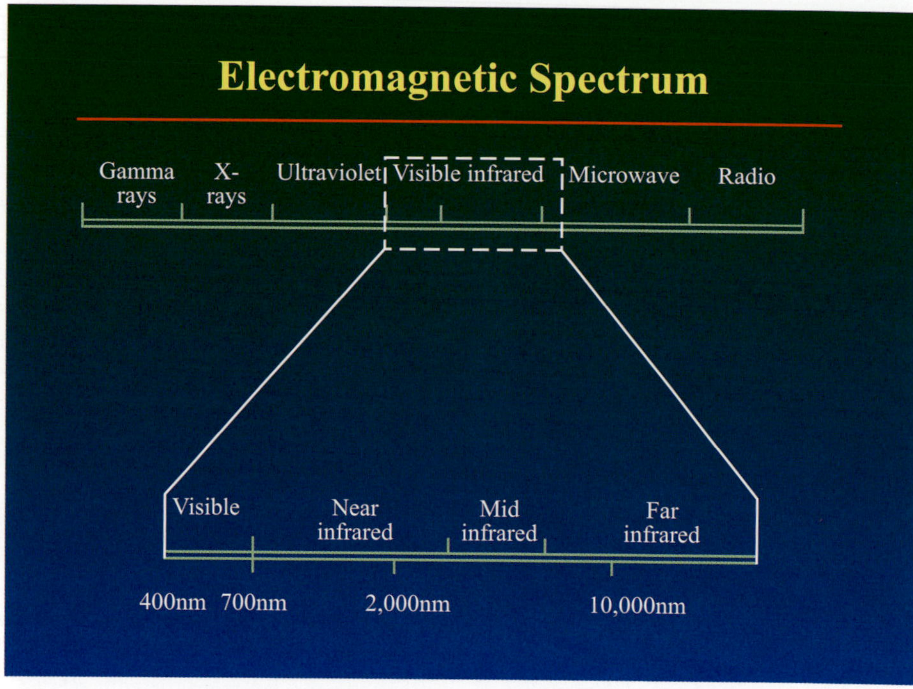

Figure 1.1. Electromagnetic spectrum (EMR) utilized in dermatologic laser treatments

chromophores include water, melanin, and hemoglobin. Artificial chromophores include the various dyes and inks seen in tattoos.

The entire skin is accessible to light. At an optical wavelength of about 1200 nm, about one quarter of the incident light goes entirely through the dermis.[1] In principle, then, every cell type and multicellular structure in the skin is a potential treatment target. However, according to the Grotthus-Draper law, selective photothermolysis and all associated light-activated mechanisms must begin with light absorption of a penetrating light.

Excellent progress has been seen when the EMR 'target' is the natural chromophores of hemoglobin or melanin. In tattoo removal, an exogenous pigment defines the target. There is no single laser (wavelength) that will perform every kind of laser surgery. While performing laser surgery, attention must be focused not only on the laser's potential to perform precise treatments, but also on the destructive potential of that same EMR-emitting system. It is this destructive potential that forms the basis of potential complications that may be associated with cutaneous laser surgery.

In the ultimate analysis, current laser systems all heat an absorbing target. A laser surgeon wishes to avoid excess thermal injury to tissue. There is, generally, a transitional zone between death and survival of any biologic system heated above its normal temperature. Any combination of temperature and time, corresponding to a point lying beyond the transition zone, will lead to the potential for excess tissue injury and resultant complications.

BASIC LASER PRINCIPLES

The term LASER is an acronym for the words Light Amplification by the Stimulated Emission of Radiation (Figure 1.2). Radiation may be defined as the transmission of energy from one point in space to another, with or without an intervening material absorbing medium.

Radiation can be:

I. *Particulate radiation.* Particulate radiation is a stream of material particles, such as electrons, neutrons, or other atomic fragments. This kind of radiation needs no material medium for its transmission, but can pass through various mediums, usually with some attenuation and/or change of direction. Particulate radiation requires a transfer of mass, and the energy transmitted is the kinetic energy of the moving particles. Dermatologic lasers do not fit into this category.

II. *Mechanical radiation.* Mechanical radiation is the transmission of vibrations through a material medium. Sound is an example. Mechanical radiation requires the presence of a material medium for its transmission. However, the

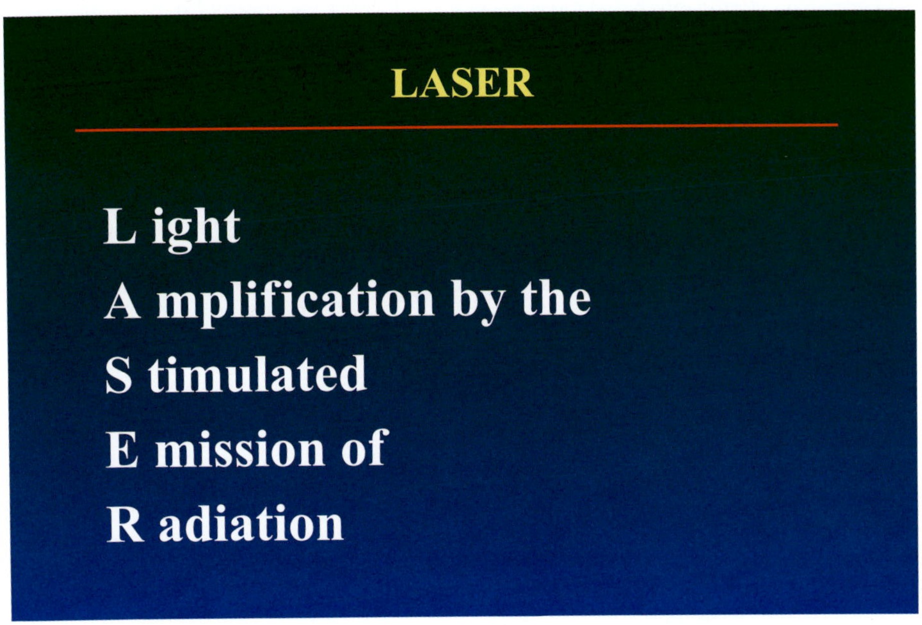

Figure 1.2. LASER (Light Amplification by the Stimulated Emission of Radiation)

medium need not move as a whole; its particles merely oscillate elastically about fixed positions, transmitting energy from one to the next. Current dermatologic lasers also do not fit into this category.

III. *Electromagnetic radiation (EMR).* EMR is what current dermatologic lasers produce. Unlike mechanical radiation, electromagnetic radiation requires no medium for its transmission, as it can travel through free space devoid of any matter whatever. It can also propagate through space-containing matter in the form of gases, liquids, or solids. Upon entering such mediums electromagnetic radiation will, in general, be changed in direction and speed of propagation.

ELECTROMAGNETIC SPECTRUM

The range of values in terms of frequency, wavelength, and/or photonic energy encountered in the natural universe is known as the electromagnetic spectrum. In terms of any one of these parameters, there may be a span of some ×20 magnitude. At the very short end of the wavelength spectrum, there are cosmic rays, and at the very long end there are radio waves.

In general, lasers generate EMR ranging in wavelengths from 100 nm to 20 000 nm (1 nm = 1×10^{-9} m). Although for simplicity these wavelengths are all called 'light', by strict definition light is only the interval from 400 nm to 700 nm. This is the light which our eyes can perceive in daylight (the visible light spectrum).

The amount of laser energy delivered per area is fluence, sometimes called the dose, usually given in J/cm^2 (joules). The rate at which energy is delivered is called power, measured in watts (W). Power delivered per unit area is therefore the rate of energy delivery per amount of skin surface. This is called the irradiance, usually given in W/cm^2. Laser exposure duration (pulsewidth) for pulsed lasers, is an extremely important term because this parameter defines the time over which energy is delivered. Finally, the laser delivery system spot size may greatly affect intensity within the skin.

BASIC ELEMENTS OF LASERS

Every laser has certain common elements of structure and function (Figure 1.3). These common elements are:

I. A material medium having the proper energy levels to produce the desired wavelengths of light. The mediums available today for lasers include hundreds of different materials grouped into three basic categories: gases, liquids, and solids.

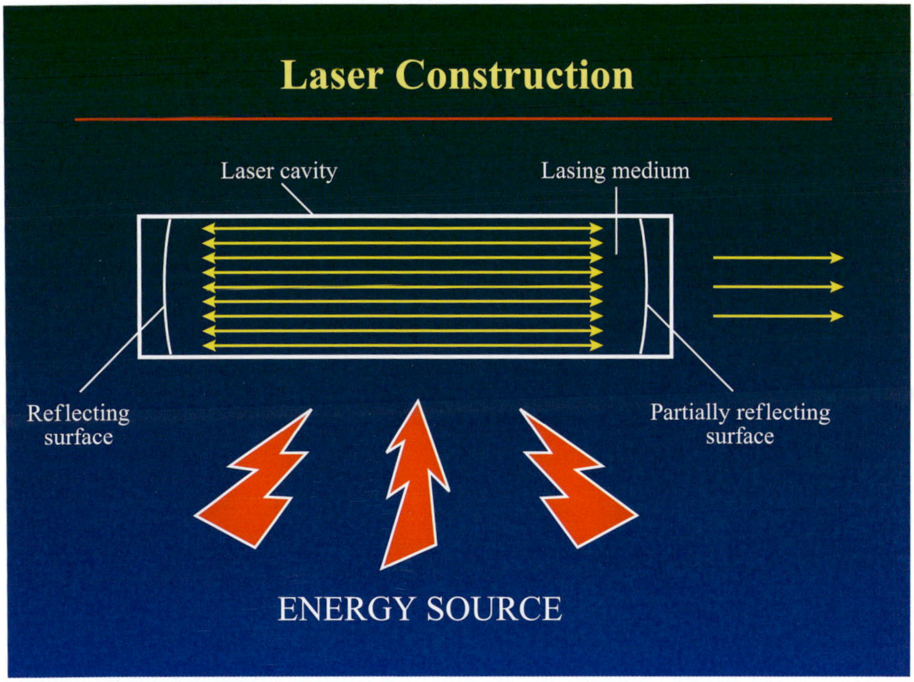

Figure 1.3. Laser structure

II. A resonant optical cavity shaped in the form of a cylinder whose length is much greater than its diameter, and having coaxial mirrors at opposite ends of it.
III. An external source of energy to provide the excitation of the atoms or molecules of the medium by the process of pumping.
IV. The delivery system which may be composed of fiberoptics or articulating mirrors. Not all wavelengths of laser light can be transmitted efficiently through a slender quartz optical fiber, the most flexible and convenient device of all. In non-invasive cosmetic laser dermatology, where laser wavelengths lie in a range from 300 nm to 2100 nm, the most commonly used delivery system is the quartz optical fiber. Wavelengths in the mid-to-far infrared (2500–20 000 nm ablative lasers) range of the spectrum must be transmitted via a series of articulating mirrors.

GENERATION OF LASER LIGHT

Laser light is generated when the laser medium is pumped by the introduction of energy from an external source. Some of the atoms or molecules in the medium will be excited into an upper level of energy. From there, one sees a possible downward radiative transition to a lower level that is above the ground level. The difference between this upper level and the original status of the laser medium determines the frequency and wavelength of the emitted laser radiation.

UNIQUE/SPECIAL PROPERTIES/ CHARACTERISTICS OF LASER LIGHT

It is now well established that laser light has three unique/special characteristics:

1. Collimation
2. Coherence
3. Monochromaticity.

Collimation: Laser-emitted rays are collimated in that they emanate from a laser, and all rays are parallel to each other. Because of this property of laser light there is no divergence or convergence of laser-emitted radiation, unless a lens or mirror is placed in front of the beam path.

Coherence: Laser-emitted irradiation is coherent in that the rays are in phase with each other in both space and time. Spatial coherence means that the crests and troughs of all the waves coincide along lines perpendicular to the rays. Temporal coherence means that the frequency, wavelength, and speed of travel are all constant.

Monochromaticity: Laser light is said to be monochromatic in that it consists of just one wavelength. In reality, no light source produces just a single wavelength, but the bandwidth variation of dermatologic lasers is generally no more than 0.1 nm.

LASER–TISSUE INTERACTION

Laser–tissue interaction leads to four fundamental optical phenomena:

1. Reflection and backscattering from the surface at impact
2. Transmission into or through the tissue
3. Absorption by the tissue
4. Scattering within and perhaps out of the tissue.

Reflection

In general, reflection shows pronounced variations within the spectral range of 400 –1500 nm. This reflection is strongly dependent on the pigments present in the absorbing tissue. However, in the ranges of 100–300 nm and 2000–40 000 nm, reflectance is 'colorblind'. The most significant practical effect of reflection of laser light from living tissue is the reduction of power density of the laser irradiation once there is actual penetration into tissue.

Transmission

Transmission is measured in terms of transmittance, which is the ratio of the intensity of a transmitted ray as it emerges distally from the absorbing tissue to that of the same ray immediately after entering the tissue.

Absorption

Absorption of laser energy leads to the conversion of the radiant laser energy into other forms of energy, such as thermal energy (heat).

Scattering

Scattering is defined as a change in direction of a light in living tissue without a change in its wavelength. Scattering is actually a composite of several distinct phenomena, such as diffuse reflection, refraction of light rays, reflectant diffraction, and resonant absorption. In the end, it is the two fundamental processes of absorption and scattering that govern all interactions of light with matter. The absorption spectra of major skin chromophores dominate most laser–tissue interactions in dermatology. When absorption occurs, the laser photons surrender energy to an absorbing chromophore. On absorption, the photon ceases to exist and the absorbing chromophores then become excited.

Optical penetration in skin is governed by a combination of absorption and scattering. From the ultraviolet (UV) through the near infrared (IR) spectrum, both absorption and scattering tend to be stronger at shorter wavelengths. In general, however, a gradual increase occurs in the depth of penetration into skin with longer wavelengths. The most penetrating wavelengths are in the 650–1500 nm, red, and near infrared region. Far infrared (water-absorbing) wavelengths penetrate significantly less.

THEORY OF SELECTIVE PHOTOTHERMOLYSIS

The concept of selective photothermolysis (SP) was conceived in 1983,[2] to explain the laser treatment of pediatric port wine stains.[3] Initially, laser wavelengths were chosen at the peak of oxyhemoglobin's yellow absorption band (577 nm). This maximized light absorption in the superficial blood vessels relative to epidermal melanin.

At the time, dye lasers were the only technology producing 577 nm light. They provided the first evidence for effective and safe treatment of pediatric port wine stains.[4]

This theory of SP has been proposed to explain the laser-induced injury that is confined to microscopic sites of selective light absorption in the skin with minimal damage to the adjacent tissues. To achieve this selective effect, lasers need to fulfill three requirements:

1. They should emit a wavelength that is highly absorbed by the targeted structure.
2. They should produce sufficiently high energies to inflict thermal damage to the target.
3. The time of tissue exposure to the laser should be short enough to limit the damage to the target without heat diffusion to the surrounding tissues.

This theory revolutionized cutaneous laser therapy. A new generation of highly selective pulsed lasers that conformed to these principles was developed in the late 1980s and early 1990s. These lasers were successfully employed in clinical practice for the treatment of various disorders. SP remains the basis of low-risk laser treatment of photoaging skin, benign pigmented lesions and tattoos, unwanted hair, and the cutaneous vascular lesions seen within both medical and cosmetic laser dermatology. However, as will be seen in this book, the risk of complications with all lasers will always remain.

EXTENDED THEORY OF SELECTIVE PHOTOTHERMOLYSIS

The concept of selective photothermolysis (SP) emphasizes both the selective damage and minimal light energy requirements seen with current laser technology.[2] However, the use of such a short pulsewidth may become inapplicable when the target absorption is non-uniform over its area. This may be seen when the actual target exhibits weak or no absorption, yet other surrounding portions of the target exhibit significant absorption. If this is the case, the weakly absorbing part of the target chromophore has to be damaged by heat diffusion from the highly pigmented/strongly absorbing portion of the chromophore (the heater or absorber). Such non-specific thermal damage evokes the concept of thermal damage time (TDT). The TDT of a target is the time required for irreversible target damage with sparing of the surrounding tissue. For a non-uniformly absorbing target structure, the TDT is the time it takes for the outermost part of the target to reach a target damage temperature through heat diffusion from the heated chromophore.

According to the concept of extended SP, target damage can still be selective even though the TDT is many times as long as the thermal relaxation time (TRT) of the actual target.

This new extended theory of selective thermal damage of non-uniformly pigmented structures in biological tissue postulates that the target is destroyed by heat diffusion from the absorbing chromophore to the target but not by direct heating from laser irradiation as is seen with SP.[5] This theory has been applied to the treatment of both unwanted hair and some vascular lesions. With the extra thermal effect needed to comply with this concept, complications can arise.

LASER COMPLICATIONS

Complications can arise after any laser procedure. Each chapter in this book will evaluate the potential problems associated with distinct broad categories of cutaneous laser procedures.

LASER RESURFACING

It is reasonable to assume that any means of depth-controlled destruction could be used to treat photoaged skin. Like chemical peels and dermabrasion, laser resurfacing is used to destroy the skin to a controlled depth. One would, therefore, expect a strong correlation between the duration and extent of wound-healing and clinical efficacy. Differences in efficacy between the applications of different lasers should relate to factors affecting the wound-healing response. Both efficacy and duration of wound-healing are related to the total anatomic depth of necrosis, including residual thermal damage.[6] With superficial injury there will be faster healing; but lower efficacy may be observed.

The mechanisms of tissue damage during laser resurfacing include removal by vaporization of a layer near the surface, thermal coagulation of extracellular matrix proteins in a residual layer, and a deeper zone of sub-lethal thermal injury. In addition, some photomechanical damage may occur in the case of Er:YAG (Erbium: Yttrium-Aluminum-Garnet) laser irradiation.

Type I collagen fibrils are known to contract rapidly at temperatures of 55–60°C and to shrink to as much as one third of their original length.[7,8] It is hypothesized that the post-laser repair of this tightened collagen scaffolding results in preservation of the heat-induced collagen contraction. Because new collagen is formed during the heating process the shortened collagen fibrils lead to a new tightened overall structure.

The use of high-energy pulsed and scanning carbon dioxide (CO_2; 10 600 nm), and Er:YAG (2940 nm) lasers allows clinicians to remove rhytides and other effects of photodamage (Figures 1.4–1.7). Too much thermal damage or any process that interferes with the normal re-epithelialization process may lead to the complications described in Chapter 2 of this book.

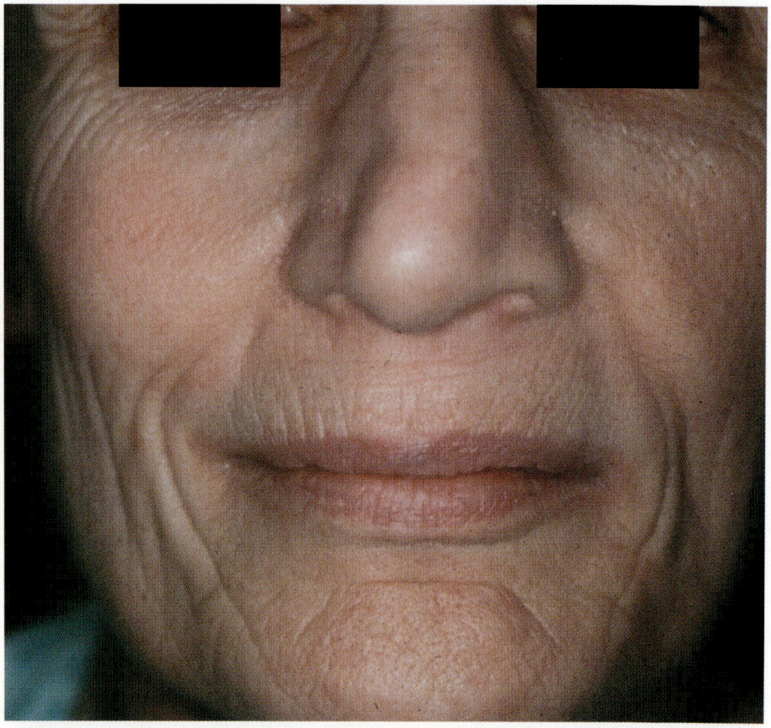

Figure 1.4. Before CO_2 laser resurfacing

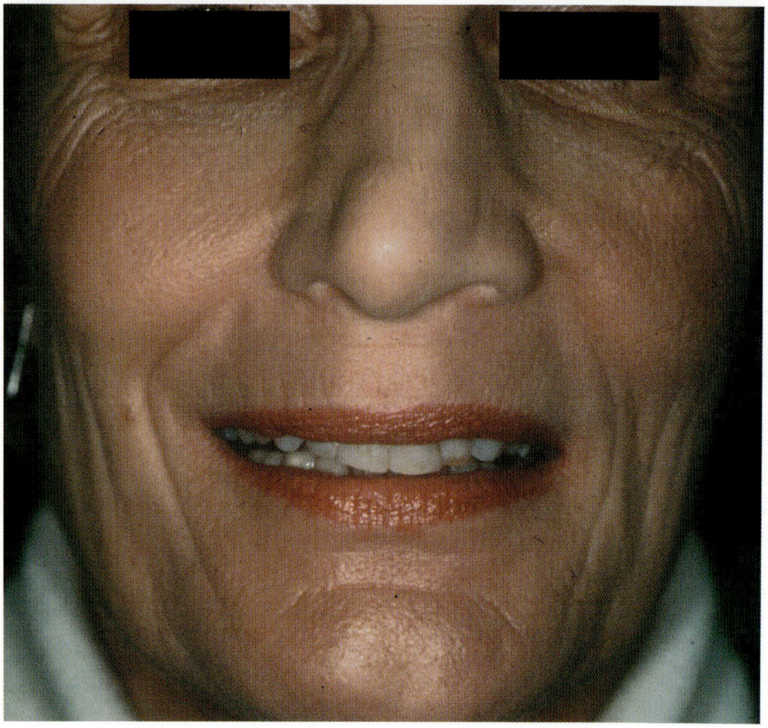

Figure 1.5. After CO_2 laser resurfacing

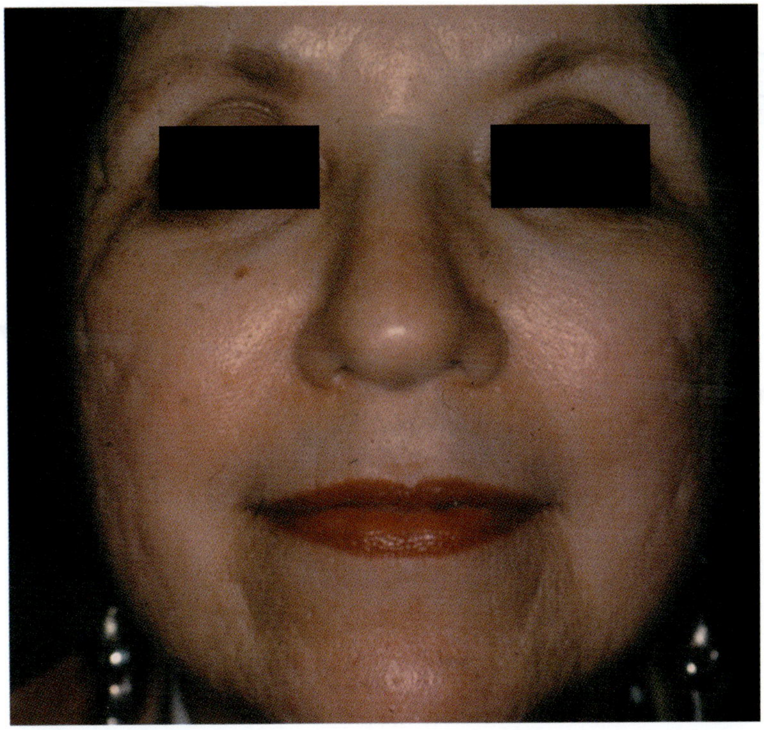

Figure 1.6. Before Er:YAG laser resurfacing

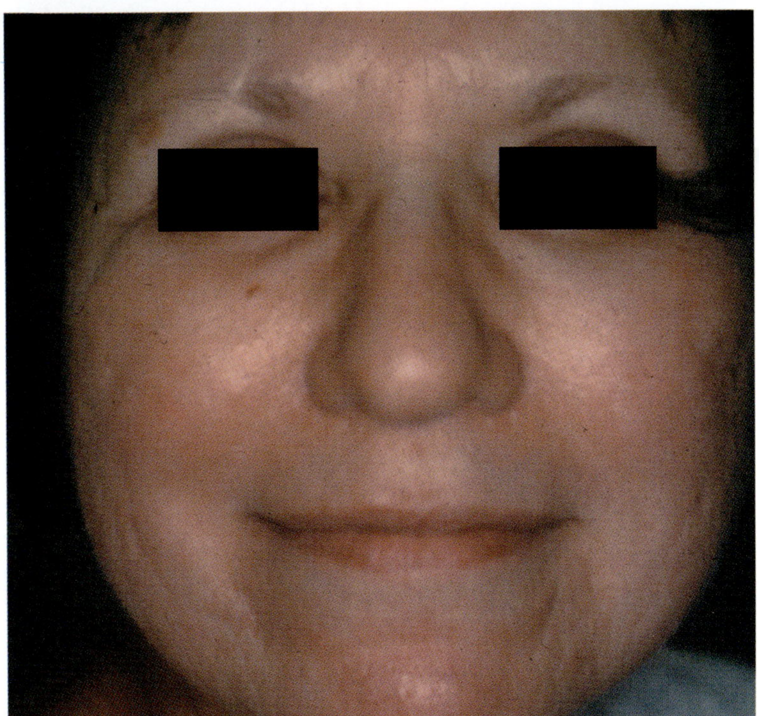

Figure 1.7. After Er:YAG laser resurfacing

Carbon Dioxide Laser

The 10 600 nm wavelength of the CO_2 laser is preferentially absorbed by water, having an extinction coefficient of about 30 μm (1 μm = 1×10^{-6} m).[9,10] The thermal relaxation time of the absorbing layer of tissue has been calculated to be less than 1 millisecond.[11] If the laser–tissue interaction time is confined to this time period, or less, by rapid pulsing of the laser or by rapid scanning of a continuous beam, then a layer of tissue will be rapidly vaporized, leaving a layer of residual thermal necrosis measuring only 50–100 μm.[10–12]

When the CO_2 laser interacts with tissue, there are three distinct zones of tissue alteration correlating with the degree of tissue heating. (1) The zone of direct impact results in vaporization of intracellular water and tissue ablation. (2) Underlying this zone is a layer of irreversible thermal damage and denaturation resulting in tissue necrosis. (3) Below this layer is a zone of reversible, non-lethal thermal damage. It is in this last zone of reversible thermal damage in which collagen shrinkage occurs. This accounts for the visible tissue tightening observable as the CO_2 laser interacts with the dermis.

Er:YAG Laser

The Er:YAG laser wavelength of 2940 nm closely corresponds to an absorption peak of water. This laser wavelength is approximately 10-fold better absorbed by water than is the 10 600 nm wavelength of the CO_2 laser.[13] The efficient superficial absorption, when coupled with a short pulse duration (250–350 microseconds; μs), allows Er:YAG lasers to ablate even fine layers of tissue, with significantly less Er:YAG laser-induced collateral thermal damage than is seen with a CO_2 laser. A single pass with an Er:YAG laser may ablate 10–30 μm and leave a zone of thermal necrosis of only 5–15 μm.[14,15] With such a small zone of thermal injury, little tissue desiccation occurs, and each subsequent pass produces very similar effects. Therefore, unlike the CO_2 laser, there is not a significantly diminished return with each subsequent pass of the laser. With less non-selective thermal damage, the Er:YAG laser when used superficially, achieves more rapid healing and a significantly lower rate of complications. However, when this laser is aggressively used, significant penetration into the skin can occur because of its minimal laser-induced thermal effect. In this case, the Er:YAG laser can potentially induce the same or even higher risk of scarring than is seen with a CO_2 laser.

Non-ablative lasers and light sources do not remove the epidermis. Their thermal effect is also markedly lessened as compared to the CO_2 laser. However, since their basic mechanism is still one of heat induction, complications can also arise from these systems. In addition, because some of the non-ablative systems are used with protective epidermal cooling, problems can arise when the cooling impacts on highly pigmented skin.

Non-ablative Skin Systems

Recently, skin cooling has been combined with mid-infrared lasers to produce an 'upside-down' burn/heating, in which the dermis reaches a much higher temperature than the epidermis. This technique has been employed to treat photoaged skin without inducing the obvious wound seen after ablative laser resurfacing.

Improvement after non-ablative treatment may result from:

1. Photothermal heating that leads to fibroblast activation, collagen remodeling, and subsequent increased pro-collagen III expression; and/or
2. Vascular activation with endothelial disruption leading to cytokine activation and subsequent collagen remodeling.

The mid-infrared lasers (1064–1540 nm) with deeply penetrating wavelengths can be coupled with surface cooling to stimulate new collagen production by gentle dermal heating. This creates a thermal wound which may activate migration of fibroblasts and neocollagenesis rather than inducing the immediate collagen contraction seen after CO_2 laser resurfacing. The epidermal cooling prevents the thermal wound from also damaging the epidermis. Lasers that remodel through vascular activation show all the characteristics of the vascular lesion lasers described below.

Non-ablative Radiofrequency

Recently, non-ablative radiofrequency (RF) has been used to produce immediate collagen contraction with a single treatment. This volumetric heat-inducing radiofrequency source uses simultaneous contact cooling for epidermal preservation. Much akin to the non-ablative lasers, such RF sources can be associated with complications.

LASER TREATMENT OF TATTOOS AND PIGMENTED LESIONS

The first pigment-specific laser, a ruby laser, was used in 1961. Since that time, laser physicians have successfully treated many pigmentary abnormalities within the skin. Properly chosen wavelengths of light used with appropriate pulse durations can selectively alter pigmented cells and disrupt exogenous and endogenous pigment in a manner that leaves the adjacent skin totally intact.

Targeting cutaneous pigmentation with lasers is dependent on several parameters, such as the nature of the targeted pigment (endogenous or exogenous pigment), its absorption characteristics, its distribution in tissue (intracellular or extracellular), and its anatomic location in the skin (epidermis, dermis, or both). Melanin, the main chromophore in most epidermal and dermal pigmented lesions, has a broad absorption spectrum extending from the ultraviolet range through the visible and near infrared spectra (Figure 1.8).[16] Across this wide range of absorbing wavelengths, any laser with sufficient energy levels can target melanin. To be most effective and avoid adverse effects, it is necessary to use wavelengths that both avoid absorption by other skin chromophores and penetrate to the desired depth. An ideal 'selective' window for targeting melanin lies between 630 nm and 1100 nm, where there is good skin penetration and preferential absorption of melanin over oxyhemoglobin.

Pigment specificity of lasers is not only dependent on wavelength but also on pulsewidth. Although the subcellular events that characterize the interaction between lasers and pigmented cells are not entirely known, the primary site of laser-induced pigment damage is most likely the melanosome, the intracellular organelle in which melanin is synthesized and stored.[17] Electron microscopic studies have demonstrated that melanosomes targeted by short-pulsed lasers exhibit membrane disruption and disorganization of their internal content.[18] With an estimated thermal relaxation time that ranges from 250 nanoseconds to 1000 nanoseconds, depending on their size, melanosomes require sub-microsecond laser pulses (<1 microsecond) for their selective disruption. Pulse durations of 40–750 nanoseconds (Q-switched lasers) are able to disrupt melanosomes, but longer pulse durations, in the millisecond domain,

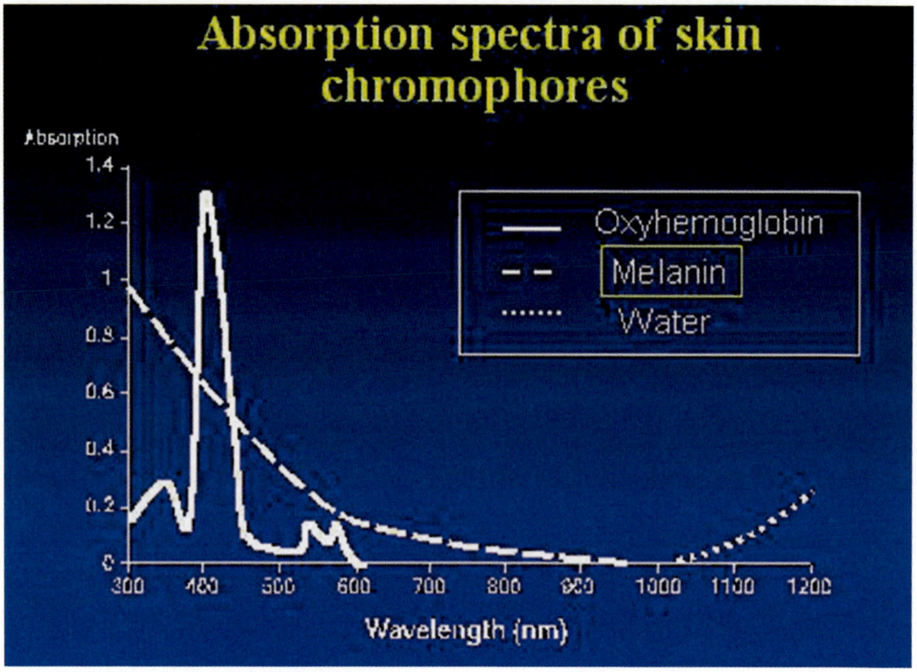

Figure 1.8. Melanin absorption curve

do not appear to cause specific melanosome damage.[19] Action spectrum studies,[20,21] comparing the effectiveness of different laser wavelengths in inducing pigment injury in guinea pig skin have shown similar melanosome alterations to that seen in humans but with substantial differences in threshold doses and depth of penetration. Shorter wavelengths (<600 nm) damage pigmented cells with lower energy fluences, while longer wavelengths (>600 nm) penetrate deeper into the skin yet need more energy to induce melanosome disruption. In addition, shorter wavelengths can damage only superficial pigmented lesions, leaving deeper structures intact, while longer wavelengths can target pigmented lesions in the dermis, such as nevus of Ota, and many tattoos.

Mechanism of Laser–Tattoo Interaction

Tattoos consist of insoluble, sub-micrometer-sized pigmented particles that are phagocytosed by dermal cells.[22] Treatment with short-pulsed lasers results in fragmentation of tattoo particles and selective death of pigment-containing cells.[23] The released pigment is then removed through transepidermal elimination, rephagocytosed by dermal macrophages, or eliminated through lymphatic drainage.

The physical mechanisms of laser–tattoo interaction are not well understood.[24,25] This is because the size of the tattoo particles is too small, and the laser duration too short, to make direct observations of the tattoo pigment break-up process feasible.

Laser-energy deposition in tattoo particles must be both heat- and stress-confined in order to fracture the tattoo particles. When these conditions are satisfied, a strong stress (i.e. acoustic or pressure) wave is generated inside the tattoo particle. Fracture occurs when the strength of the tensile or compressive component of the stress wave exceeds the corresponding strength limit of the particle. The efficiency for causing fracture increases with decreasing laser pulselength. However, this efficiency fails to further increase if the pulselength decreases below the stress confinement time.

The maximal temperature reached inside a treated tattoo particle is about 900°C at the end of a 35 picosecond pulse. This is well below the melting point for graphite. However, because the temperature of the tattoo particle reaches a value well above the boiling point of water, a cavitation bubble is formed in the tissue around the particle. As the bubble expands, the shear stress at the bubble surface increases and may cause collateral damage to the soft tissue immediately surrounding the tattoo particle. This could be the cause of empty vacuoles in the ash-white lesions seen throughout the dermis after laser treatment of tattoos.[26] Too much collateral damage may lead to the complications described in Chapter 3 of this book.

Lasers with longer pulse durations (millisecond lasers and light sources) are less efficient in generating the required tensile stress for breaking tattoo particles. They may also generate excessive heat with a resultant chance of complications.

Lasers used in Pigmented Lesion/Tattoo Treatments

Short-pulsed, Q-switched lasers (pulse duration <1 microsecond) have become the standard for the treatment of many pigmented skin disorders and tattoos (Figures 1.9–1.12). These Q-switched lasers operate through an extremely fast electromagnetic switch that allows build-up of excessive energy in the laser cavity. This energy is released in the form of a powerful pulse, sufficiently short in duration to selectively target sub-cellular organelles, such as melanosomes and tattoo particles. There are three short-pulsed pigment selective lasers in clinical use today. They are the Q-switched ruby laser (694 nm, 25–40 nanoseconds), the Q-switched alexandrite laser (755 nm, 50–100 nanoseconds), and the Q-switched Nd:YAG laser (1064 nm, 5–10 nanoseconds), which can be frequently doubled to emit a green light at 532 nm of the same pulse duration.

Pigment non-specific lasers, such as the CO_2 laser (10 600 nm) and the Er:YAG laser (2940 nm), are primarily used in laser skin resurfacing but may also remove superficial pigmented lesions as a secondary event. Continuous-wave and quasicontinuous-wave millisecond-emitting 511–694 nm laser irradiation produces selective pigment removal at these wavelengths. However, in the absence of reproducible nanosecond-induced spatial confinement of thermal injury, these millisecond systems carry a higher risk for textural and pigment changes compared with pulsed lasers. Pigment removal can also be achieved with a filtered flashlamp that generates an intense, polychromatic, visible to infrared millisecond-pulsed light at variable pulsewidths and intervals. With the placement of cut-off filters, specific wavelengths are selected that can target a variety of skin disorders. These systems do not usually generate the immediate post-treatment wound that is seen with Q-switched lasers, but they are also not as user-friendly as the nanosecond Q-switched systems.

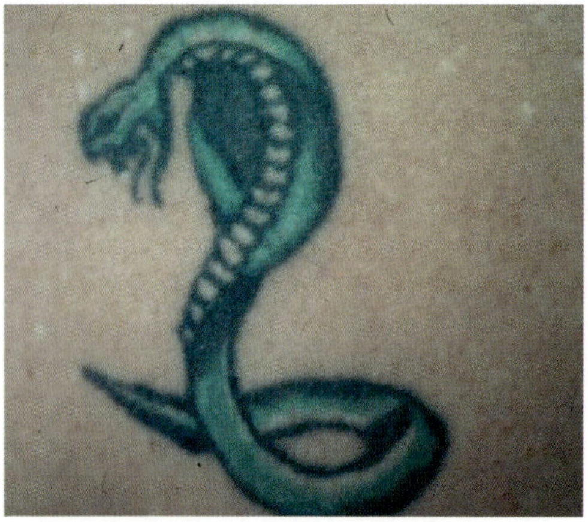

Figure 1.9. Tattoo before treatment with Q-switched laser

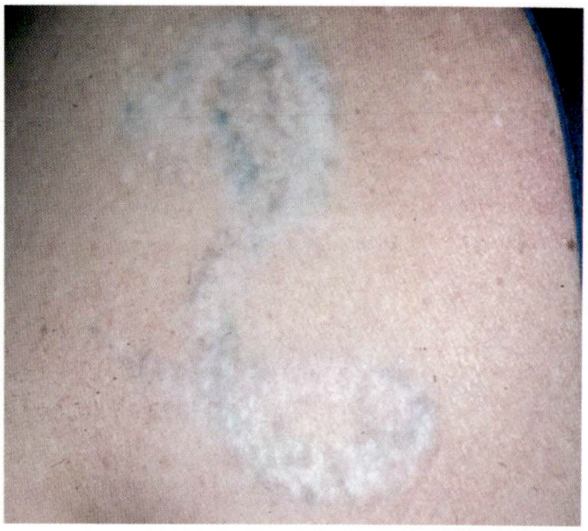

Figure 1.10. Tattoo after eight treatments with Q-switched laser

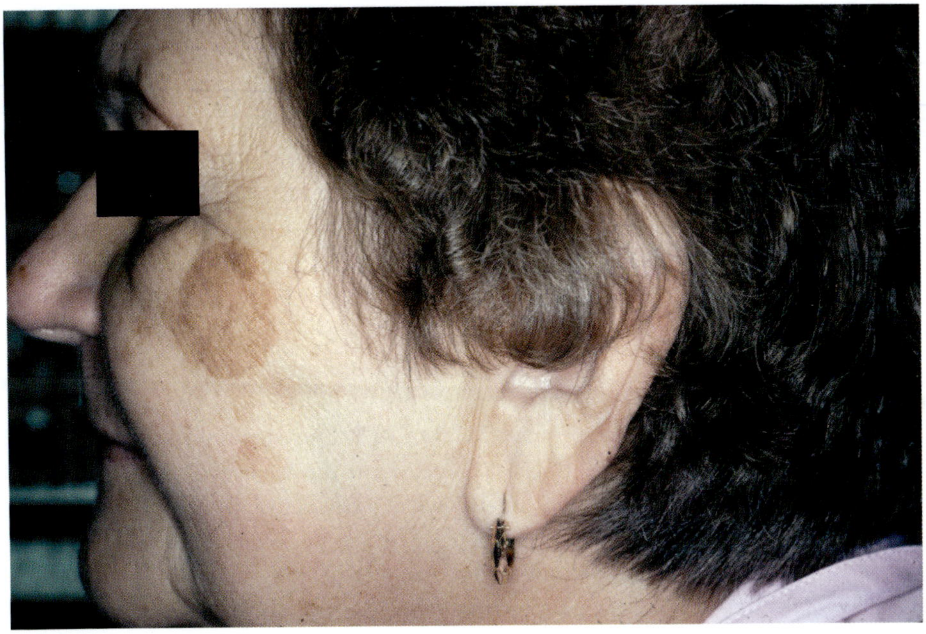

Figure 1.11. Solar lentigines before treatment with a Q-switched laser

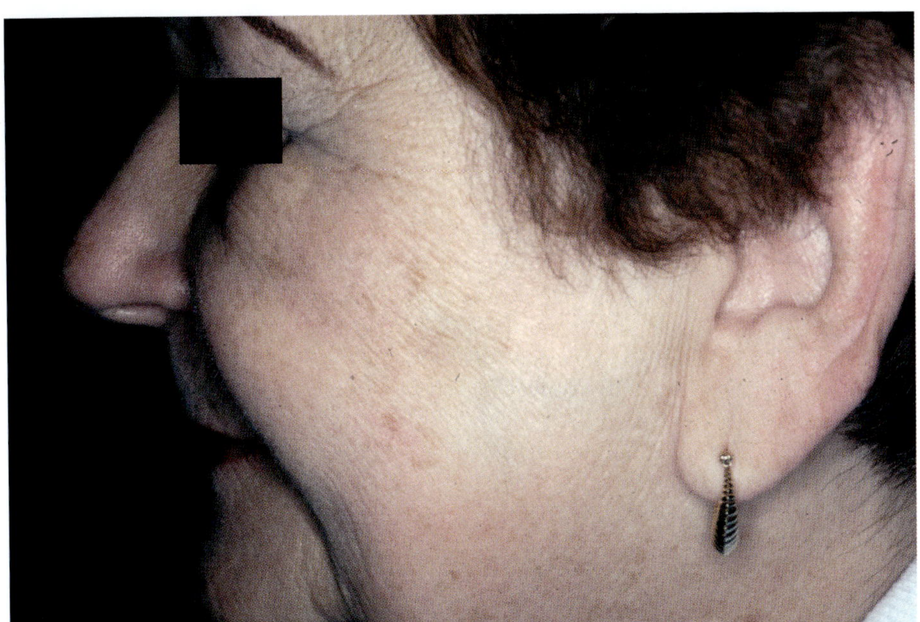

Figure 1.12. Solar lentigines after treatment with a Q-switched laser

LASER TREATMENT OF UNWANTED HAIR

Although the exact mechanism of action of laser hair removal is unknown, the use of laser and light source devices is based on the theory of selective photothermolysis.[2]

Laser hair removal utilizes light to cause thermal or mechanical damage of hair follicles. To achieve hair growth delay, it is sufficient to either damage matrix cells of anagen hair follicles, coagulate blood vessels of the papilla, or possibly to destroy part of the outer root sheath (ORS).[27] For permanent hair follicle damage, it is necessary to damage stem cells that are located in the bulge area at the interface of the ORS and the connective tissue sheath.[28] One can also irreversibly damage a hair follicle at the level of the dermis by replacing it with connective tissue.

The matrix cells produce the hair shaft. The matrix cells also contain melanosomes that produce hair melanin (Figure 1.13). The concentration of melanin in the matrix cells is significantly higher than it is in the hair shaft. This melanin is distributed uniformly and densely in the matrix cells. Thus, for a pulsewidth longer than the thermal relaxation time (TRT) of individual melanosomes (1 microsecond), the matrix cells act as a uniformly pigmented target. This is a typical example of a target where the theory of selective photothermolysis (SP) theory is applicable (Figures 1.14 and 1.15). For selective and effective treatment, the energy and pulsewidth have to be significantly shorter than the TRT of the matrix cells.

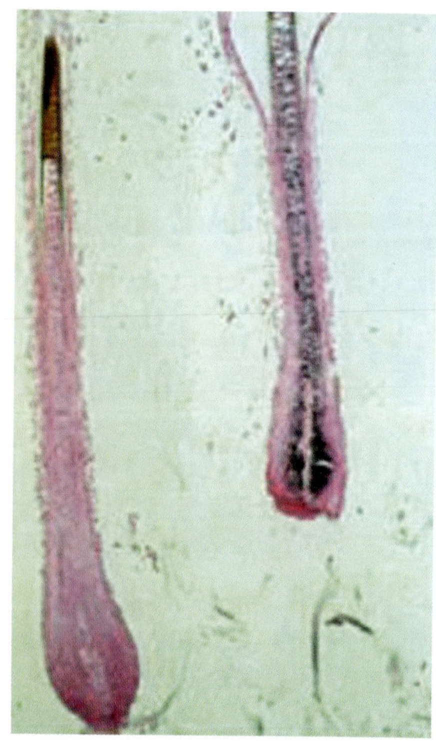

Figure 1.13. Hair follicle containing melanin-absorbing chromophore

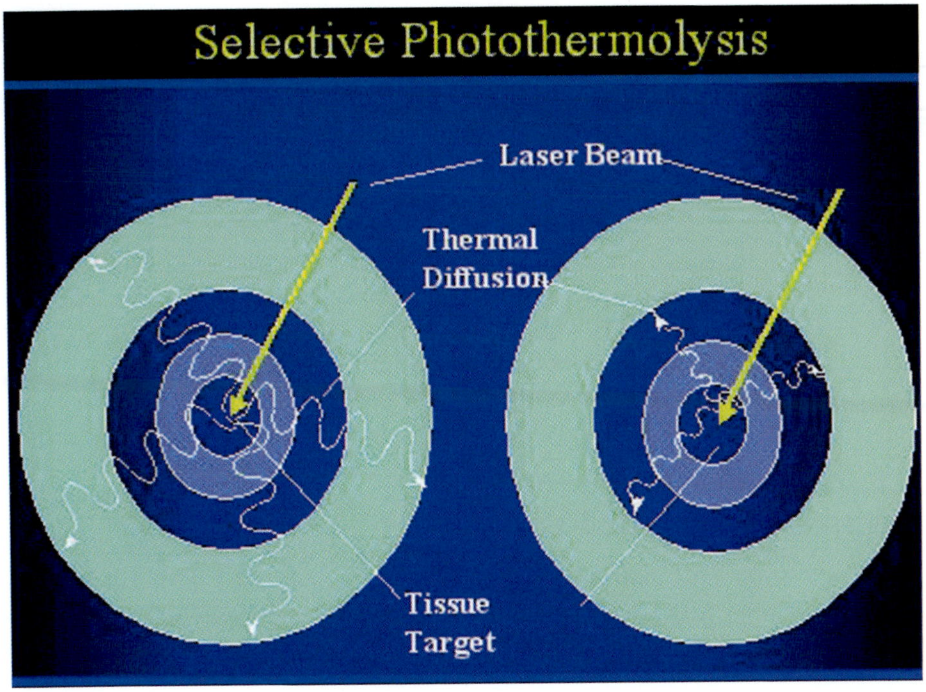

Figure 1.14. Selective photothermolysis (SP) of target tissue (hair) and resultant thermal diffusion

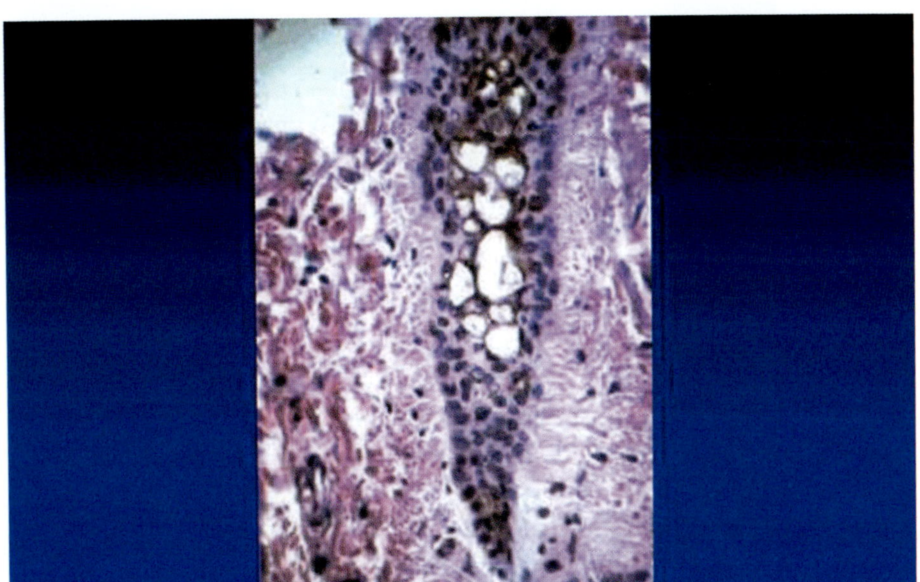

Figure 1.15. SP and resultant vacuolization produced in laser-treated hair

Another theoretical method of halting hair shaft growth is to coagulate blood vessels in the papilla. The loop of blood vessels in the papilla is located in the center of the matrix cell dome. Blood absorption is significantly lower than melanin absorption in the neighboring matrix cells because of the small vessel size. So the most effective method of papilla blood vessel coagulation is to utilize heat diffusion from the matrix cells that absorb light. In this scenario, the extended theory of SP may be applicable.

Finally, although stem cells in the basal cell layer of the lower isthmus ORS do not have pigment that can effectively absorb light in the therapeutic hair removal window (600–1200 nm),[27] these stem cells can be damaged by heat diffusion from the melanin-rich hair shaft or an artificial chromophore inside the internal root sheath (IRS).

Lasers used for Hair Removal

Ruby (694 nm), alexandrite (755 nm), diode (810 nm), Nd (Neodymium):YAG (1064 nm) lasers, as well as intense pulsed light systems (550–1100 nm) all emit light that is absorbed by hair containing melanin as well as epidermal melanin

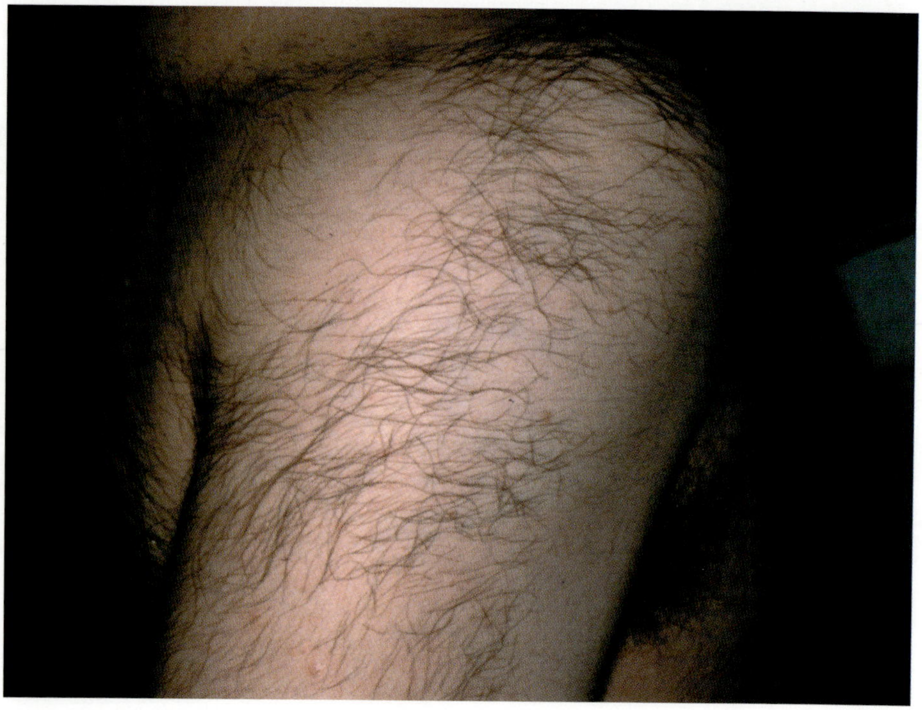

Figure 1.16. Hair before laser hair removal

(Figures 1.16 and 1.17). The longer the wavelength, the deeper is the penetration. Conversely, the shorter the wavelength the greater is the melanin absorption. Thus, longer wavelength systems tend to be less absorbed by epidermal melanin and generally are safer in darker complexioned individuals. In addition, hair removal systems are generally coupled with some sort of cooling system that is also epidermis-protective. It is the heat that is required for hair removal, or the overproduction of this thermal effect, that may lead to the complications described in Chapter 4 of this book.

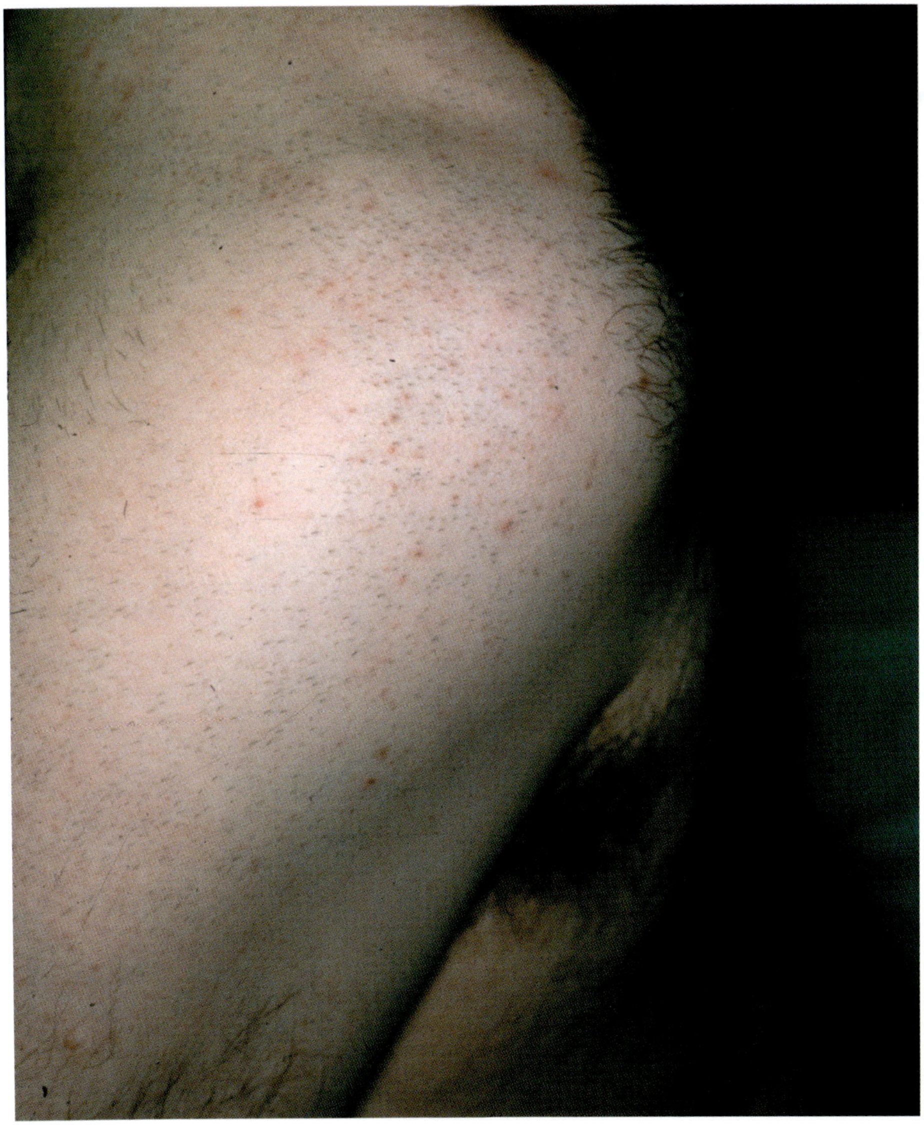

Figure 1.17. Decrease in hair after six treatments of laser hair removal

LASER TREATMENT OF VASCULAR LESIONS

Lasers have been used to treat vascular lesions since the early 1970s. It was not until the development of the pulsed dye laser in the late 1980s that the first cosmetically reproducible results were easily achieved. Recent development of longer wavelength, longer pulse duration, pulsed lasers, and light sources have improved outcome significantly. Basic requirements for a laser or light source to treat vascular lesions are:

1. a wavelength that is proportionately better absorbed by the target (hemoglobin) than surrounding chromophores;
2. an ability to penetrate to the full depth of the target blood vessel;
3. sufficient energy to damage the vessel without damaging the overlying skin; and
4. an exposure duration long enough to slowly coagulate the vessel and its lining without damaging the surrounding tissue.

The choice of laser wavelength(s), fluence determination, and pulse duration of light exposure are all related to the size, flow, depth, and type of treated targeted vessel. The correct choice of treatment parameters is aided by an understanding of the histology of target vessels. Lasers with larger spot size-delivering handpieces penetrate deeper into tissue and optimize fluence delivery to the target.

Over the last two decades, there has been a steady progression toward longer wavelength and longer pulse duration vascular lasers.[29–31] The slower incorporation of energy emitted by these longer pulse duration lasers allows for a gradual, diffuse vascular necrosis as opposed to the early more rapid pulse duration vascular lasers that produce a more explosive phase change (vaporization), with a pressure wave phenomenon causing vessel wall rupture.

For vascular lesions, the exposure time should be long enough to conduct heat from the red blood cell-filled lumen to the entire blood vessel wall. Merely coagulating the endothelium is insufficient because a direct correlation exists between the permanent eradication of a vein and degree of vessel wall injury. Greater success is expected as the depth of the vessel wall damage progresses from the endothelial cell layer intima and media to the adventitia.[32–35]

Large-diameter vessels require a longer pulse duration to allow sufficient time for an even diffusion of heat throughout the cylindrical vessel lumen.[30] Consistent with the above findings, the trend towards longer pulsewidths has been driven by the desire to eliminate purpura as an immediate complication of pulsed dye laser treatment. Purpura results from a combination of intravascular hemorrhage (immediate), thrombosis, and vasculitis (delayed). Pulsewidths greater than 10 milliseconds produce little or no immediate purpura. However, such long pulse duration lasers may still cause delayed vasculitis. Patients must still be warned that 'bruising' can appear several days after treatment. Of note, the millisecond non-laser pulsed light systems work in a similar manner to the millisecond vascular lasers.

A new generation of longer wavelength and long-pulse duration, near infrared lasers (755–1064 nm) has emerged for the treatment of some telangiectasia and leg

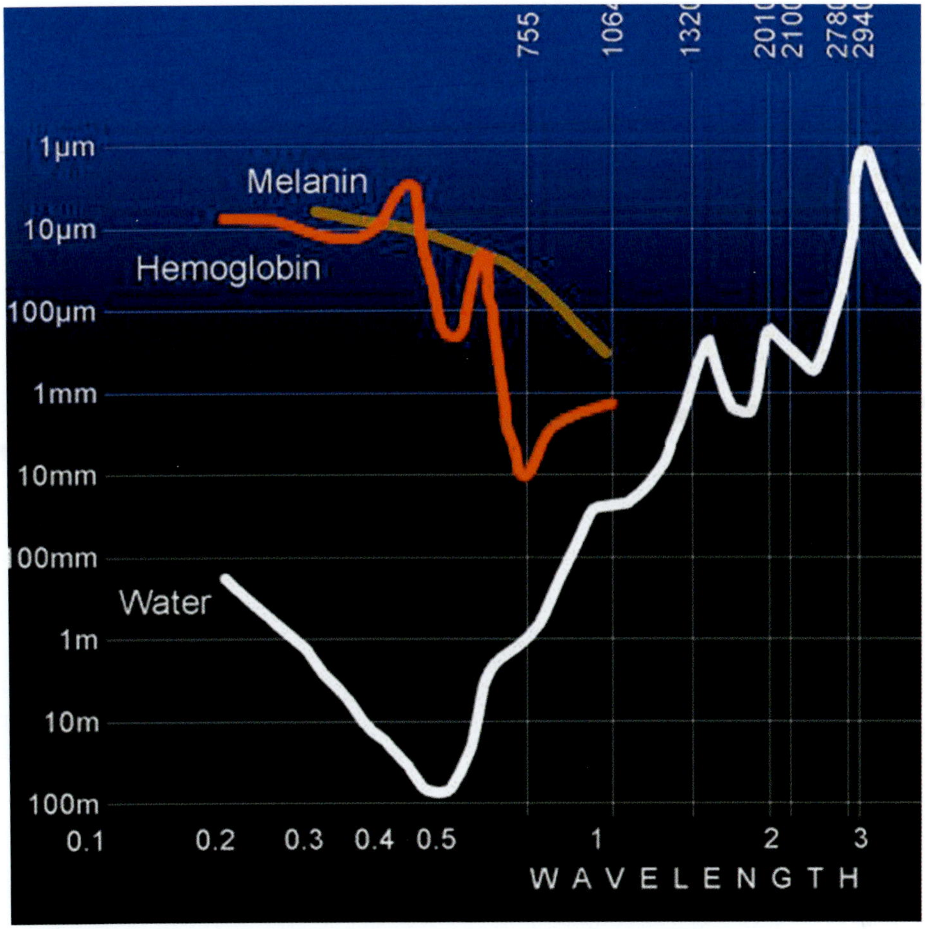

Figure 1.18. Hemoglobin absorption curve

veins (Figure 1.18).[36–38] Deeper vessels require a longer wavelength to allow penetration to their depth. However, even with deeper penetrating wavelengths, pulse durations must be matched to the vessel size. As the depth and size of the vessel changes, so do the absorption characteristics.

Several studies have demonstrated that heating induces hemoglobin modification.[39,40] The change is due to oxidative reactions with formation of met-hemoglobin (Met-Hb). When blood is subject to heat, the first observable event is Met-Hb formation, followed by distorted heme protein formation and protein denaturation.[39,41] Even under mild heating (50–54°C), Met-Hb is formed from oxygenated hemoglobin (HbO_2) and hemoglobin (Hb). This phenomenon is responsible for the change in blood absorption after laser irradiation.[42] Met-Hb has an absorbance about ×4.75 higher than that of HbO_2, and Met-Hb has an absorbance about ×20 higher than that of Hb.[43]

This phenomenon may explain why the longer wavelengths (e.g. infrared lasers such as Nd:YAG) are efficient in treating leg veins (Figures 1.19 and 1.20). Because the energy required to treat such vessels, and the associated required depth of penetration, complications may occur with the use of these lasers. Complications seen with these vascular lasers are described in Chapter 5.

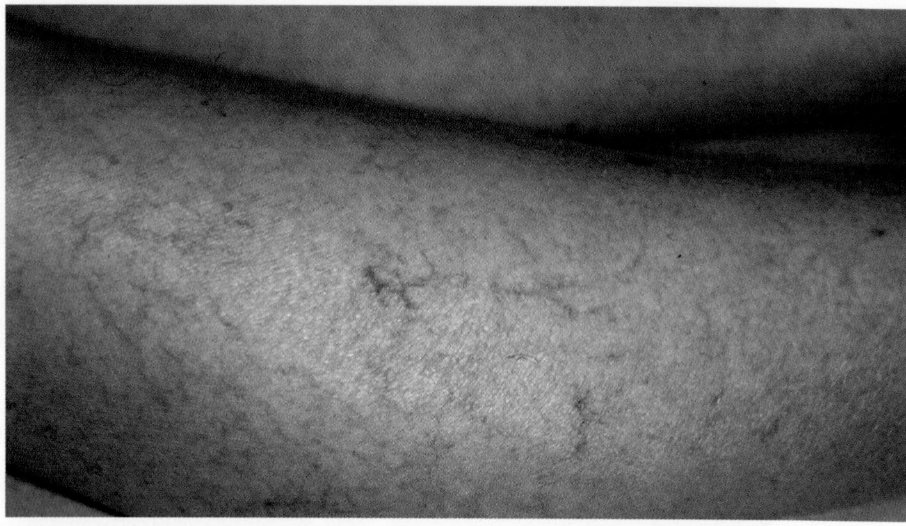

Figure 1.19. Leg veins before treatment with the 1064 nm Nd:YAG laser

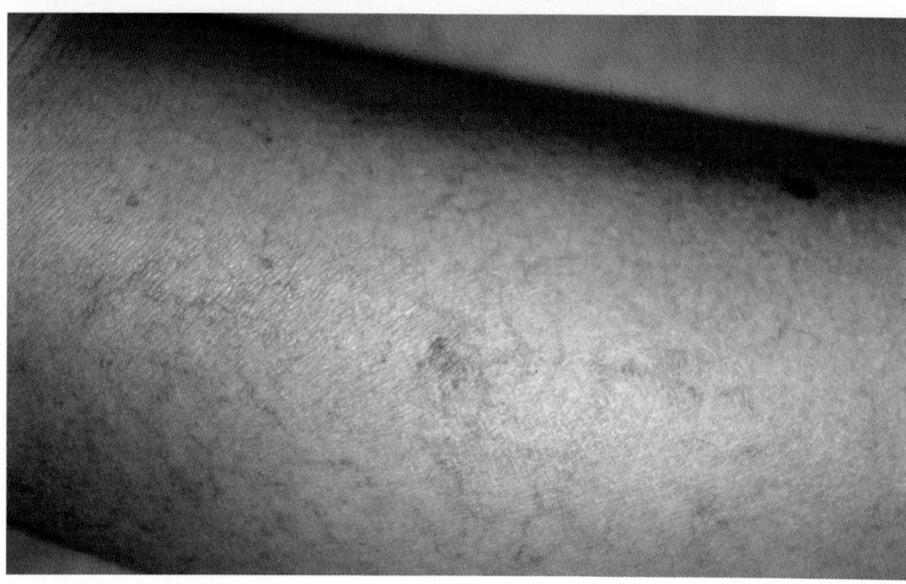

Figure 1.20. Some improvement in leg veins after treatment with the Nd:YAG laser

CONCLUSION

Cutaneous laser surgery has allowed physicians to treat photoaging skin, pigmented lesions and tattoos, unwanted hair, and a variety of vascular lesions. A thorough understanding of laser–tissue interaction should lead to a decreased likelihood of most of the complications described in this book.

REFERENCES

1 Anderson RR. Lasers in dermatology – A critical update. J Dermatol 2000;27:700–705.

2 Anderson RR, Parrish JA. Selective photothermolysis: Precise microsurgery by selective absorption of pulsed radiation. Science 1983;220:524–527.

3 Anderson RR, Parrish JA. Microvasculature can be selectively damaged using dye lasers: a basic theory and experimental evidence in human skin. Lasers Surg Med 1981;1:263–266.

4 Morelli JG, Tan OT, Garden J et al. Tunable dye laser (577 nm) treatment of port wine stains. Lasers Surg Med 1986;6:94–99.

5 Altshuler GB, Anderson RR, Smirnov MZ, et al. Extended theory of selective photothermolysis. Lasers Surg Med 2001;29:416–432.

6 Khatri KA, Ross V, Grevelink JM, Anderson RR. Comparison of erbium:YAG and carbon dioxide lasers in resurfacing of facial rhytides. Arch Dermatol 1999;135:391–397.

7 Gilchrest BA. Skin aging and photoaging. Dermatol Nurs 1990;2:79–82.

8 Goldfarb MT, Ellis CN, Weiss JS, Voorheer JJ. Topical tretinoin therapy: its use in photoaged skin. J Am Acad Dermatol 1989;21:645–650.

9 Clark SD, Kobayashi DK, Welgus HG. Regulation of the expression of tissue inhibitor of metalloproteinases and collagenase by retinoids and glucocorticoids in human fibroblasts. J Clin Invest 1987;80:1280–1288.

10 Drake LA, Dinehart SM, Farmer ER, et al. Guidelines of care for photoaging/photodamage. DermatologyWorld/Guidelines 1995;November (Suppl):11–13.

11 Fisher GJ, Datta SC, Tauar HS, et al. Molecular basis of sun-induced premature skin aging and retinoid antagonism. Nature 1996;379:335–339.

12 Fitzpatrick RE, Goldman MP, Satur NM, et al. Pulsed carbon dioxide laser, trichloracetic acid, Baker-Gordon phenol, and dermabrasion: A comparative clinical and histological study of cutaneous resurfacing in a porcine model. Arch Dermatol 1996;132:469–471.

13 Hale GM, Querry MR. Optical constants of water in the 200 nm to 200 m wavelength region. Appl Optics 1973;12:555–563.

14 Hohenleutner U, Hohenleutner S, Saumier W, et al. Faster effective skin ablation with an Er:YAG laser: Determination of ablation rates and thermal damage zones. Lasers Surg Med 1997;20:242–247.

15 Kaufman R, Hibst R. Pulsed erbium:YAG laser ablation in cutaneous surgery. Lasers Surg Med 1996;19:324–330.

16 Anderson RR, Parrish JA. The optics of human skin. J Invest Dermatol 1981;77:13–19.

17 Polla LL, Margolis RJ, Dover JS, et al. Melanosomes are a primary target of Q-switched ruby laser irradiation in guinea pig skin. J Invest Dermatol 1987;89:281–286.

18 Dover JS, Polla LL, Margolis RJ, et al. Pulse width dependence of pigment cell damage at 694 nm in guinea pig skin. SPIE Lasers Med 1986;712:200–205.

19 Watanabe S, Flotte T, Margolis R, et al. The effects of pulse duration on selective pigmented cell injury by dye lasers. J Invest Dermatol 1987;88:532.

20 Anderson RR, Margollis RJ, Dover JS, et al. Selective photothermolysis of cutaneous pigmentation by Q-switched Nd:YAG laser pulse at 1064, 532, and 355 nm. J Invest Dermatol 1989;93:28–32.

21 Sherwood K, Murry S, Kurban A, Tan O. Effects of wavelength of cutaneous pigment using pulsed irradiation. J Invest Dermatol 1989;92:717–720.
22 Ort RJ. Tattoos and their treatments. Med Surg Dermatol 1998;5:265–268.
23 Taylor CR, Anderson RR, Gange RW, et al. Light and electron microscopic analysis of tattoos treated by Q-switched ruby laser. J Invest Dermatol 1991;97:131–136.
24 Sheeban-Dare RA, Cotterill JA. Lasers in dermatology. Br J Dermatol 1993;129:1–8.
25 Zelickson BD. Laser tattoo removal. Lasers in dermatology. Bio-optics and treatment of human skin. Optical Society of Am Tech Digest Series 1997;15:42–47.
26 Ferguson JE, Andrew SM, Jones CJP, et al. The Q-switched neodymium:YAG laser and tattoos: a microscopic analysis of laser tattoo interactions. Br J Dermatol 1997;137:405–410.
27 Dierickx CC, Grossman MC, Farinelli WA, Anderson RR. Permanent hair removal by normal-mode ruby laser. Arch Dermatol 1998;134:837–842.
28 Sun T, Cotsarelis G, Lavker RM. Hair follicle stem cells: the bulge activation hypothesis. J Invest Dermatol 1991;96 (suppl 5):77S–78S.
29 Garden JM, Tan OT, Kerschmann R, Anderson RR, Parish JA. Effects of dye laser pulse duration on selective cutaneous vascular injury. J Invest Dermatol 1986;87:653–657.
30 Dierickx CC, Casparian JM, Venugopalan V, Farinelli WA, Anderson RR. Thermal relaxation of port wine stains vessels probed in vivo: the need for 1–10 millisecond laser pulse treatment. J Invest Dermatol 1995;105:709–714.
31 Hsia J, Lowry JA, Zelickson B. Treatment of leg telangiectasias using a long pulsed dye laser at 595 nm. Lasers Surg Med 1997;20:1–5.
32 Goldman MP, Kaplan RP, Oki LN, Cavender PA, Strick RA, Bennett RG. Sclerosing agents in the treatment of telangiectasias: comparison of the clinical and histologic effects of intravascular polidocanol, sodium tetradecyl sulfate, and hypertrophic saline in the dorsal rabbit ear vein model. Arch Dermatol 1987;123:1196–1201.
33 Hanschell HM. Treatment of varicose veins. Br Med J 1947;2:630.
34 Goldman MP. A comparison of sclerosing agents: clinical and histologic effects of intravascular sodium morrhuate, ethanolamine oleate, hypertonic saline (11.7%) and Sclerodex in the dorsal rabbit ear vein. J Dermatol Surg Oncol 1991;17:354–362.
35 Martin DE, Goldman MP. A comparison of sclerosing agents: clinical and histologic effects of intravascular sodium tetradecyl sulfate and chromated plycerine in the dorsal rabbit ear vein. J Dermatol Surg Oncol 1990;16:18–22.
36 McDaniel DH, Ash K, Lords J, Newman J, et al. Laser treatment of spider leg veins: clinical evaluation of a new long-pulsed alexandrite laser. Dermatol Surg 1999;21:52–58.
37 Min RJ, Navarro L. 810 nm diode laser treatment of facial telangiectasias. Lasers Surg Med Suppl 2000:12:104.
38 Rogachefsky AS, Silapunt S, Goldberg DJ. Nd:YAG Laser (1064nm) irradiation for lower extremity telangiectases and small reticular veins: Efficacy as measured by vessel color and size. Dermatol Surg 2002; 28:220–223.
39 Alves OC, Wajnberg E. Heat denaturation of metHb and HbNO: e.p.r. evidence for the existence of a new hemichrome. Int J Biol 1993;15(5):273–279.
40 Seto Y, Kataoka M, Tsuge K. Stability of blood carbon monoxide and hemoglobins during heating. Forensic Sci Int 2001;121(1–2):144–150.
41 Barton JK, Frangineas G, Pummer H, Black JF. Cooperative phenomena in two-pulse, two-color laser photocoagulation of cutaneous blood vessels. Photochem Photobiol 2001;73(6):642–650.
42 Randeberg L, Daae Hagen A, Svaasand L. Optical properties of human blood as a function of temperature. In: Bartels KE, ed. Lasers in Surgery: Advanced Characterization, Therapeutics and Systems: XII. Bellingham, WA: SPIE; 2002:20–28.
43 Kuenstner JT, Norris KH. Spectrophotometry of human hemoglobin in near infrared region from 1000 to 2500 nm. J Near Infrared Spectroscopy 1994;2:59–65.

2 COMPLICATIONS IN LASER RESURFACING

KEY POINTS

(1) Both carbon dioxide (CO_2) and Er:YAG (Erbium:Yttrium-Aluminum-Garnet) laser resurfacing may be associated with complications
(2) CO_2 laser-induced complications follow from both the laser-induced ablative wound and thermal effect caused by this laser
(3) Er:YAG laser-induced complications follow from the laser-induced ablative wound
(4) Complications arising from non-ablative technology are generally related to either too much heat or too much epidermal cooling

INTRODUCTION

Throughout the ages, various attempts to beautify the skin have evolved. Techniques include the application of animal oils, salt, alabaster, Turkish fire exfoliation, and urine-bathed pumice stones.[1]

Aging effects on the skin are generally characterized as resulting from both intrinsic as well as extrinsic processes. Intrinsic aging refers to those processes that result purely from the passage of time.[2] Extrinsic aging is due primarily to the effects of environmental ultraviolet (UV) radiation.[3]

Photodamage accounts for more than 90% of the unwanted changes in skin appearance of sun-exposed areas. These changes vary from fine to coarse skin textural changes. In severe photodamage, one can see atrophy, irregular pigmentation, scaling and roughness of the skin surface, telangiectasia, and sallowness, as well as early predilection to bruising.[2,4,5]

Facial skin aging has been associated with negative views of body image, self-esteem, and self-confidence.[6–9] Reversal of photoaging has become a constant goal pursued by the public, the medical profession, and the cosmetic industry.

Recent advances in laser technology using the carbon dioxide (CO_2) and Erbium: YAG (Er:YAG) lasers have made these lasers very popular for resurfacing of photodamaged skin.[1,10–14]

Water is the major absorbing chromophore for both the 10 600 nm CO_2 and 2940 nm Er:YAG laser wavelengths. The Er:YAG laser's wavelength is absorbed by water 10 times more readily than is seen with the CO_2 laser. Because of this absorption, skin injury with an Er:YAG laser could conceivably be more precise and superficial than with a CO_2 laser. Conversely, CO_2 lasers, being less absorbed by water, lead to a greater thermal effect.

The mechanisms of tissue damage following laser resurfacing include removal by superficial vaporization, CO_2 laser-induced thermal coagulation, thermal denaturation of extracellular matrix proteins, and a deeper zone of sub-lethal thermal injury. In addition, some photomechanical damage may occur in the case of Er:YAG irradiation.

Both Er:YAG and pulsed CO_2 lasers are effective for the treatment of photodamage, with important differences related to the lesser residual thermal injury induced by the Er:YAG laser. Despite these differences, depth of injury is the most significant factor in both clinical results and risk of morbidity from both of these lasers.

Non-ablative technology has been touted as generally safer, albeit less effective, than ablative laser treatments. Nevertheless, these modalities generally promote some thermal effect. Some non-ablative technologies are also utilized with significant epidermal cooling devices. The thermal and/or cooling effect of these machines may also be associated with rare complications.

Laser resurfacing can deliver consistently good results with a reasonable safety profile. Laser resurfacing may also have a better risk/benefit ratio than is seen with other non-laser ablative modalities. Like every other treatment procedure for skin rejuvenation, however, laser resurfacing can induce its share of complications.

Prevention of some complications is best managed by pre-treatment patient education.

Complications following cutaneous laser resurfacing range widely from the expected post-treatment morbidity (with eventual clinical improvement) to permanent disfigurement.

Numerous studies have demonstrated that a certain percentage of patients will experience complications following laser resurfacing.[15–18]

Adverse effects, and complications of cutaneous laser resurfacing, range in severity from mild to severe.[19] Mild reactions include prolonged erythema, acne or milia formation, contact dermatitis, and pruritis. Moderate complications include viral, bacterial, or fungal infections, post-inflammatory hyperpigmentation, and delayed onset of hypopigmentation. The most serious complications, and fortunately the most rare, include hypertrophic scarring and disseminated infection.

HYPERPIGMENTATION

Post-inflammatory hyperpigmentation (PIH) is the most common adverse effect seen with cutaneous laser resurfacing, occurring in approximately 35–40% of patients with Fitzpatrick skin types I–III, and virtually 100% of those with darker skin phototypes (Fitzpatrick skin types IV–VI).[17,19–21] PIH generally begins in the malar region and then extends laterally and centrally. Although it is transient and treatable, it is not completely preventable (Figures 2.1 and 2.2).

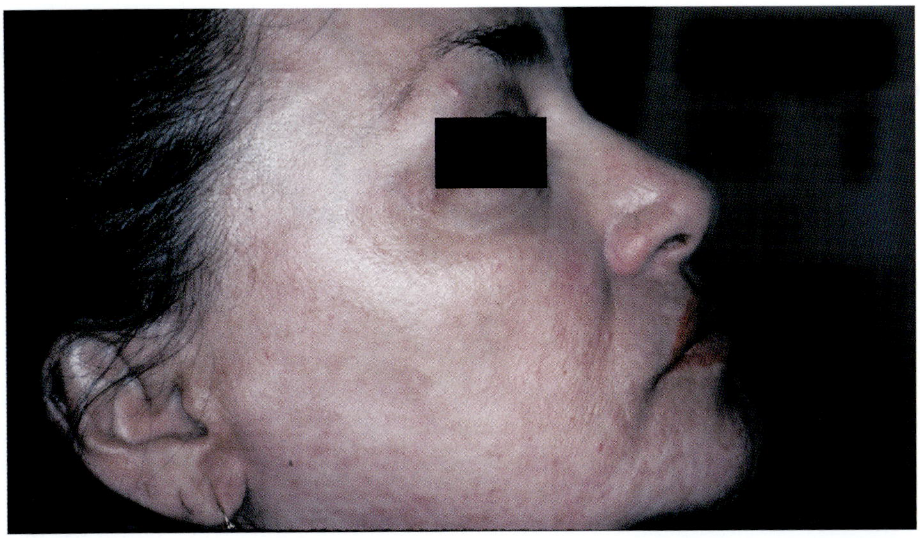

Figure 2.1. Post-inflammatory hyperpigmentation 6 months after CO_2 laser resurfacing

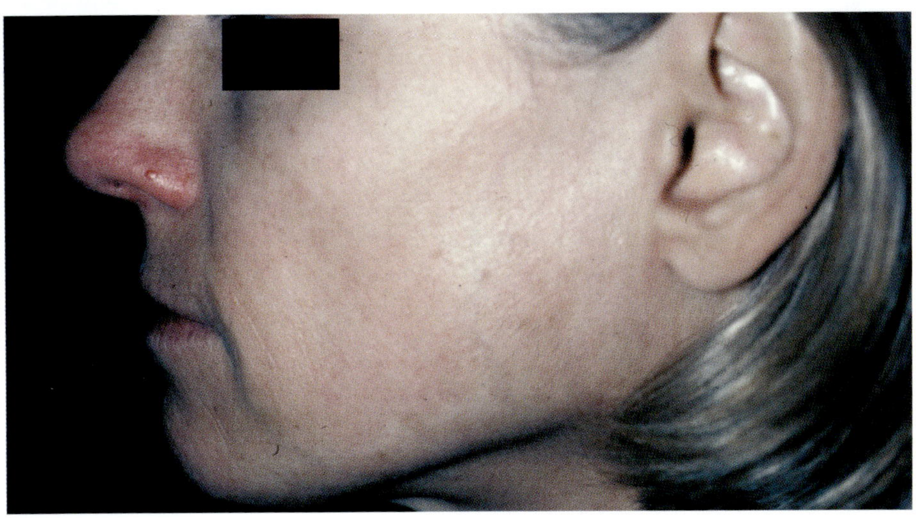

Figure 2.2. Post-inflammatory hyperpigmentation 6 months after Er:YAG laser resurfacing

The cause of PIH is poorly understood. It can occur with any disruption of the skin. In general, the risk parallels the degree of the patient's natural color or pigment; the darker the color, the greater the potential risk of hyperpigmentation.

Although post laser-induced hyperpigmentation is more likely to occur following exposure to ultraviolet (UV) light, it may occur in the complete absence of any sun exposure. Any procedure that creates prolonged erythema, dramatically increases the risk of increased pigmentation. It is postulated that estrogens may stimulate melanogenesis, and patients with high endogenous estrogen levels or using exogenous estrogens (e.g. use of oral contraceptives), may be at higher risk. Patients who are suntanned have a much higher risk of post-operative hyperpigmentation, presumably because of melanocytic stimulation.

Hyperpigmentation usually manifests within the first month following treatment, and generally spontaneously resolves during the next several months. Since this cutaneous reaction pattern is often so conspicuous, many patients seek medical intervention to speed its resolution.

PIH may also occur after non-ablative laser treatment. Such PIH is most commonly caused by a cryogen injury that may occur with over-zealous use of the epidermal protecting cryogen spray associated with some non-ablative devices. It may also result from the thermal effect of these devices (Figures 2.3–2.22).

Treatment must not be overly aggressive to lessen the incidence of PIH. There has been considerable debate about pre-treatment of the skin before laser resurfacing. Some studies have not found pre-treatment with hydroquinone and/or retinoic acid at all useful in preventing post-operative hyperpigmentation. There is also no theoretical basis upon which such treatment should be helpful.

Pre-operative hydroquinone only inhibits the synthesis of melanin in melanocytes, which will inevitably be removed in the first laser resurfacing pass. The melanocytes responsible for post-inflammatory pigmentation are deep in the bases of the appendages and are not affected by pre-operative use of hydroquinones. After resurfacing, melanocytes at the appendageal level will migrate to the surface and will concurrently be activated to produce and release increased amounts of melanin. It is only when they have reached the epidermal surface that they are susceptible to topical hydroquinones.

Pre-treatment with retinoic acid is largely a hold-over from the chemical peel literature. It is well accepted that topical retinoic acid thins the epidermis, allowing chemical peel solutions to penetrate more easily and evenly.[22] This has little relevance to laser resurfacing. Topical retinoic acid also does not appear to influence the penetration depth of laser resurfacing.

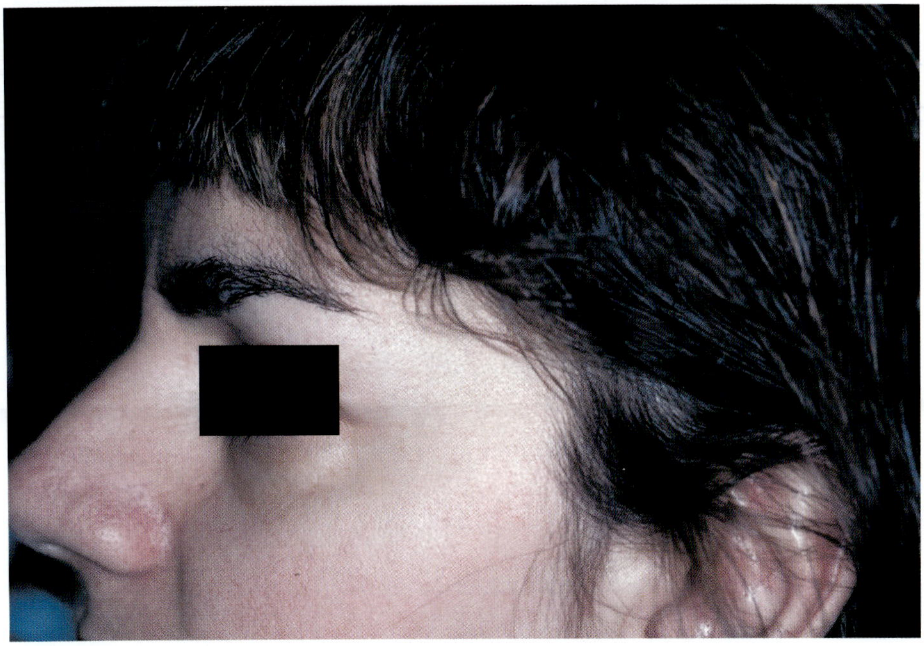

Figure 2.3. Before non-ablative treatment with an intense pulsed light source

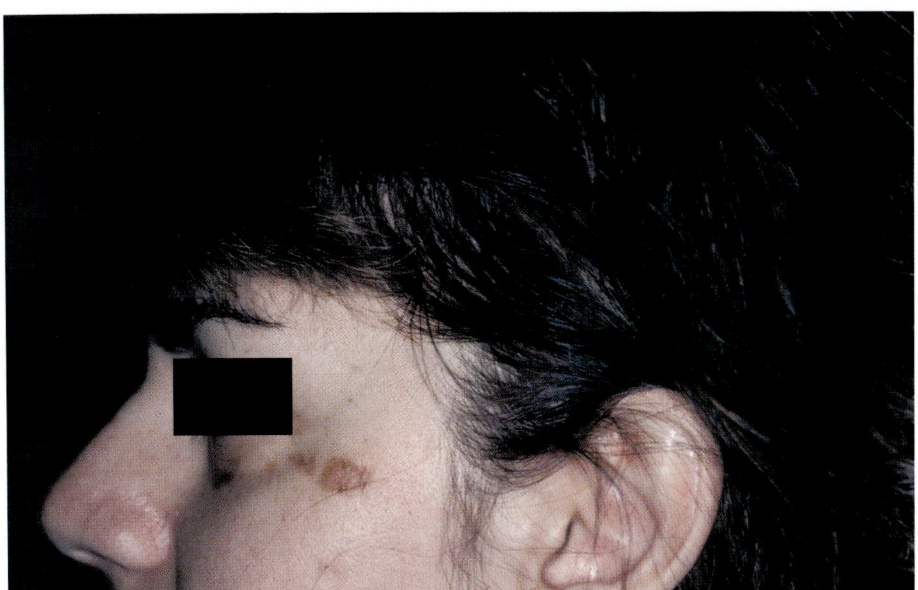

Figure 2.4. Post-inflammatory hyperpigmentation 3 months after intense pulsed light treatment

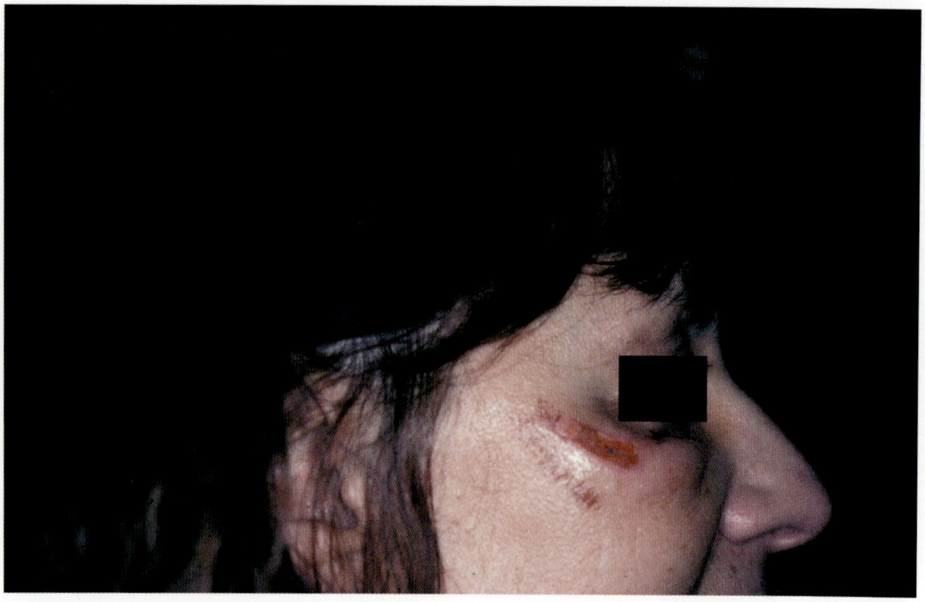

Figure 2.5. Crusting 2 weeks after non-ablative intense pulsed light treatment

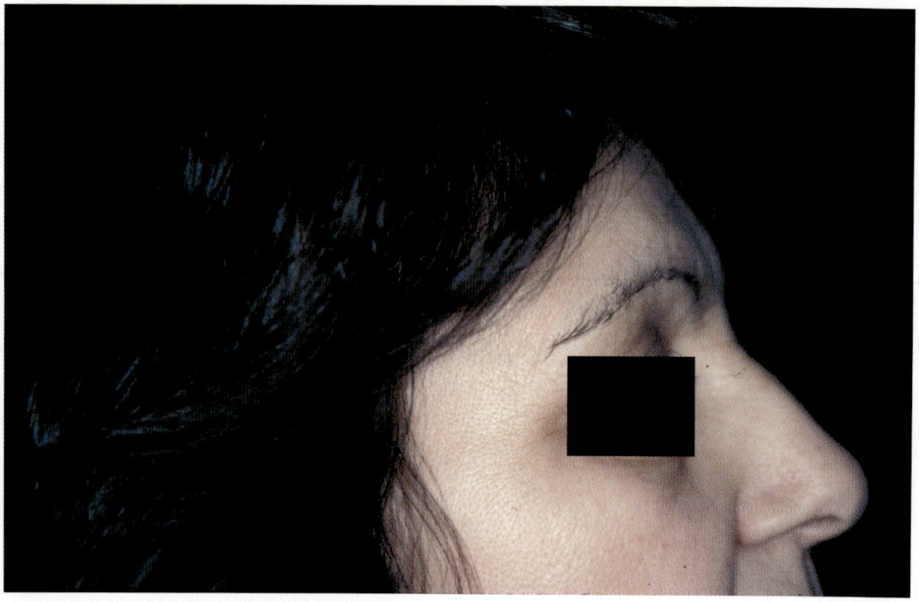

Figure 2.6. Minimal post-inflammatory hyperpigmentation 3 months after non-ablative intense pulsed light treatment: patient in Figure 2.5

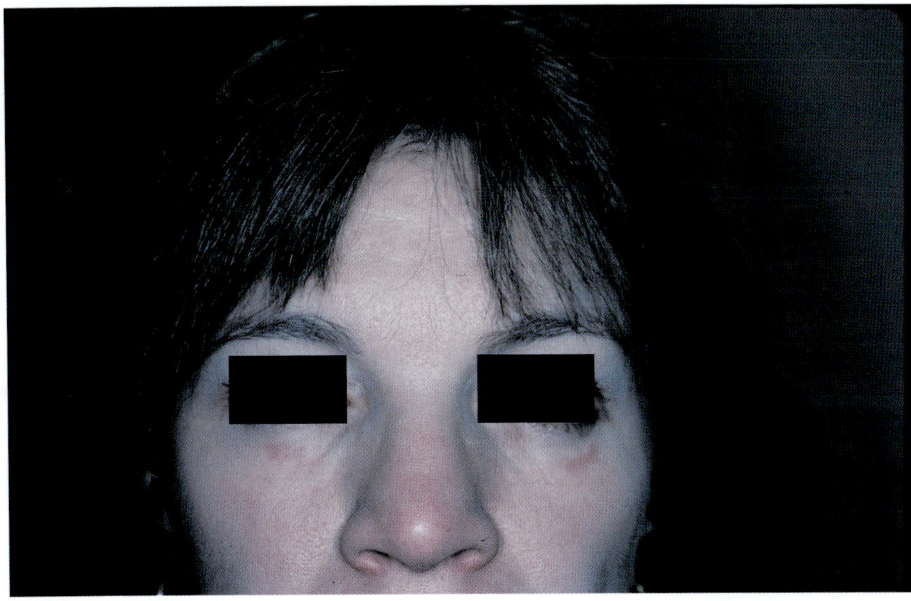

Figure 2.7. Post-inflammatory hyperpigmentation 3 months after intense pulsed light treatment

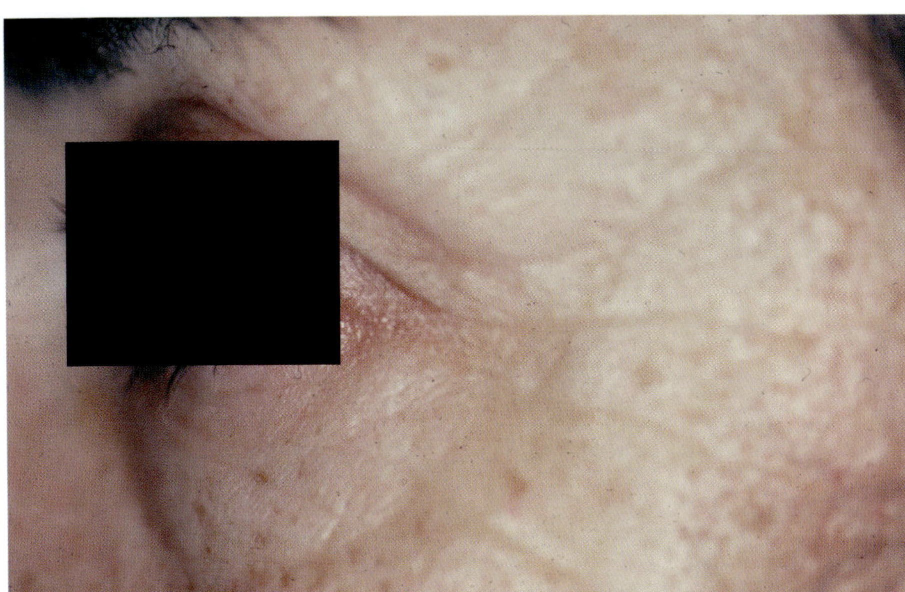

Figure 2.8. Before 1450 nm diode non-ablative treatment

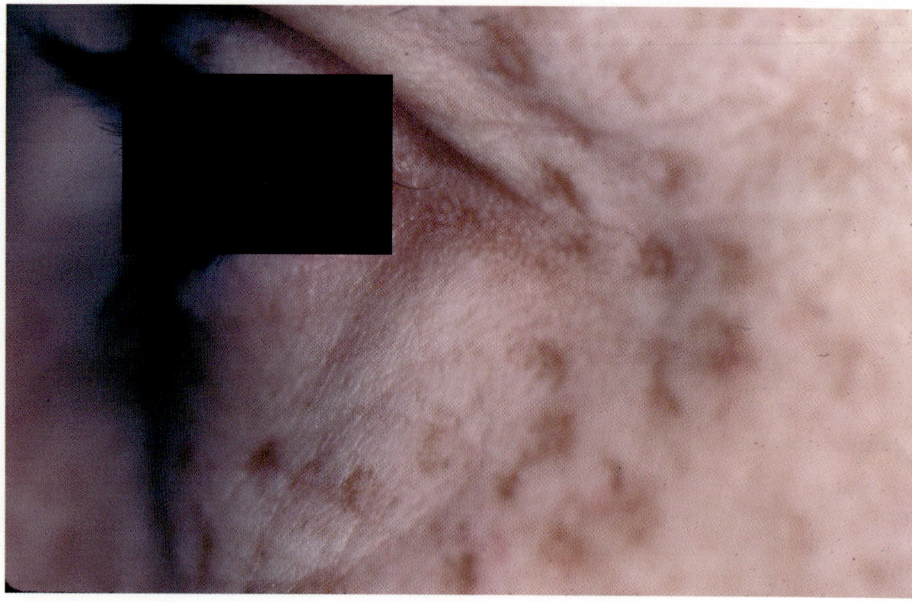

Figure 2.9. Post-inflammatory hyperpigmentation 3 months after 1450 nm diode laser non-ablative treatment

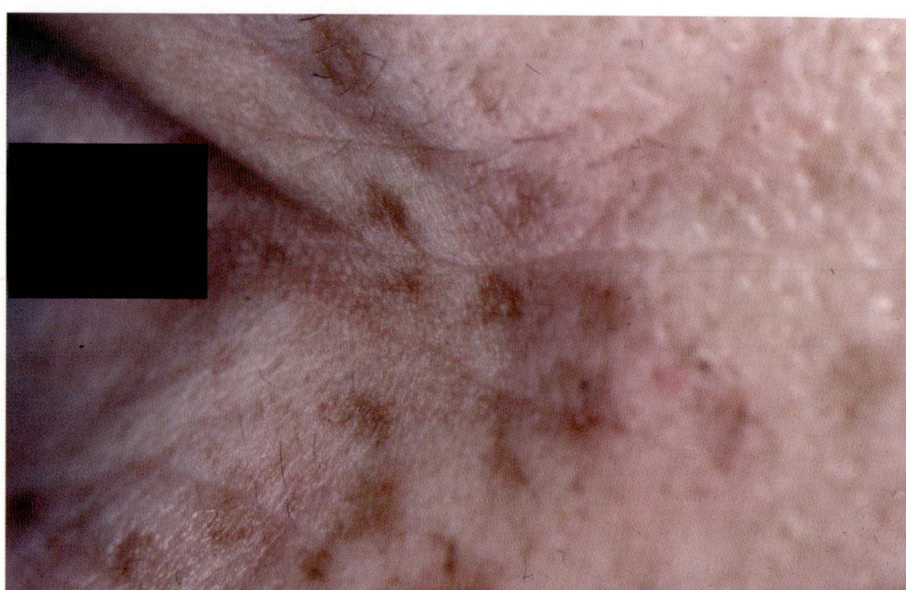

Figure 2.10. Post-inflammatory hyperpigmentation 3 months after 1320 nm Nd:YAG laser non-ablative treatment

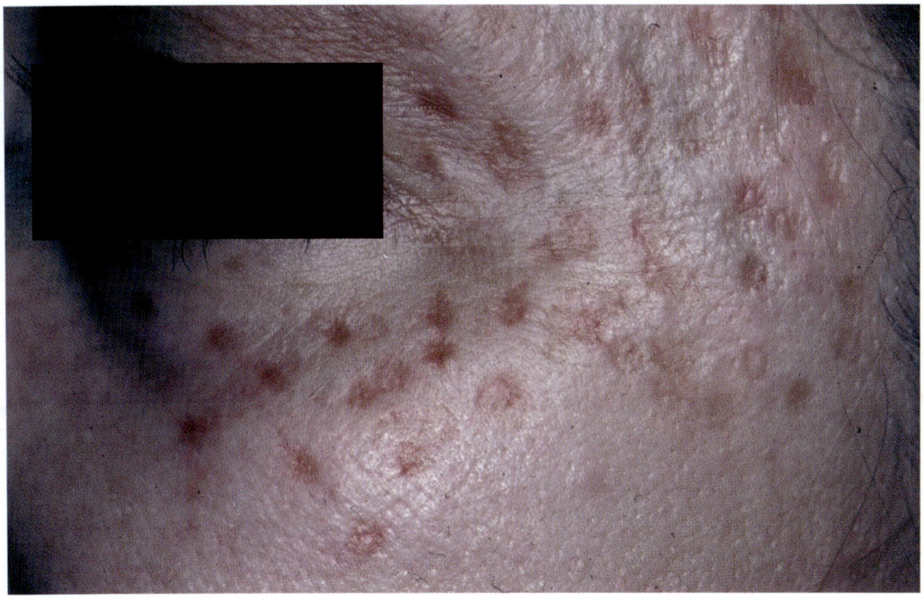

Figure 2.11. Extensive post-inflammatory hyperpigmentation 2 months after 1450 nm diode laser non-ablative treatment

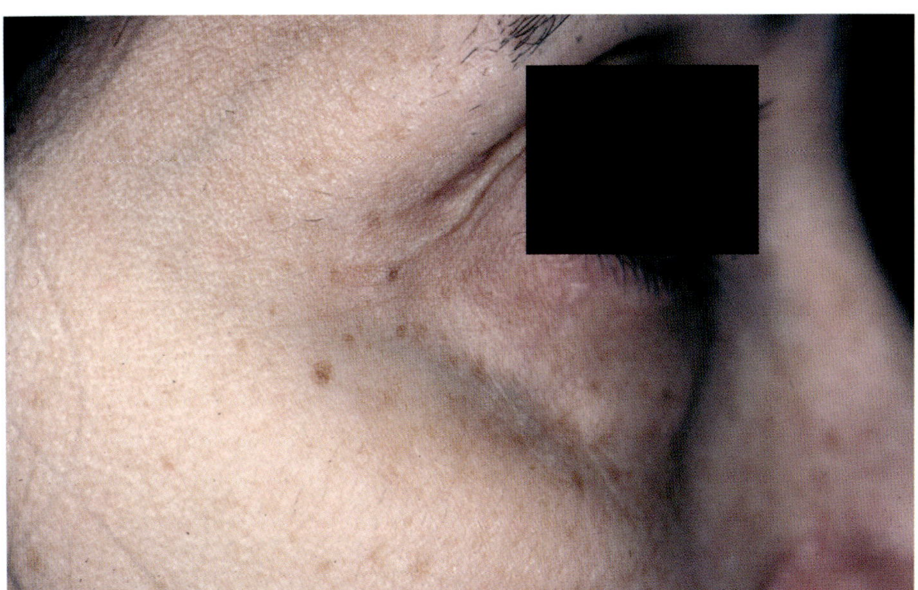

Figure 2.12. Before 1450 nm diode laser non-ablative treatment

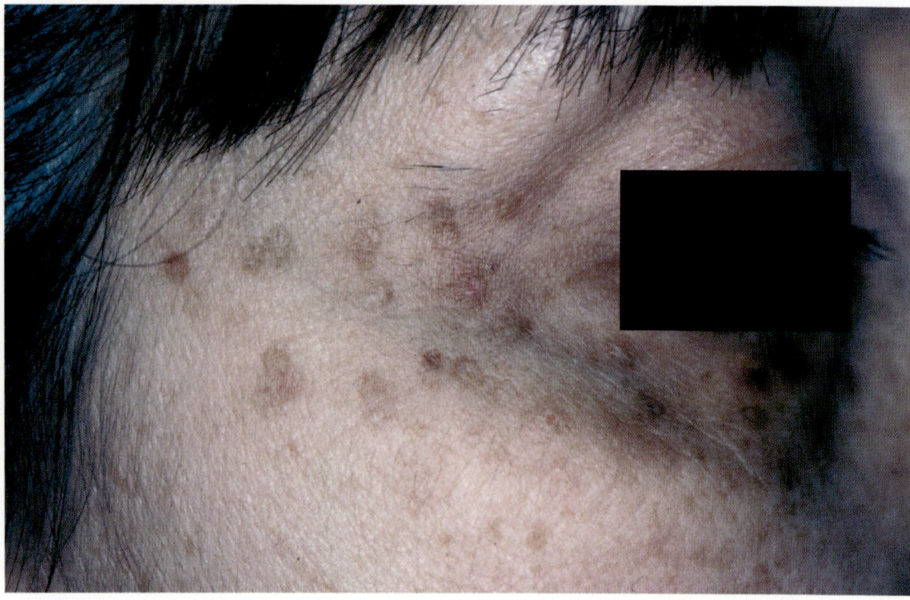

Figure 2.13. Post-inflammatory hyperpigmentation 5 months after 1450 nm diode laser non-ablative treatment

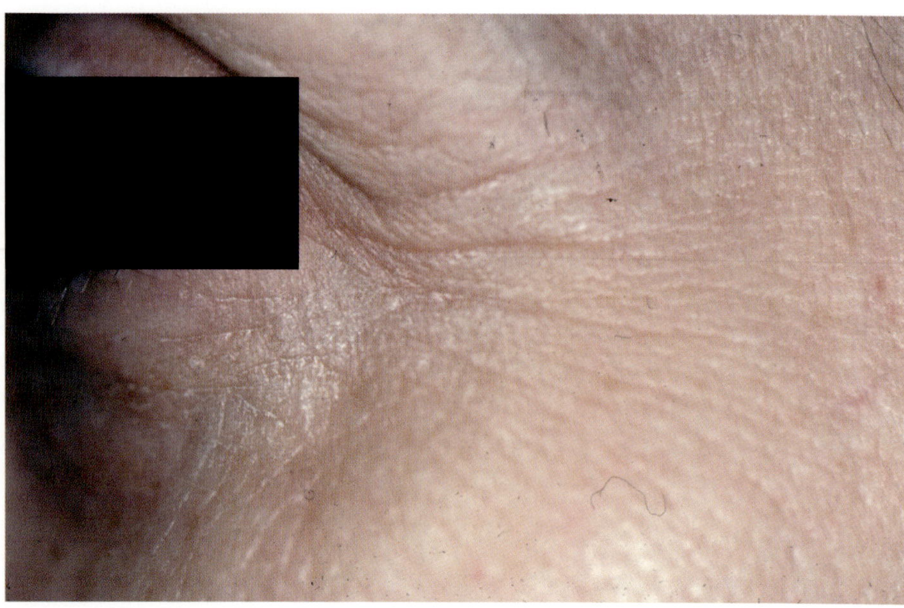

Figure 2.14. Before 1320 nm Nd:YAG laser non-ablative treatment

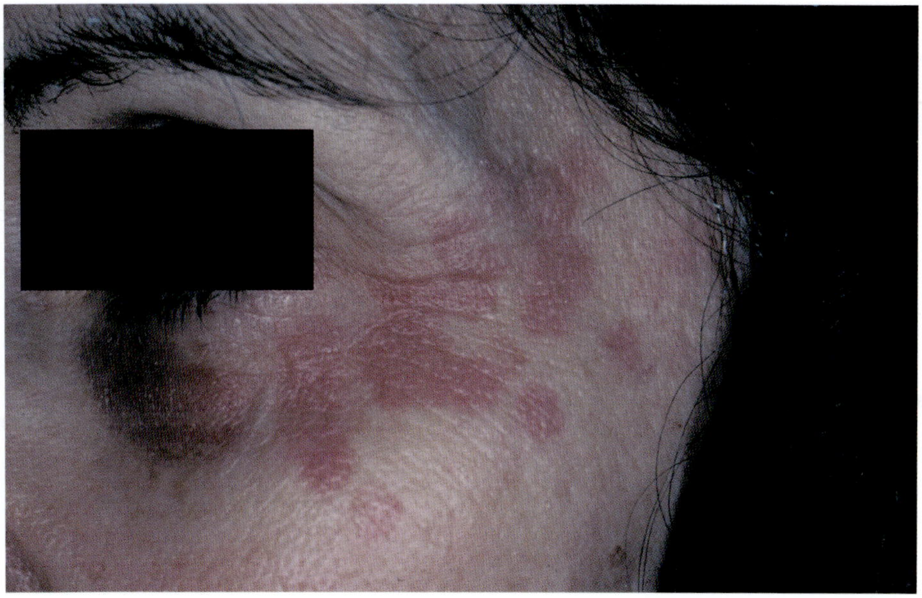

Figure 2.15. Extensive erythema immediately after 1320 nm Nd:YAG laser treatment. Generally this does not lead to permanent pigmentary changes

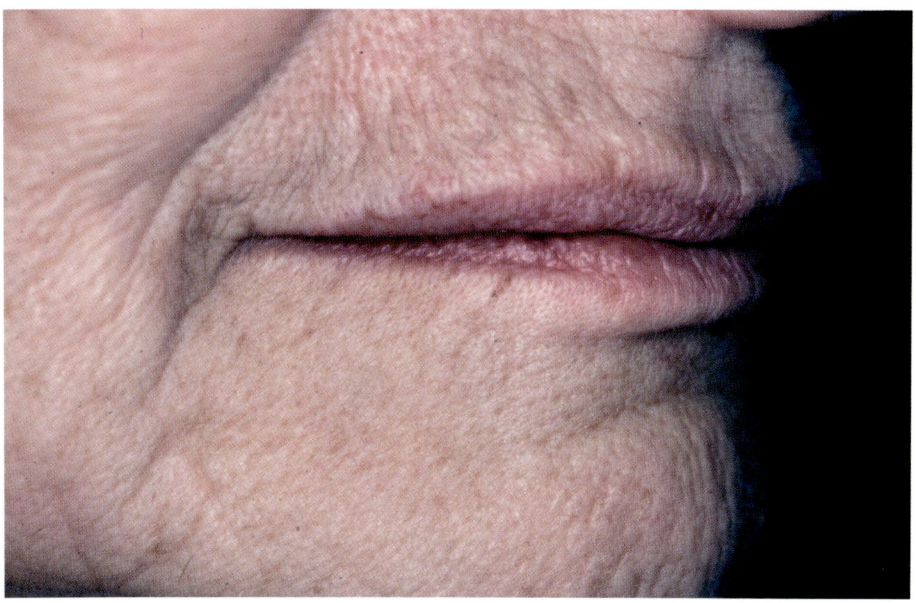

Figure 2.16. Before 1320 nm Nd:YAG laser non-ablative treatment

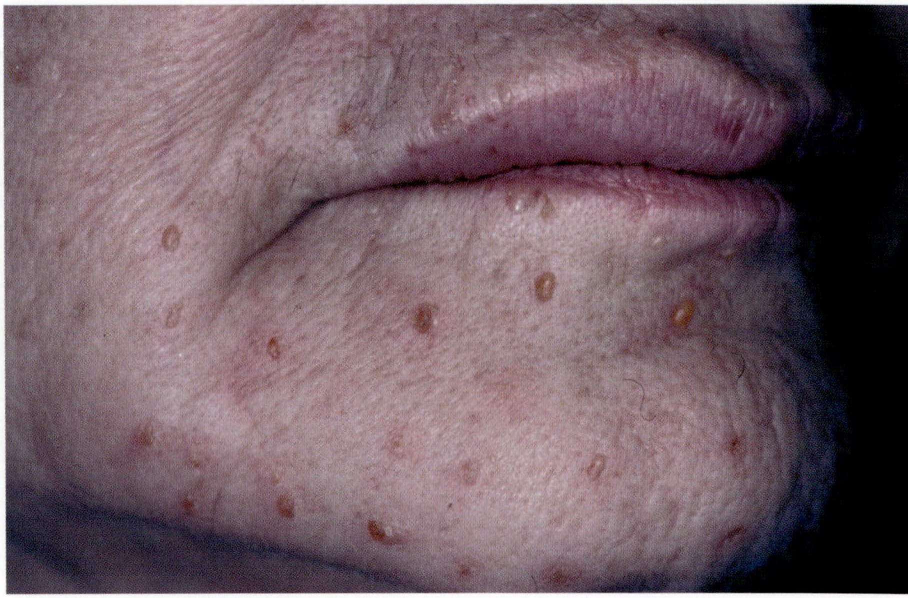

Figure 2.17. Blistering after 1320 nm Nd:YAG laser treatment. This may lead to pigmentary changes

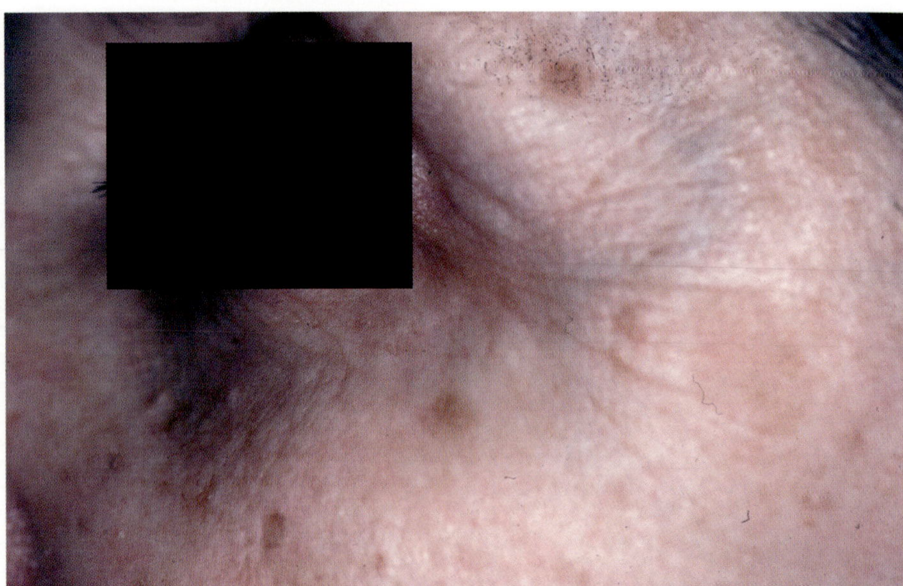

Figure 2.18. Before 1320 nm Nd:YAG laser non-ablative treatment

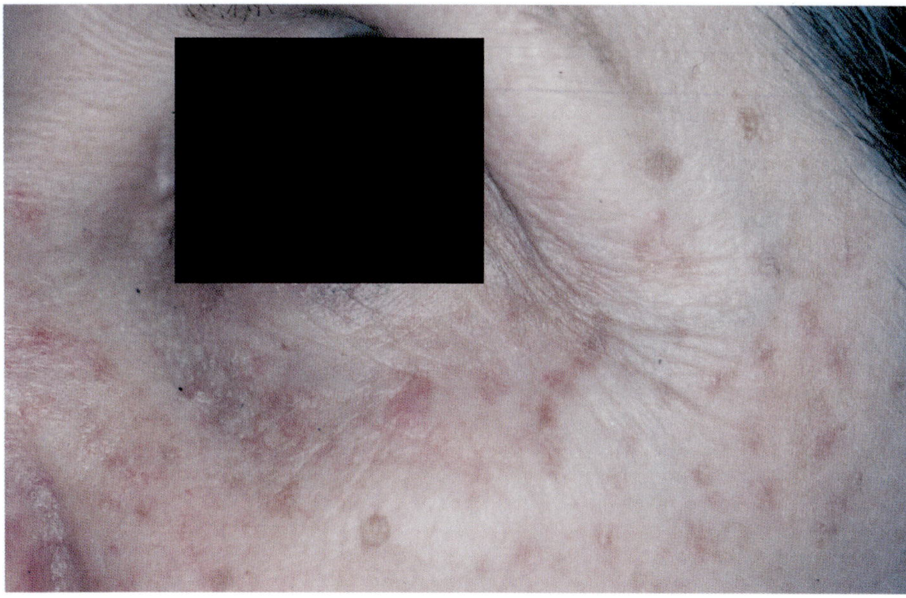

Figure 2.19. Post-inflammatory hyperpigmentation 3 months after 1320 nm Nd:YAG laser non-ablative treatment

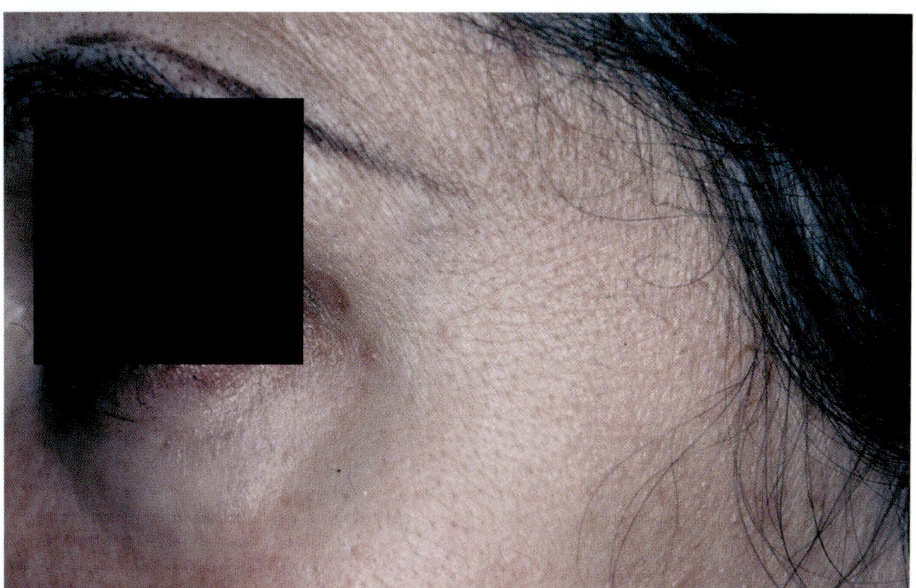

Figure 2.20. Before 1320 nm Nd:YAG laser non-ablative treatment

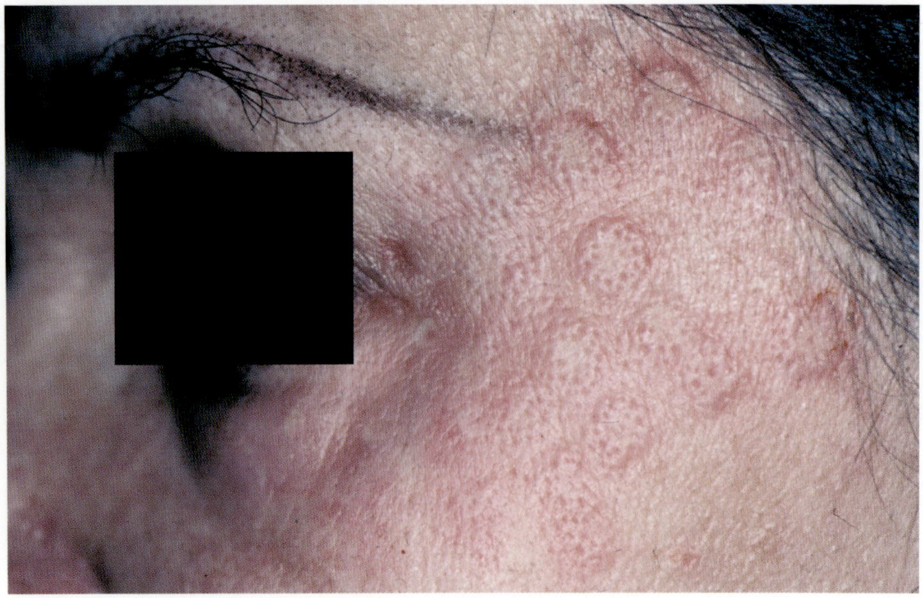

Figure 2.21. Early blistering after 1320 nm Nd:YAG laser treatment

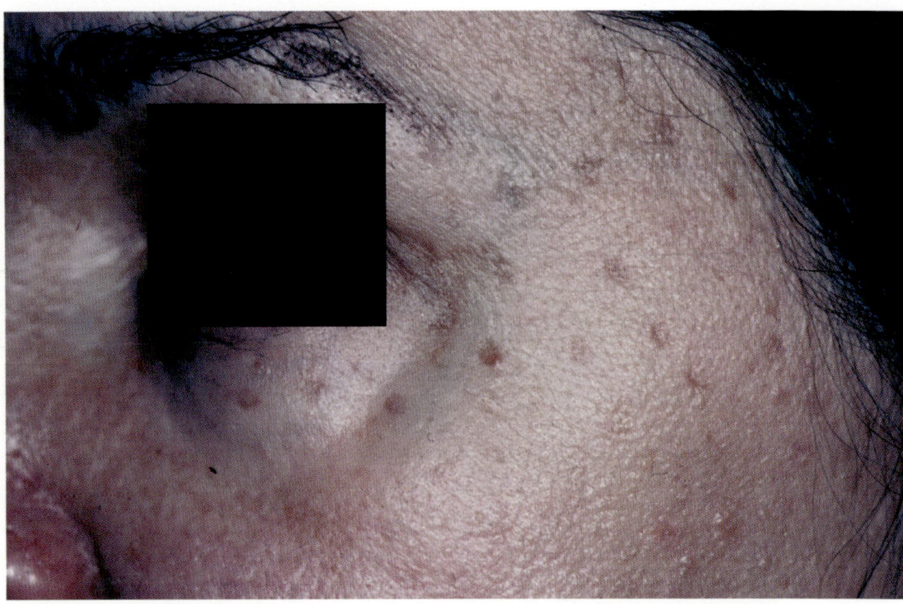

Figure 2.22. Post-inflammatory hyperpigmentation 3 months after 1320 nm Nd:YAG laser non-ablative treatment

HYPOPIGMENTATION

Whereas hyperpigmentation is an early, transient complication of laser resurfacing, hypopigmentation appears to be delayed and may rarely be permanent. Hypopigmentation occurs in up to 16% of ablative laser-treated patients,[15–18] and has been reported in Fitzpatrick skin types I–IV (Figures 2.23 and 2.24).

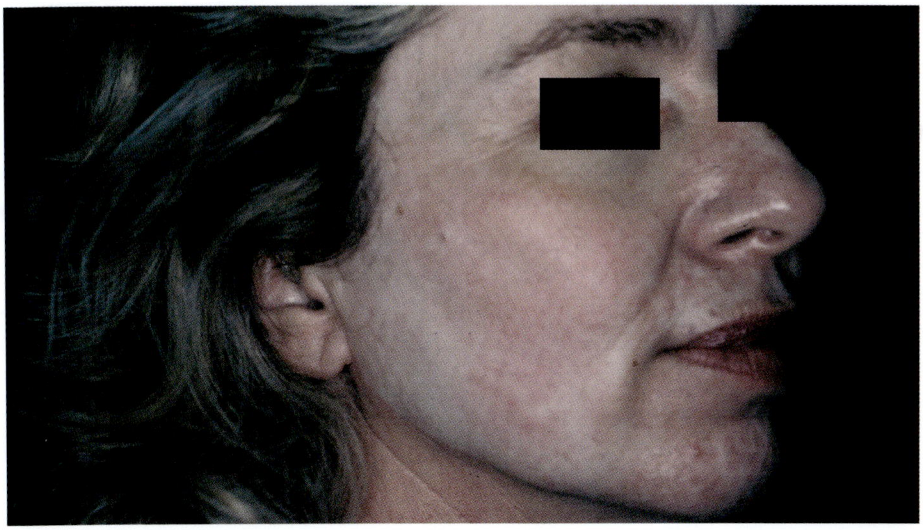

Figure 2.23. Post-inflammatory hypopigmentation 9 months after CO_2 laser resurfacing on the face

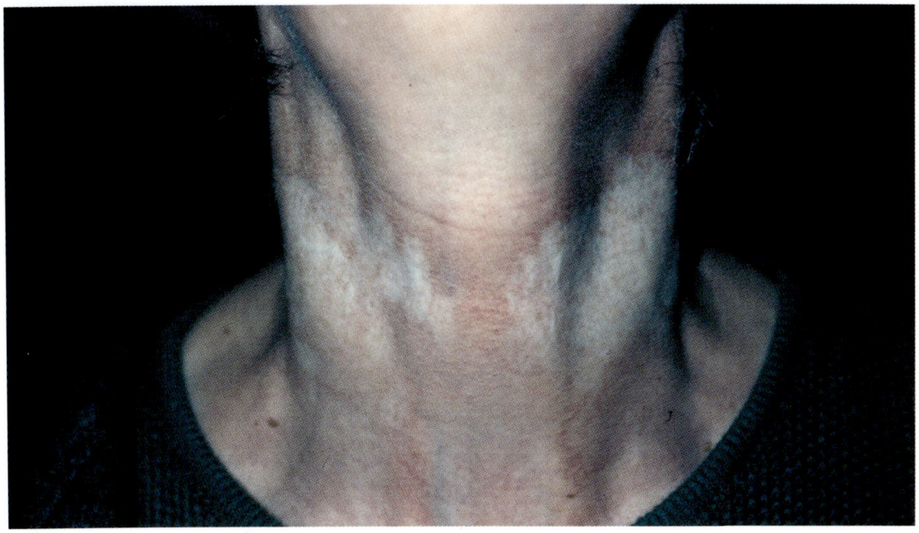

Figure 2.24. Post-inflammatory hypopigmentation 12 months after CO_2 laser resurfacing on the neck

It should be noted that post-operative hypopigmentation had not been reported in initial laser resurfacing studies. These studies all had limited follow-up periods.[23–30]

Recent reports of laser resurfacing complications show a higher incidence of delayed hypopigmentation.[31,32] Hypopigmentation does not usually become evident until several months after resolution of post laser-induced erythema. This clinical loss of pigmentation has been noted as early as 3 months and as late as 10 months, with an average of 6.75 months after treatment.

Often, the delayed hypopigmentation occurs after a period of time in which the skin appears normal. It is difficult, however, to predict who is at greatest risk for hypopigmentation, as this complication may be seen in a variety of skin types.

A common factor among the subset of patients with delayed permanent hypopigmentation is the significant degree of pre-laser photodamage to their skin. Patients at risk are generally bronzed with scattered solar lentigines. In addition to these risks, the risk of hypopigmentation after laser resurfacing is directly related to the depth of laser penetration and degree of thermal injury imparted to the tissue. Additional risk factors include prior dermabrasion, phenol peeling, and patients with a tendency to develop hypopigmented scars. Focal persistent post-treatment erythema may also correlate with the appearance of hypopigmentation 6–12 months after the laser procedure.

Hypopigmentation can be more evident in patients undergoing *localized* CO_2 laser resurfacing. Resurfacing of whole cosmetic units is less likely to produce sharp clinically obvious demarcation zones. However, hypopigmentation occurs equally, but is less clinically apparent in patients having full-face procedures.

Hypopigmentation can also become quite noticeable when the neck is laser resurfaced. Because sebaceous glands and hair follicles on the neck are fewer in number than those seen on the face, laser vaporization in this area may result in delayed wound healing, fibrosis, and loss of pigment cells.

Although there is no difference in the numbers of melanocytes by MART-1 immunohistochemical staining in laser-induced hypopigmentation, there does appear to be a significant decrease in epidermal melanin as determined by Fontanna-Mason staining.[33]

Despite the many theories to explain post laser resurfacing-induced delayed hypopigmentation, the exact cause of this phenomenon is poorly understood.

According to Weinstein,[34] hypopigmentation is due to laser-induced dermal fibrosis, which creates opacification of the papillary dermis. As the new collagen bundles mature and become organized, they form tighter bundles than those seen with the original collagen configuration. Although this is largely responsible for the 'tightening' of the skin that occurs after CO_2 laser resurfacing, it also alters the light reflectance of the skin, leading to the loss of luminescence.

Patients with lighter skin have a relatively transparent epidermis due to the paucity of melanin within this layer, so dermal fibrosis is more clearly noted. Darker-skinned patients with a less transparent epidermis have a lesser noted incidence of dermal opacification.

In addition, the greater the depth of resurfacing, the denser is the post-healing fibrosis. With this, the dermis appears more opaque and consequently paler. Hypopigmentation is, therefore, more likely to be clinically apparent when resurfacing is deeper, such as is seen in patients with acne scars and deeper rhytides. This is true for all ablative resurfacing procedures, and is not exclusive to the CO_2 laser. Once delayed hypopigmentation occurs, it is likely to be permanent.

Alster has expressed a different view about the etiology of delayed hypopigmentation.[20] She has suggested that this complication may be caused by damage to follicular melanocytes resulting from overly aggressive laser treatment; or it may simply be an unmasking of pre-existing hypopigmentation resulting from earlier trauma (e.g. dermabrasion and phenol peeling).

She also notes that what is perceived as a 'complication' may simply represent only a return to the constitutive pigment of the skin. According to this theory, the underlying fibroplasia seen after laser therapy can change the hue of the skin to a whitish color even with normal melanization.[35]

According to Alster, true hypopigmentation would be rare. Most cases of skin lightening represent 'relative hypopigmentation' caused by the removal of photodamaged skin (appearing as pale skin adjacent to non-treated dyspigmentation).

SCARRING

Although transient 'scarring' occurs in up to 2.8% of resurface-treated patients, fewer than 1% experience permanent scarring.[15,17,18] Of physicians using the CO_2 laser, 64% have seen at least one case of hypertrophic scarring.[36] Any cause of delayed complete epidermal re-epithelialization, 14–21 days after laser resurfacing, significantly increases the chances of scarring (Figures 2.25–2.36).

Focal areas of intense erythema and induration are the first signs of impending scar formation. This must be recognized early and treated promptly to avoid permanent sequelae. Hypertrophic scarring and textural changes are rare but represent serious complications following cutaneous laser resurfacing. Although there are individual differences with respect to scar propensity, most scars seen after laser resurfacing appear to be a result of either poor technique and/or post-operative infections.

Scarring, usually of the atrophic variety, may also be induced by the thermal effect of non-ablative devices. The use of either too low or too high a delivered fluence, stacking or overlapping of pulses, and/or an excessive number of laser passes all may result in excessive tissue damage.

By delivering a fluence below the threshold of skin ablation, heat conduction will occur before the tissue is completely ablated. This creates a heat sink with thermal injury occurring below the intended level. Because collagen is so heat-sensitive, complete dermal destruction and scarring may result. Similarly, if laser pulses are overlapped or stacked without removing ablated tissue and rehydrating the underlying skin, a heat sink will occur, causing focally increased heat penetration.

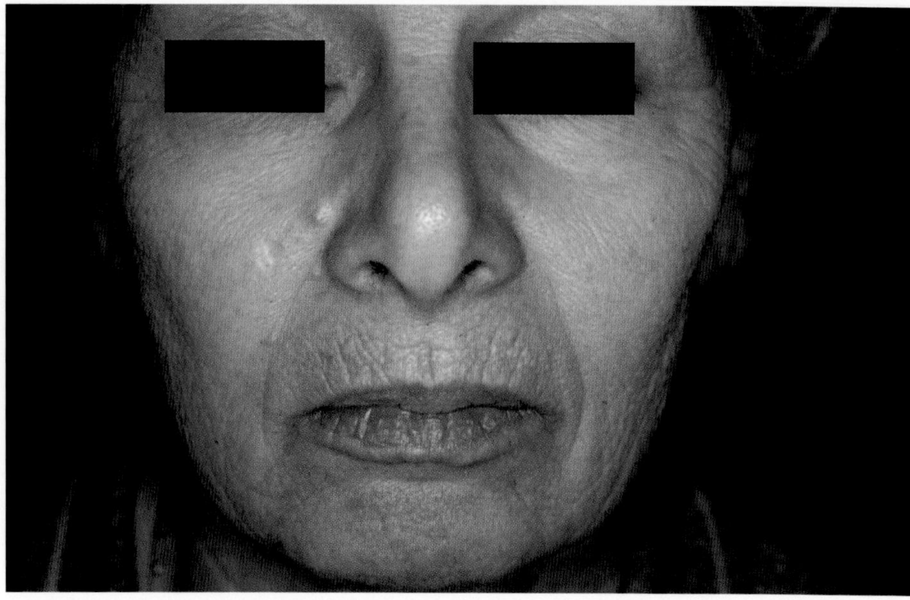

Figure 2.25. Before Er:YAG laser resurfacing

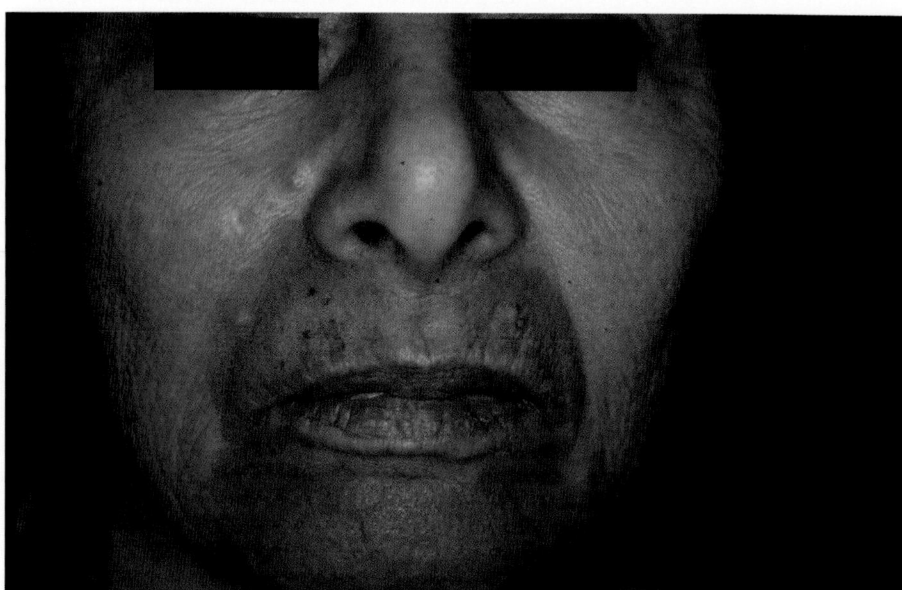

Figure 2.26. Immediately after Er:YAG laser resurfacing

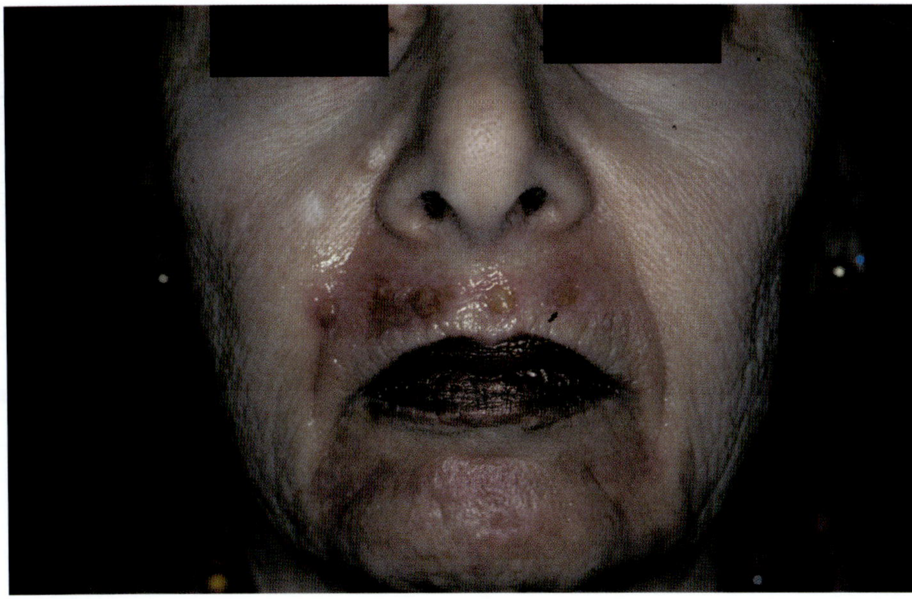

Figure 2.27. Non-healing 2 weeks after Er:YAG laser resurfacing

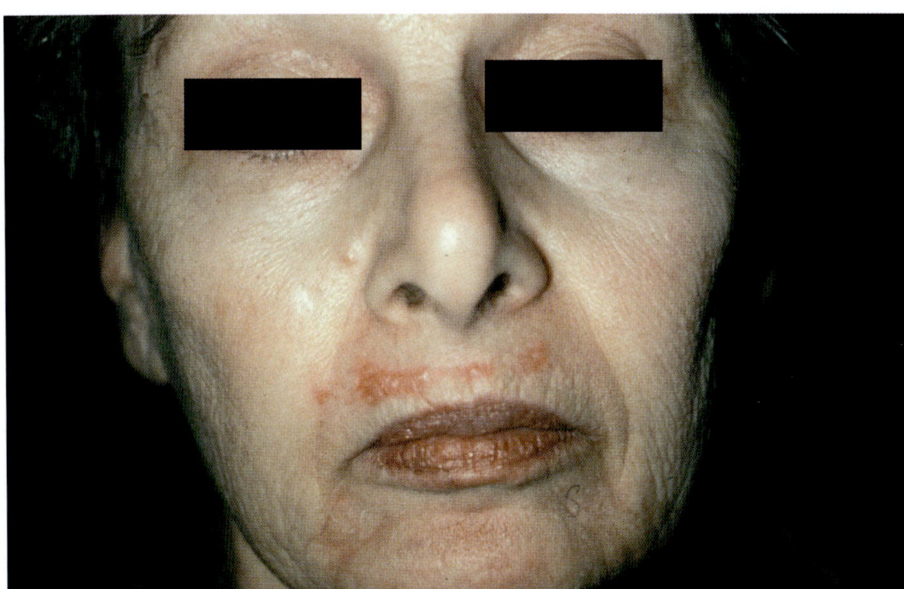

Figure 2.28. Hypertrophic scarring 4 months after Er:YAG laser resurfacing

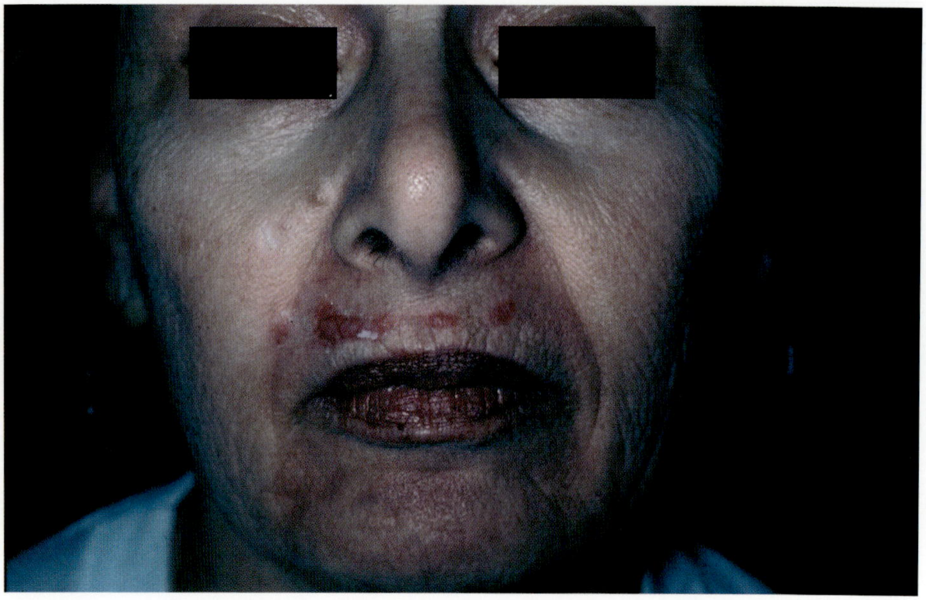

Figure 2.29. Hypertrophic scarring 6 months after Er:YAG laser resurfacing

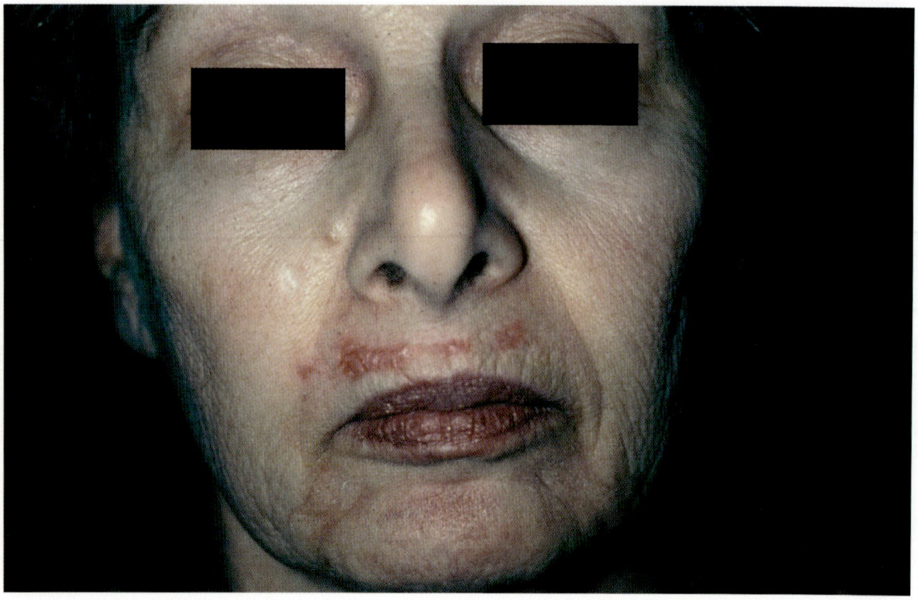

Figure 2.30. Hypertrophic scarring 8 months after Er:YAG laser resurfacing

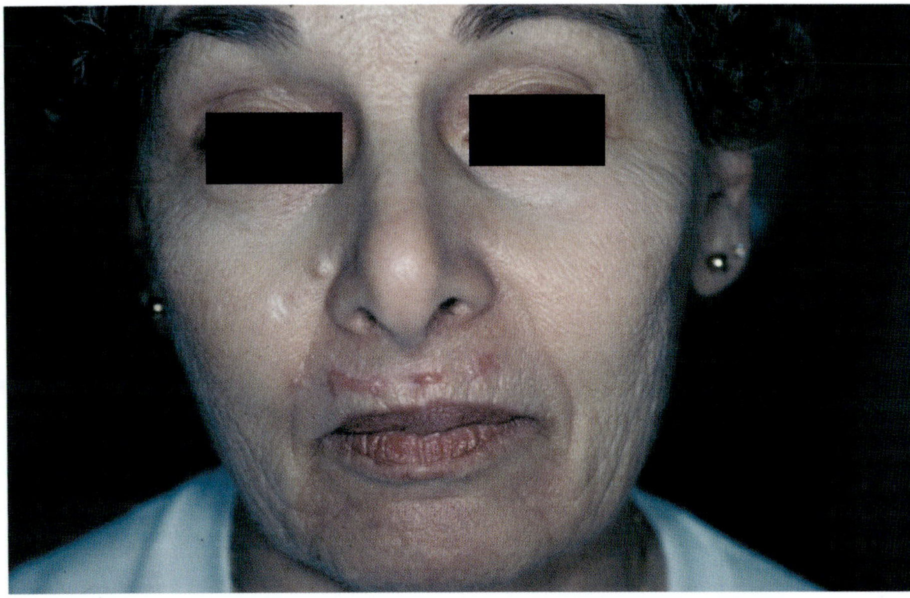

Figure 2.31. Hypertrophic scarring 10 months after Er:YAG laser resurfacing

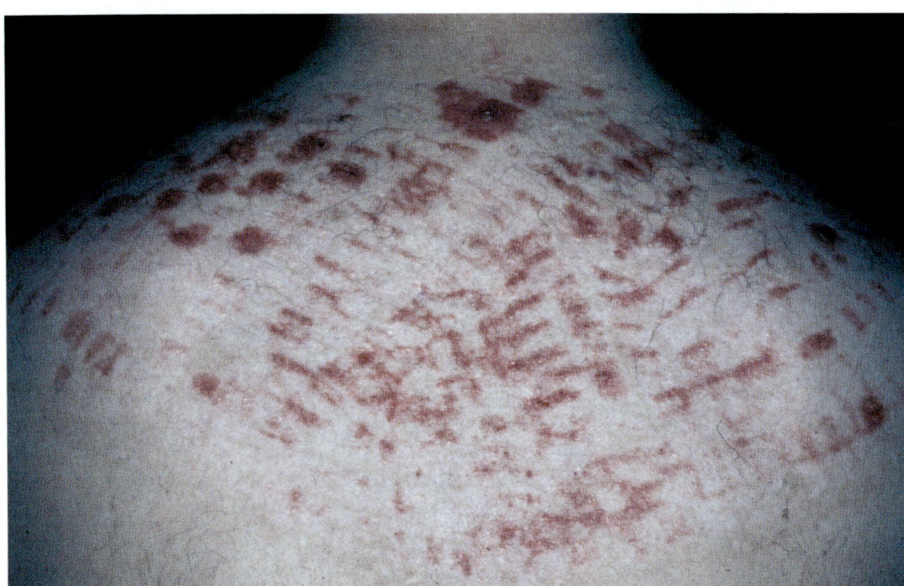

Figure 2.32. Hypertrophic scarring of the back 1 year after CO_2 laser resurfacing

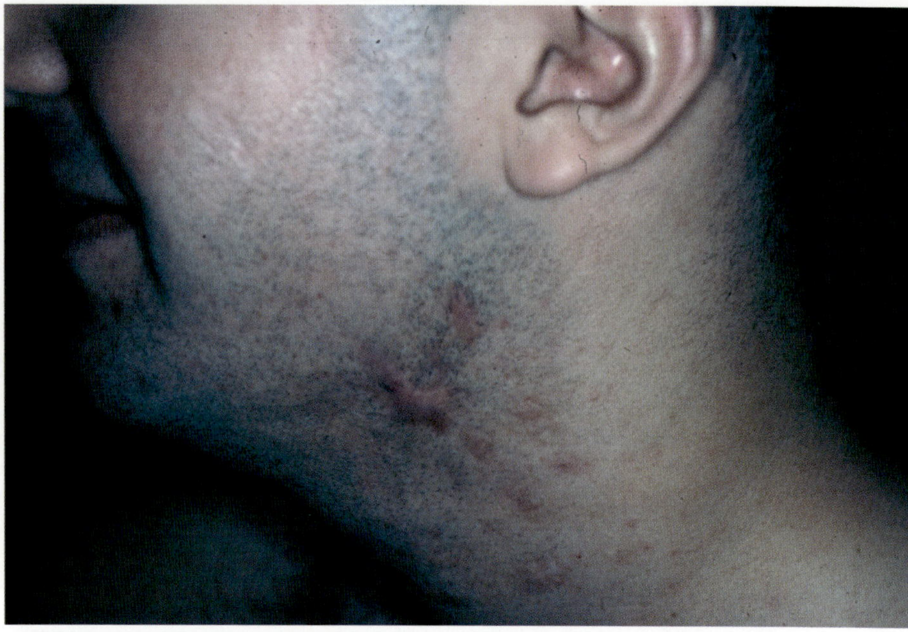

Figure 2.33. Hypertrophic scarring of the neck 1 year after CO_2 laser resurfacing

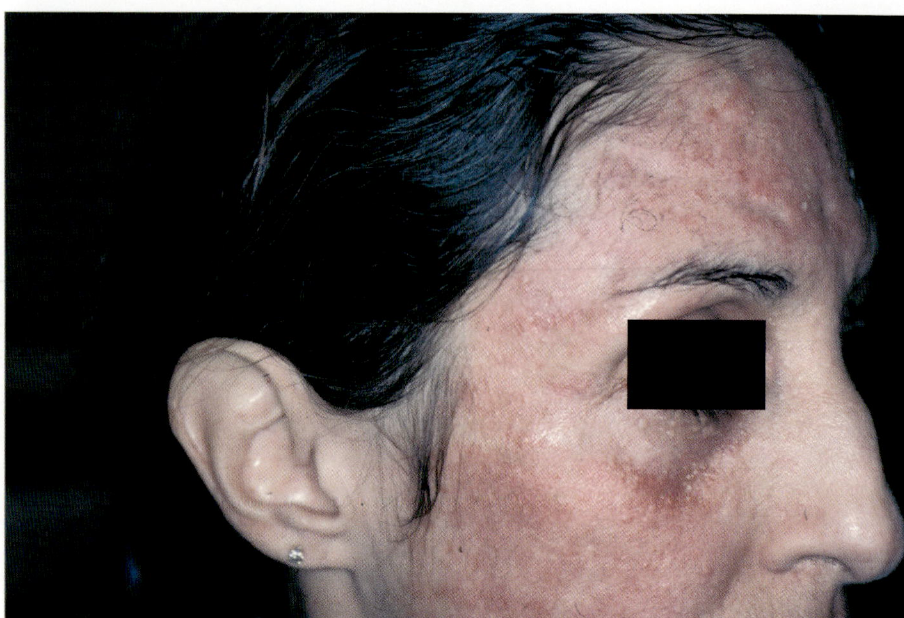

Figure 2.34. Hypertrophic scarring of the face 1 year after CO_2 laser resurfacing

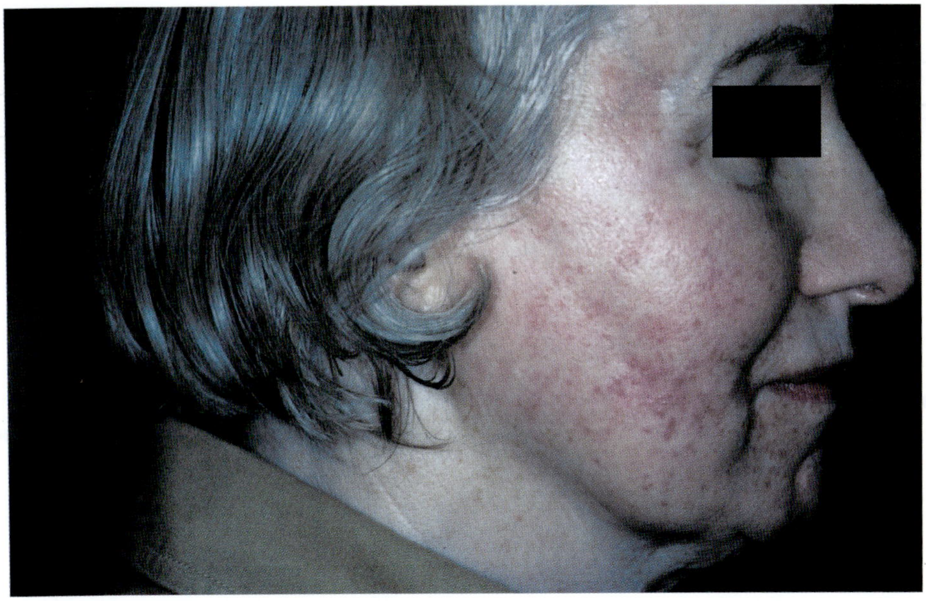

Figure 2.35. Persistent erythema and mild hypertrophic scarring 6 months after Er:YAG laser resurfacing

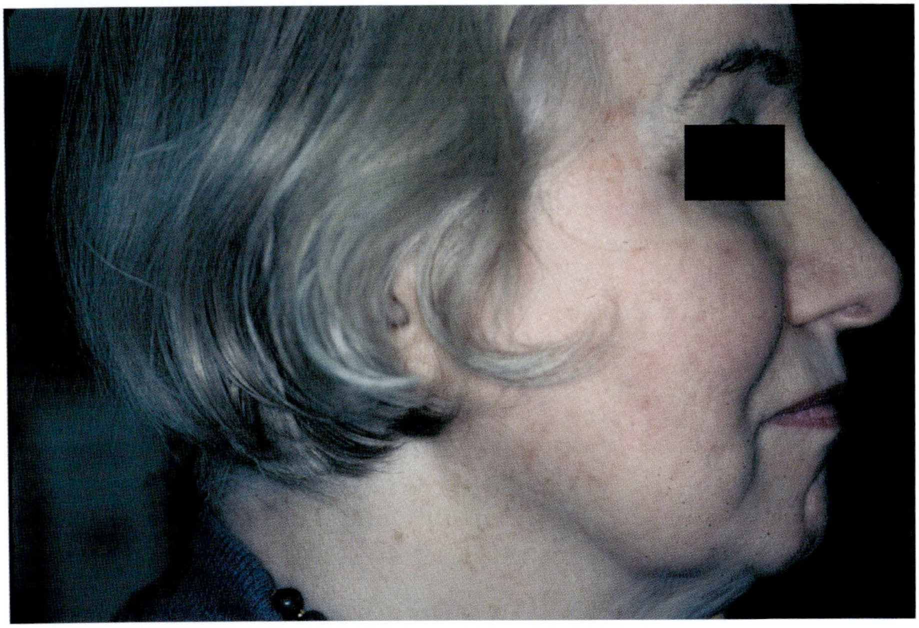

Figure 2.36. Resolution of erythema and mild hypertrophic scarring 18 months after Er:YAG laser resurfacing

This may occur if the frequency of the pulses is too rapid or the operator's hand speed is too slow. To avoid this problem, the frequency of the pulses should be reduced, so that a comfortable hand speed may be used at all times. With newer computerized scanners, this risk is lessened as the computer lays down laser pulses in a fixed pattern with fixed overlap.

Finally, repeated CO_2 laser passes will dehydrate and coagulate the dermal collagen, which subsequently limits the penetration of laser energy affecting both the ablative effect and the incidental thermal injury of subsequent passes. Because a large part of the heat in subsequent passes is not actually used to ablate the tissue, the thermal loading of tissue increases. With more thermal scattering now occurring in the reticular dermis, there is also a potential increase in scarring. Because the resurfaced skin heals by re-epithelialization through intact appendages, lasering the skin too deeply will destroy these appendageal reservoirs. The base of the appendages is in the mid or lower reticular dermis. Resurfacing to a greater depth increases the risk of scarring.

Isotretinoin treatment also alters appendageal structure and function. With this, the normal mechanism for re-epithelialization may be temporarily impaired. Patients who have recently been taking oral isotretinoin do not have normal appendageal function and have fragile skin. The effects of oral isotretinoin last for some time after treatment. Although the exact optimal interval between isotretinoin therapy and resurfacing is not really known, it is recommended that patients should wait at least 6–12 months after oral isotretinoin intake before undergoing an ablative laser procedure.[37–42] Because adnexal structures are diminished in patients with a prior history of radiation therapy or scleroderma (autoimmune disorder), caution should also be taken in such patients. Such patients may be at higher risk of scarring.[43]

Patients with a history of hypertrophic scars, or keloid formation may also be at higher risk for scarring. Skin that has recently been undermined, such as is seen with rhytidectomy, is characterized by diminished cutaneous circulation. Such skin should not be resurfaced for 3–6 months after rhytidectomy in order to avoid potential necrosis with resultant scarring.[43]

Certain facial areas are more prone to scar formation. Anatomic areas showing an increased incidence of scarring after aggressive laser resurfacing include the perioral, chin, neck, and mandibular regions.[15,25,40]

Patients who previously engaged in extensive electrolysis to remove unwanted lip hair may have a significant destruction of the hair follicles. Because intact appendages are necessary for resurfacing, these patients may have a significantly depleted reservoir and, therefore, are at increased risk of scarring. Patients who experience extensive post-operative contact dermatitis are also at increased risk of scarring.[44]

Localized areas of hypertrophic scarring generally begin to occur between 2 and 8 weeks post-operatively. Such scarring may also occur after non-ablative treatments (Figures 2.37–2.51).

Although patients who have an impaired blood supply, such as smokers, may have problems with delayed healing, there are no published data to suggest that laser resurface-treated patients who smoke have difficulties with re-epithelialization.

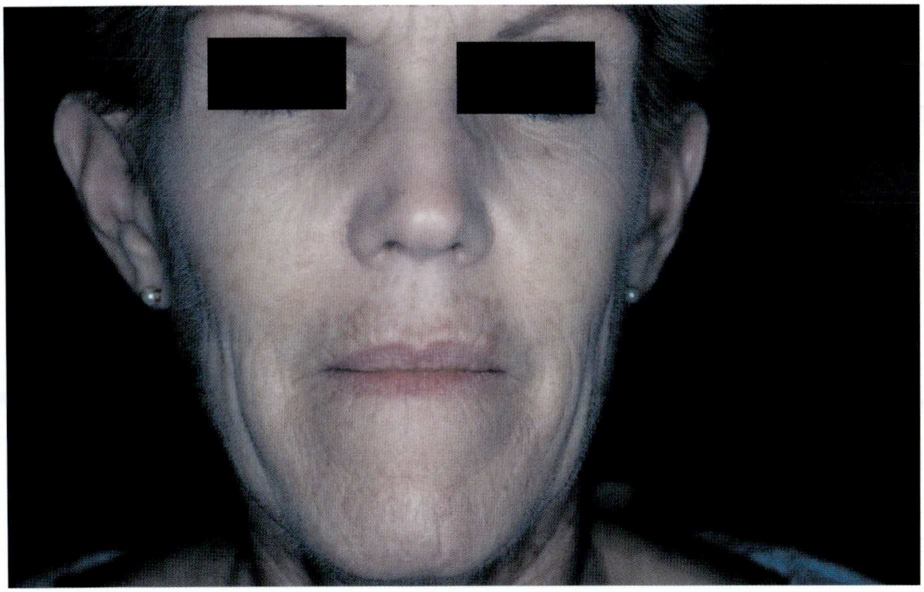

Figure 2.37. Before intense pulsed light treatment of the perioral area

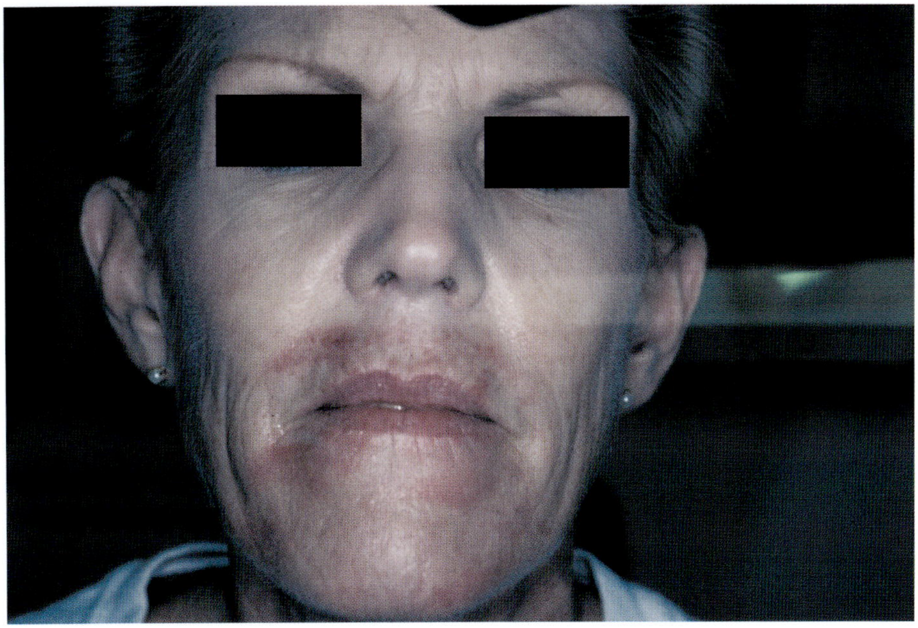

Figure 2.38. Hypertrophic scarring 3 months after intense pulsed light treatment

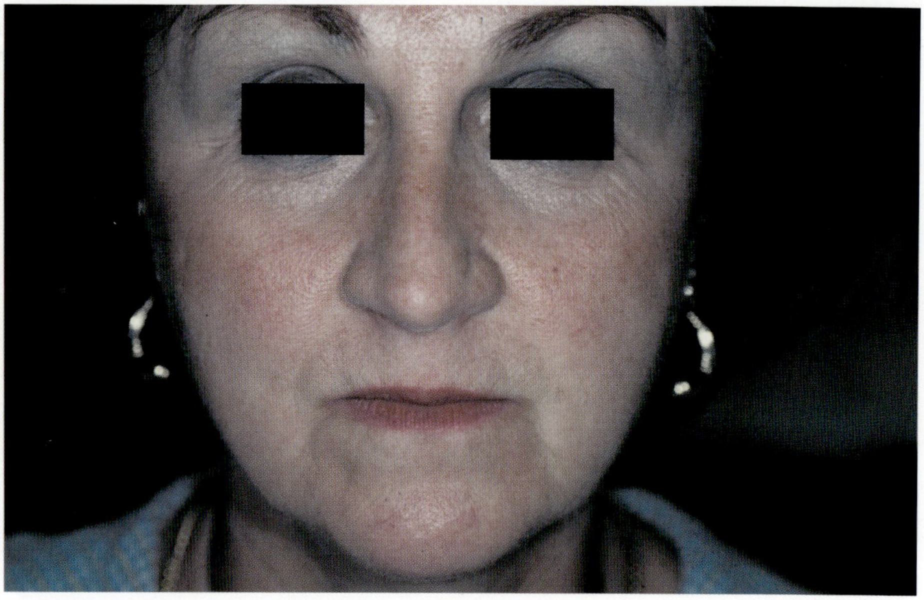

Figure 2.39. Before intense pulsed light non-ablative treatment

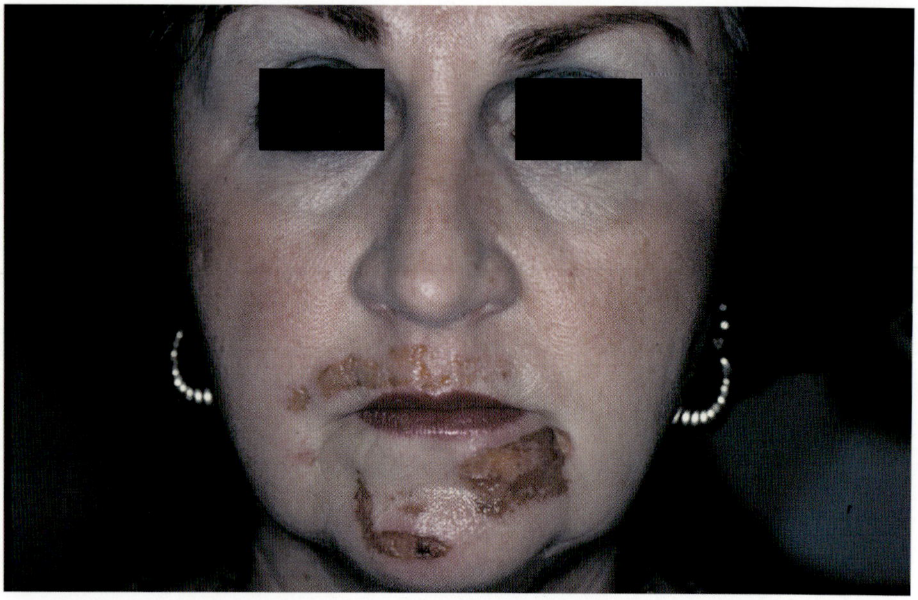

Figure 2.40. Blisters and crusting immediately after intense pulsed light non-ablative treatment. Scarring is likely to result

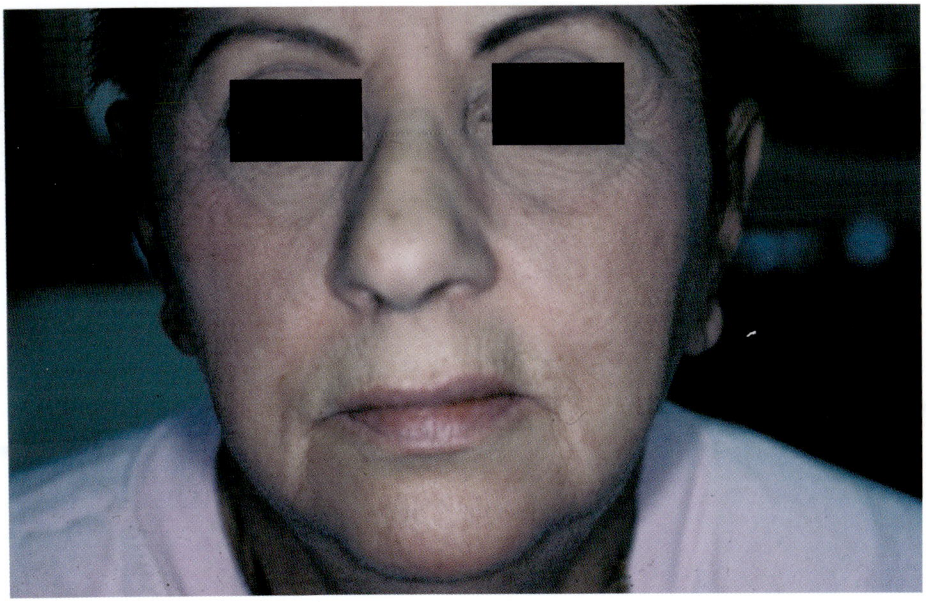

Figure 2.41. Before intense pulsed light non-ablative treatment

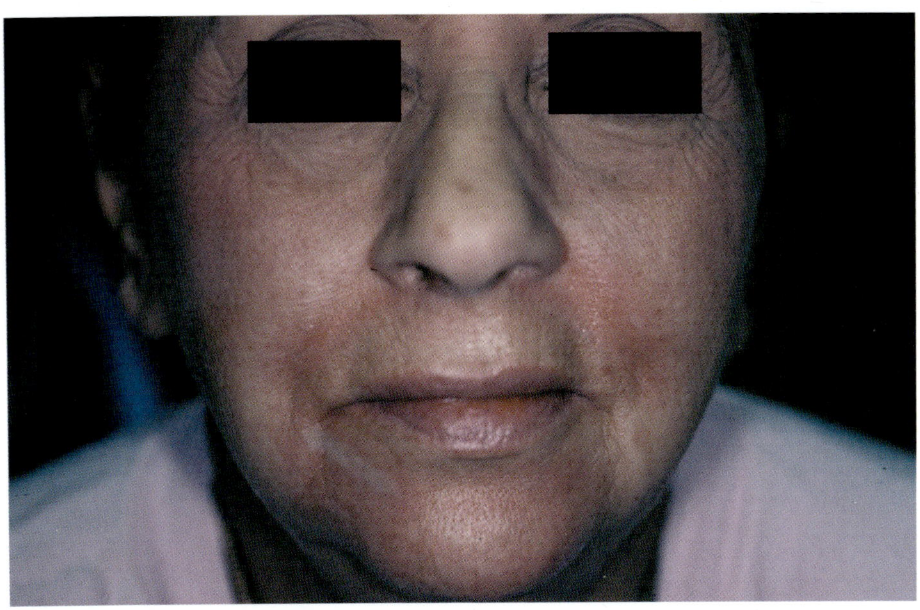

Figure 2.42. Epidermal whitening immediately after intense pulsed light non-ablative treatment. Expect to see some scarring

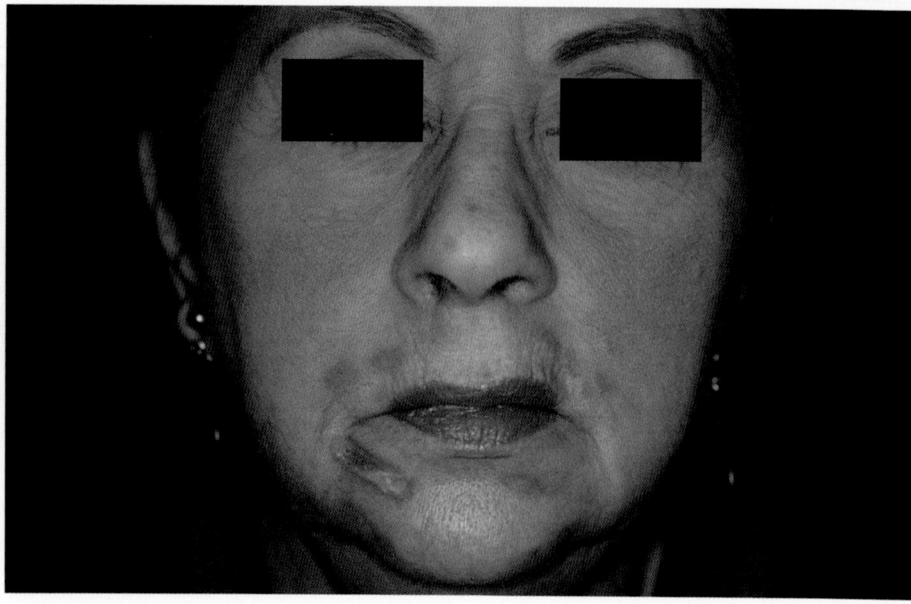

Figure 2.43. One week after intense pulsed light non-ablative treatment

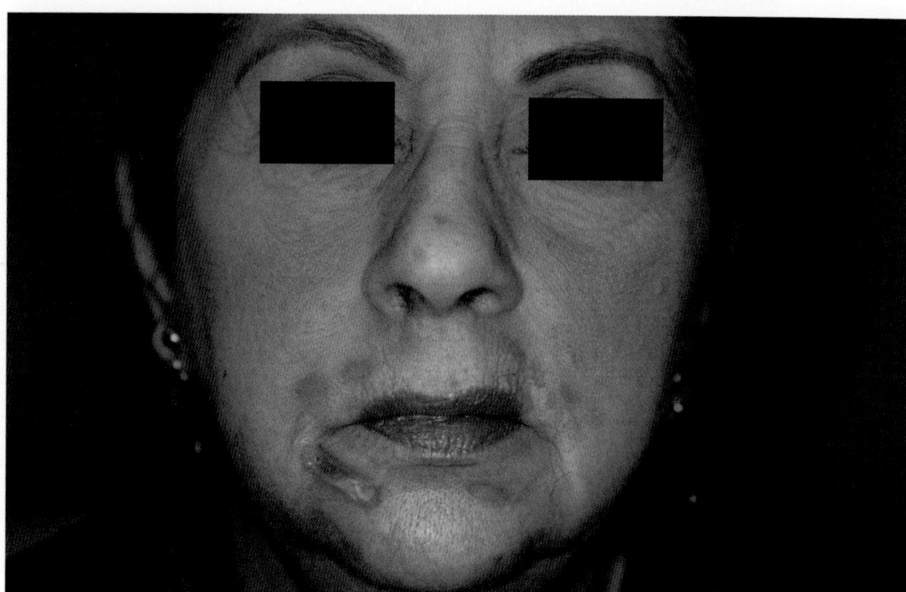

Figure 2.44. Two weeks after intense pulsed light non-ablative treatment

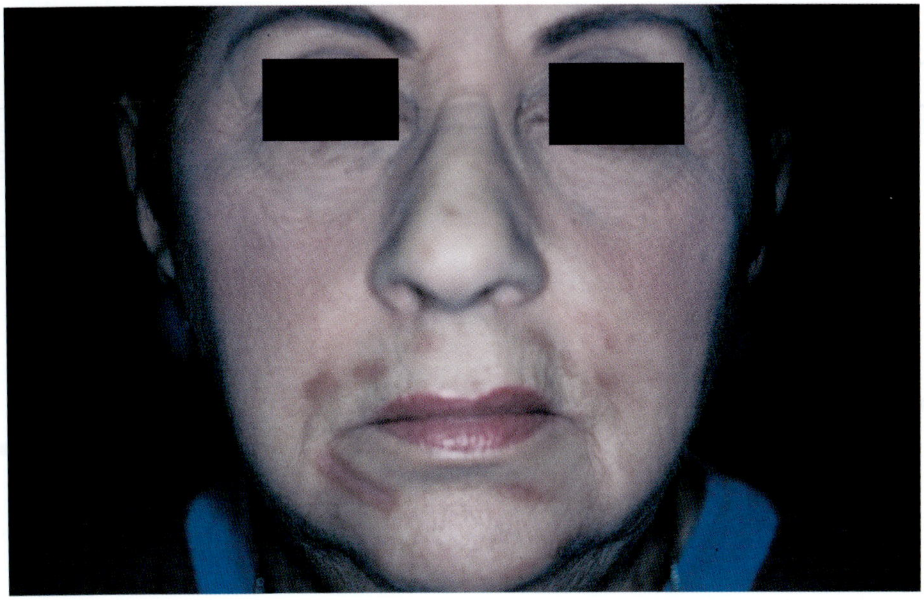

Figure 2.45. Four weeks after intense pulsed light non-ablative treatment

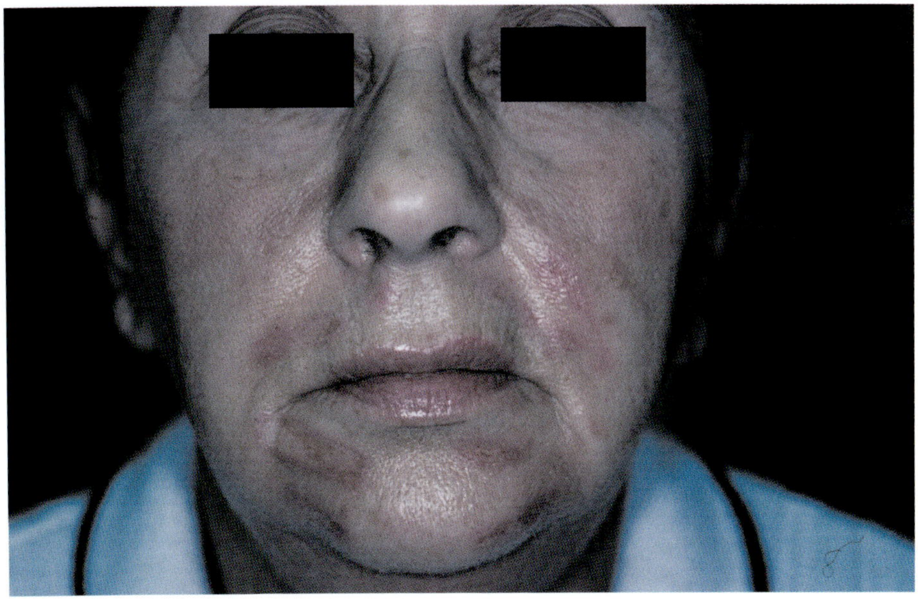

Figure 2.46. Six weeks after intense pulsed light non-ablative treatment

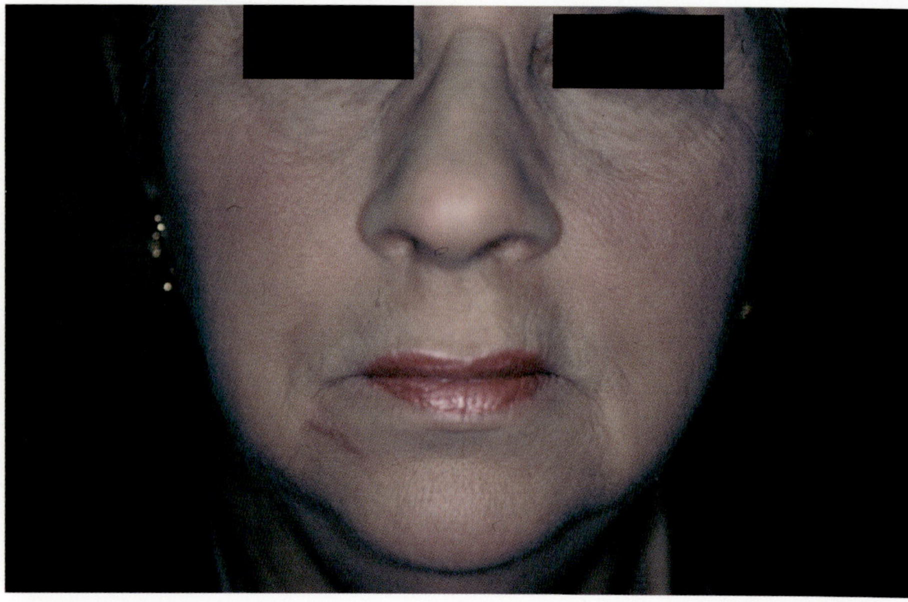

Figure 2.47. One year after intense pulsed light non-ablative treatment. Note persistent hypertrophic scarring

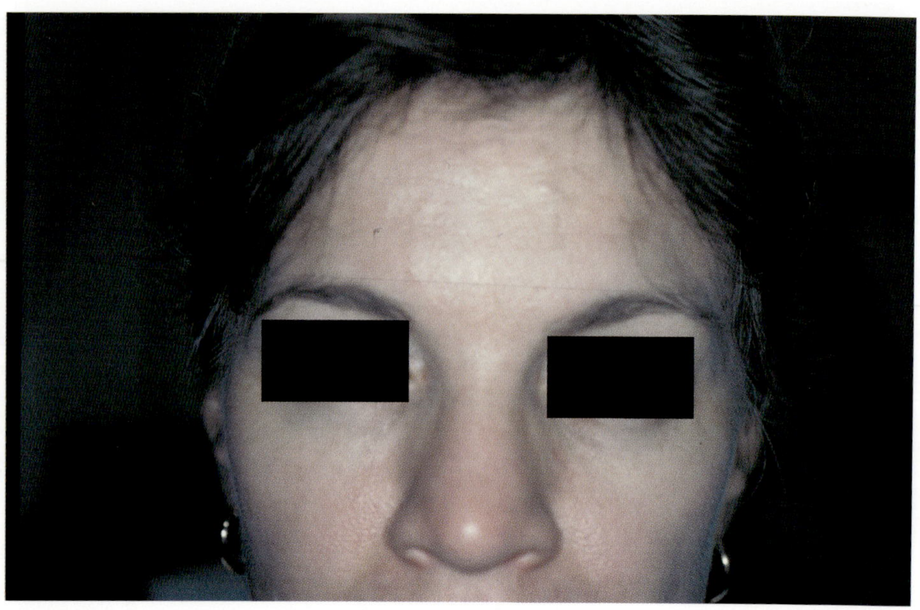

Figure 2.48. Before intense pulsed light non-ablative treatment

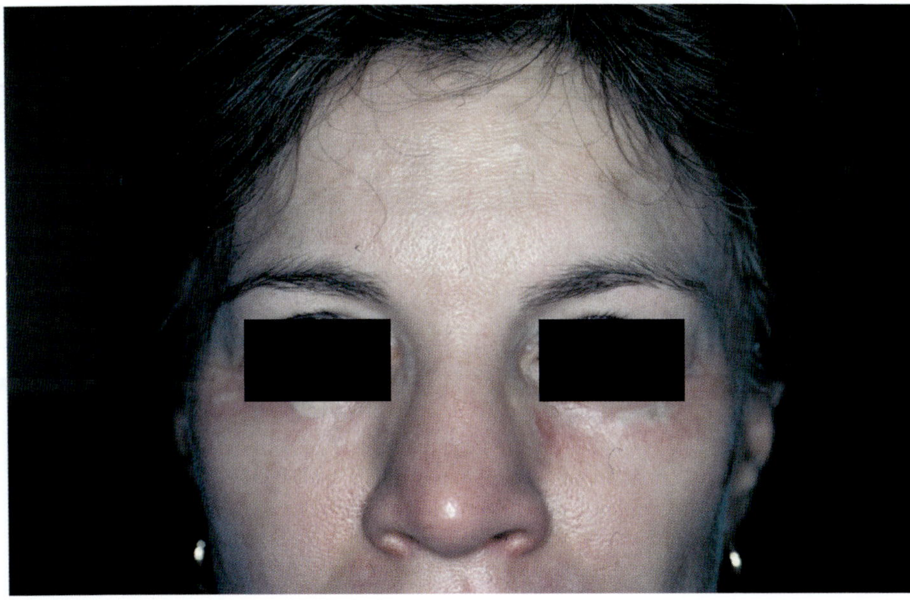

Figure 2.49. Epidermal whitening immediately after intense pulsed light non-ablative treatment

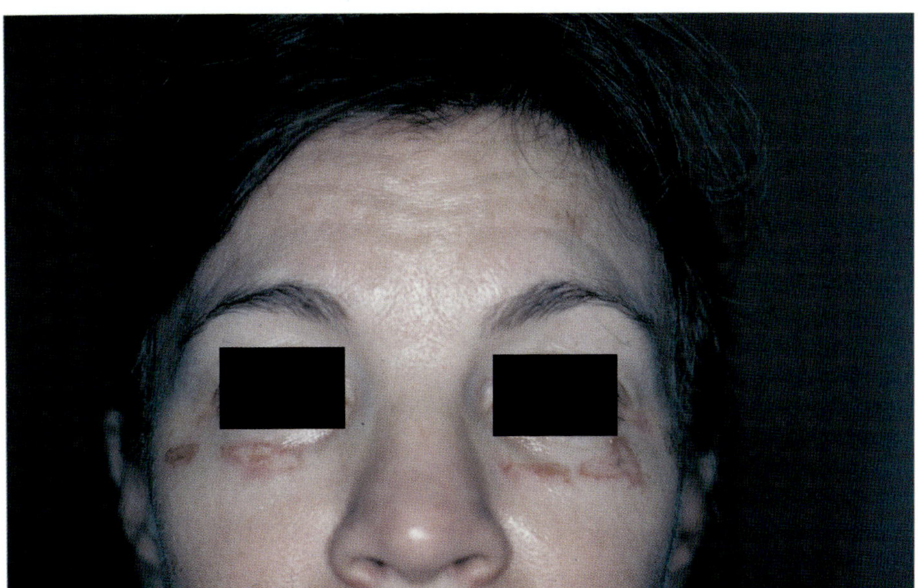

Figure 2.50. One week after intense pulsed light non-ablative treatment

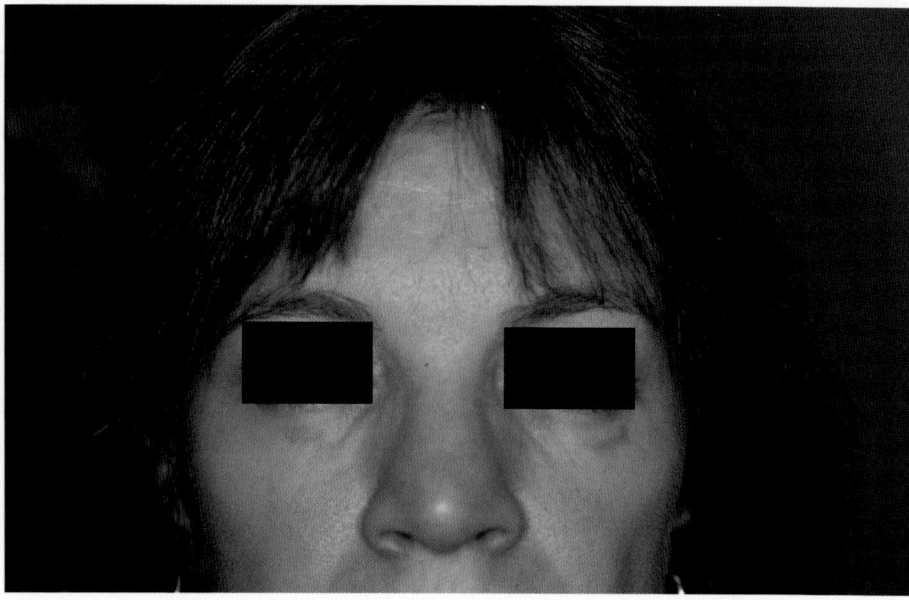

Figure 2.51. Four weeks after intense pulsed light non-ablative treatment. No scarring resulted

INFECTIONS

Viral, bacterial, and monilial infections can develop after cutaneous laser resurfacing. Such infections generally occur during the first post-operative week during the post-laser re-epithelialization process.

The thermal injury created by laser resurfacing is similar to that seen after a thermal burn. Localized immunosuppression occurs, which may predispose the patient to infection.[45]

There is also a relationship between the infection rate and the size of the ablative wound.[46] Medical conditions, such as acquired immunodeficiency syndrome and prior organ transplantation, may also predispose the patient to impaired post-operative healing, as well as increased risk for post-operative infections.[40] Pain, increased erythema, purulent discharge, crusting, or delayed wound-healing should alert the laser physician to the possibility of a superficial cutaneous infection.

Viral Infection

The most frequent infectious complication associated with laser resurfacing is the reactivation of herpes simplex virus infection (HSV).[17] It is suspected that direct laser trauma to the skin leads to latent viral activation and shedding. Herpetic outbreaks are experienced by 2–7% of all laser-treated patients, despite antiviral prophylaxis.[17,47,48] A higher percentage of those with a previous history of an herpetic infection are affected (33%), as compared with those without (5%).[47]

Herpetic outbreaks can also occur in patients treated with non-ablative devices.

Early post-ablative laser detection of HSV is often difficult because there is no intact epithelium and, rather than presenting as the characteristic intact grouped vesicles or pustules on an erythematous base, viral infection is manifest by small, superficial erosions. Symptoms of HSV reactivation include pruritis, dyesthesia, tingling, burning, or discharge from isolated foci within the treated areas. This may result in delayed re-epithelialization. Extensive eruptions can result in disseminated infection and atrophic scarring. Early lesions typically appear as a crop of small, raw, red lesions clustered as a small grouping that may progress to typical discrete white punctate lesions. More lesions may appear if the outbreak is left untreated. This infection must be recognized early and treated aggressively. (Figure 2.52).[47]

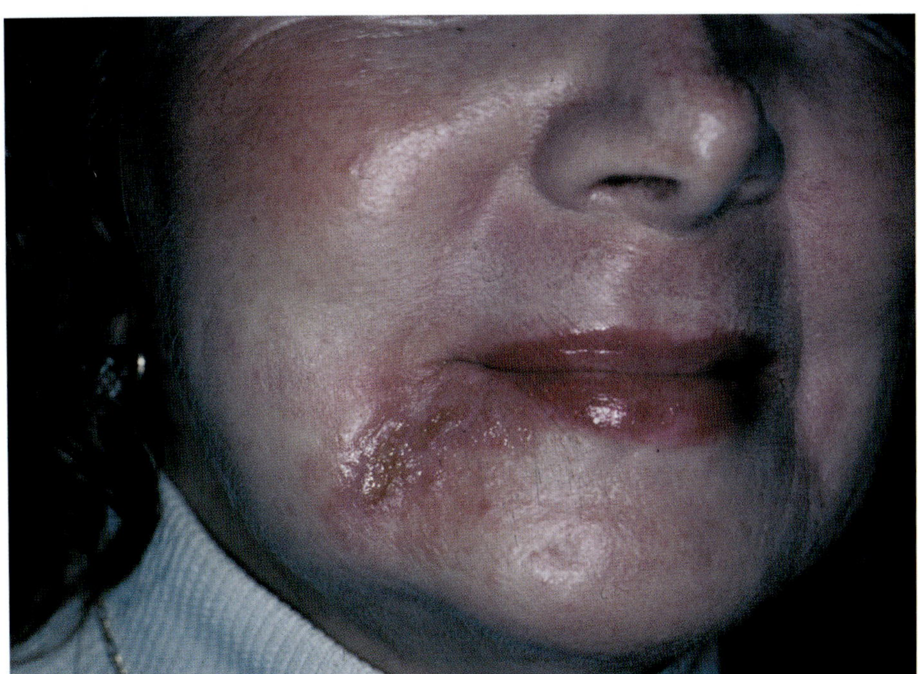

Figure 2.52. Herpetic infection after laser resurfacing

Bacterial Infection

Bacterial infections occurs in up to 5% of laser resurface-treated patients (Figures 2.53–2.55).

Infections usually occur within 2–10 days post-operatively; in 80% of the cases the onset of infection occurs during the first 7 days post-operatively. Pain and/or pruritus are common symptoms of infection. The most common sign of infection is excessive patchy erythema and patchy erosions with superficial crusts and exudates. Most superficial bacterial infections are due to Gram-positive cocci (*Staphylococcus aureus*). The relative rarity of bacterial infection is probably due to:

1. colonization of the skin with normal skin flora;
2. the excellent blood supply to the face;
3. the absence of crusting in appropriately dressed wounds; and
4. the regular washing of the wound with removal of exudate, debris, and crust.[35]

Moist wound care has been shown to enhance re-epithelialization. However, a moist wound may also provide an environment that is ideal for bacterial growth, particularly Gram-negative organisms, such as *Pseudomonas aeruginosa*. Such extremely rare infections may also occur because the use of some prophylactic antibiotics may eliminate the normal cutaneous flora.

Patients with nasal colonization of staphylococci may also be more susceptible to infection. However, it has not been proved that prophylactic topical nasal antibiotic

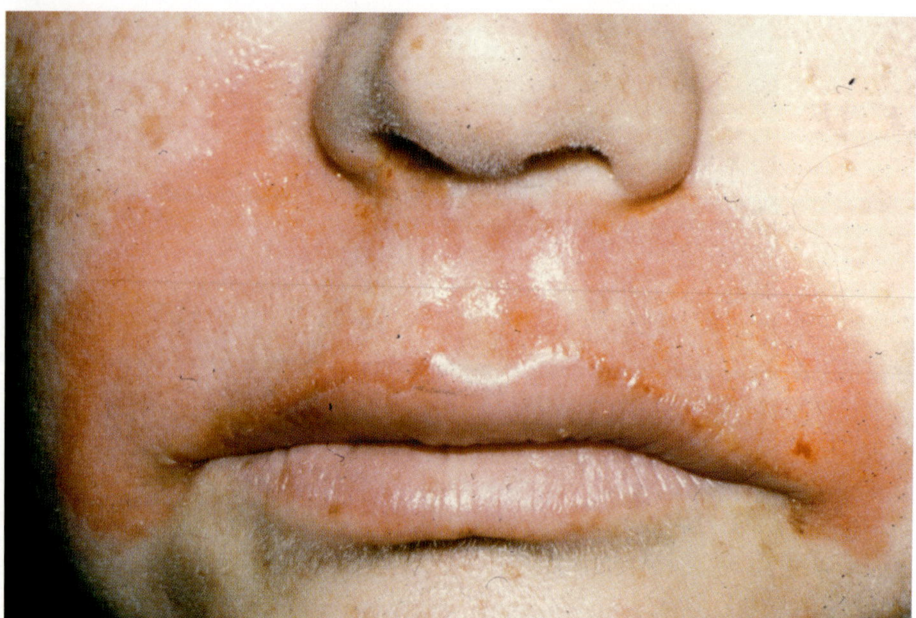

Figure 2.53. Bacterial infection one week after CO_2 laser resurfacing

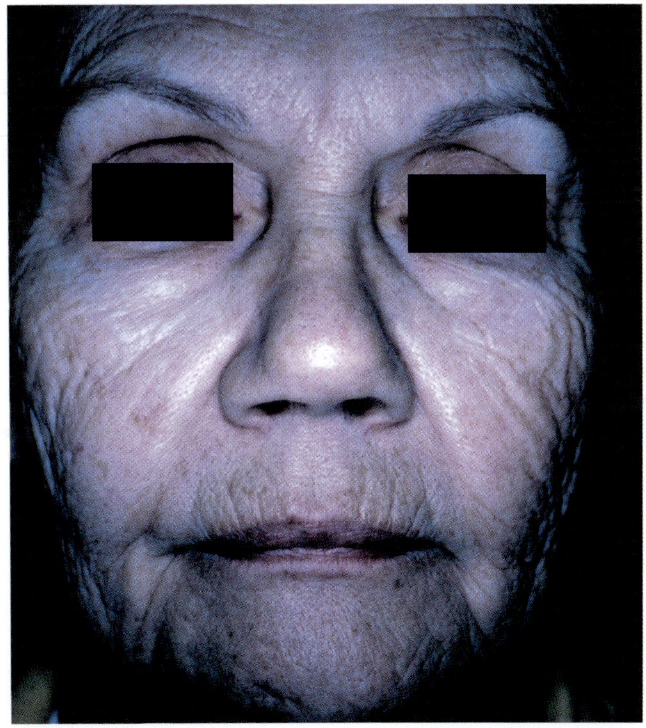

Figure 2.54. Before Er:YAG laser resurfacing

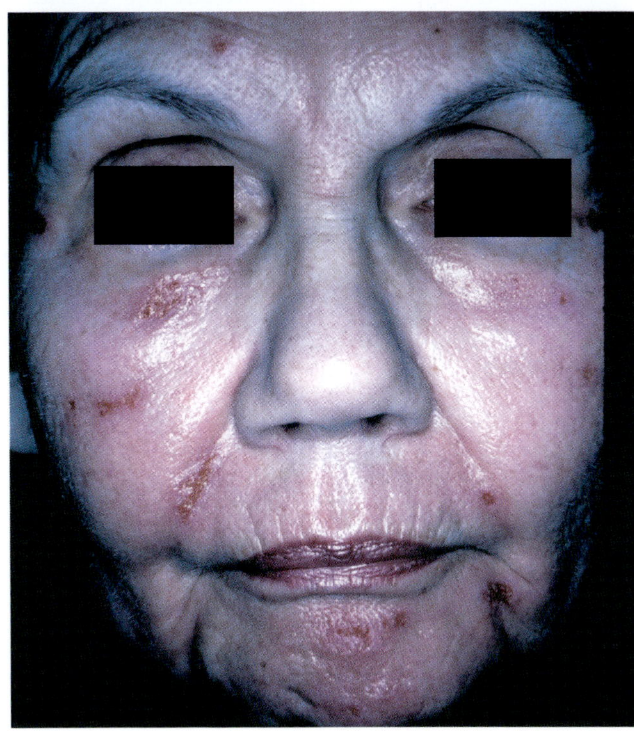

Figure 2.55. Bacterial infection one week after Er:YAG laser resurfacing

ointments decrease this risk. The use of oral prophylactic antibiotics before, during, and after laser resurfacing also remains controversial. Of interest, the cultured organisms in one study were mostly resistant to erythromycin, penicillin, and several cephalosporins. However, they were 100% sensitive to ciprofloxacin.[49] This may explain the conflicting results in the prophylactic antibiotic studies. Therefore, the correct choice of antibiotics may be useful in preventing post-laser resurfacing bacterial infections.

Although most commonly *Staph. aureus* was the offending organism, in one study, over 50% of infections were polymicrobial. In polymicrobial infections, the following organisms appear to be most commonly involved: *Pseudomonas aeruginosa* 41%, *Staph. aureus* 35%, *Staph. epidermidis* 29%, and *Candida* species 24%. Several cases involving multiple drug-resistant Gram-negative organisms have also been reported.[49]

Candidiasis

Candidal infection occurs in approximately 1% of laser resurface-treated patients (Figure 2.56).[49] Such post-operative infections may result from a post-laser moist closed wound dressing environment. They appear as soft whitish plaques similar to leukoplakia, or milia-like lesions. Such infections may present with the underlying skin appearing erythematous and eroded. Satellite lesions are characteristic of

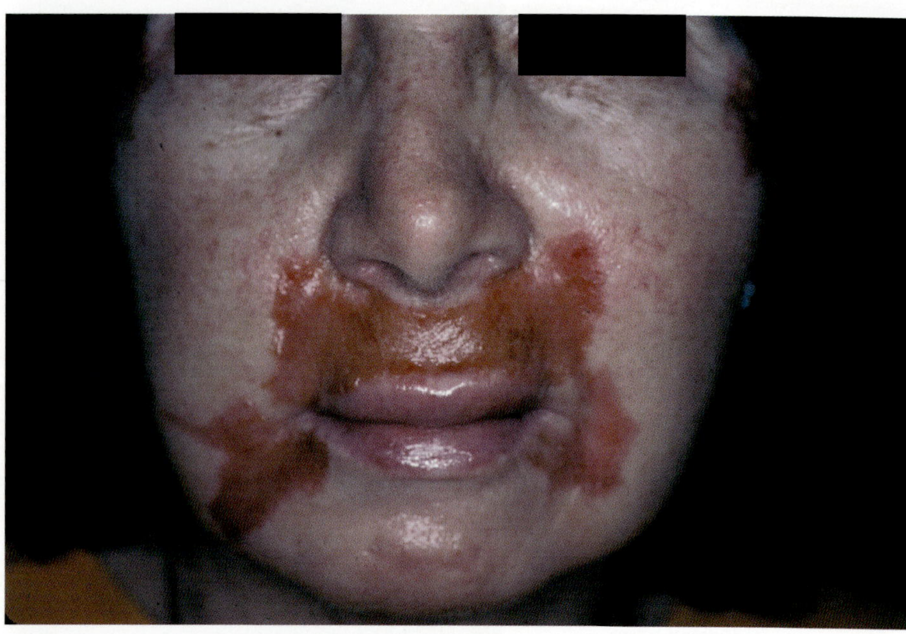

Figure 2.56. Candidiasis after laser resurfacing

monilial infections and generally extend outside of the laser treated region. Persons with increased risk of candidal infection include those with diabetes, angular cheilitis, immunosuppression, and/or vaginal candidiasis.

CONTACT DERMATITIS

Contact dermatitis is observed in up to 65% of patients after laser resurfacing.[17,20,50,51] It has been postulated that the prolonged erythema seen in some patients after laser resurfacing may be related to a contact dermatitis initiated by the post-laser resurfacing topical wound care regime.[52,53] Post-laser contact dermatitis not only results in discomfort and a prolonged recovery time for patients, but also increases the chances of prolonged post-operative erythema and hyperpigmentation. Because of the de-epithelialized state of newly resurfaced skin, the normal protective epidermal barrier is impaired, rendering the skin more susceptible to contact irritants.

Patients may react to various irritants and allergens contained within topically applied ointments, including topical antibiotics, preservatives, chemical sunscreens, fragrances, herbal and vitamin remedies, moisturizers, and cleansers. In one published study of laser resurface-treated patients, 65% of patients undergoing laser resurfacing developed contact dermatitis to several topical agents.[23] Patch testing for contact allergy was negative on normal skin which suggested a primary irritant reaction in laser-treated skin.

Topical antibiotics are probably the most common cause of post-laser resurfacing allergic contact dermatitis. Fitzpatrick and colleagues observed contact dermatitis in 39% of patients who used a regimen of polymyxin B, bacitracin, mupirocin, and hemorrhoid ointments.[24] Lowe et al. observed a 73% rate of contact dermatitis with a combination of topical ointments.[23] In addition, many patients are tempted to self-prescribe various topical herbal and vitamin preparations, including vitamin E or aloe vera-containing compounds, in an attempt to speed their recovery. These self-prescribed remedies may actually contribute to contact dermatitis.

Contact dermatitis may be difficult to recognize in newly resurfaced skin, because the epidermis is no longer present. Signs and symptoms suggestive of an irritant contact dermatitis include diffuse and intense facial erythema and/or pruritus.

Skin hypersensitivity seems to be a more common complaint in a small subset of laser resurface-treated patients. This reaction does not correlate to the depth of laser ablation, the number of passes, or a specific anatomic area. Rather, it seems to relate to the inherent atopic or allergic characteristics of patients. In some patients, the skin reaction is severe enough to require a course of systemic steroid therapy. Since the routine use of antibiotic ointments has been largely eliminated as a post-resurfacing regimen, a sharp decline in post-laser contact dermatitis has been observed.[25,26,51,54,55]

ERYTHEMA

Erythema is the most common and expected adverse event experienced by virtually all patients who undergo resurfacing with either CO_2 or Er:YAG lasers.[17,19,51,55–57] This transient erythema is the normal consequence of a natural healing process of resurfaced skin. Post-laser erythema is only considered abnormal if it persists for an extended period (Figure 2.57).

Erythema initially appears after laser resurfacing between days 8 and 11 post-operatively. It reaches its maximum intensity at about 2 weeks, and lasts for several weeks to 6 months (average 2–4.5 months) after the procedure.[17,23,27,58,59]

Post-operative erythema is thought to occur as a result of a combination of epidermal immaturity, reduced melanin absorption of light, reduced dermal optical scattering and increased blood flow secondary to the laser-induced inflammatory response.[59] The intensity, amount, and duration of erythema also appear to be proportional to the degree of residual thermal damage in the dermis.

Patients who regularly use tretinoin or glycolic acid compounds, or who have a history of acne or rosacea, are also predisposed to persistent post-operative erythema. Post-operative wound infection and contact dermatitis may also result in persistent erythema. Patients with a prior history of radiation therapy have been shown to heal more slowly and experience more post-operative erythema.[60] It should be noted that the clinical perception of erythema persists longer in patients receiving segmental localized resurfacing as compared with those undergoing full-face resurfacing.[15,17]

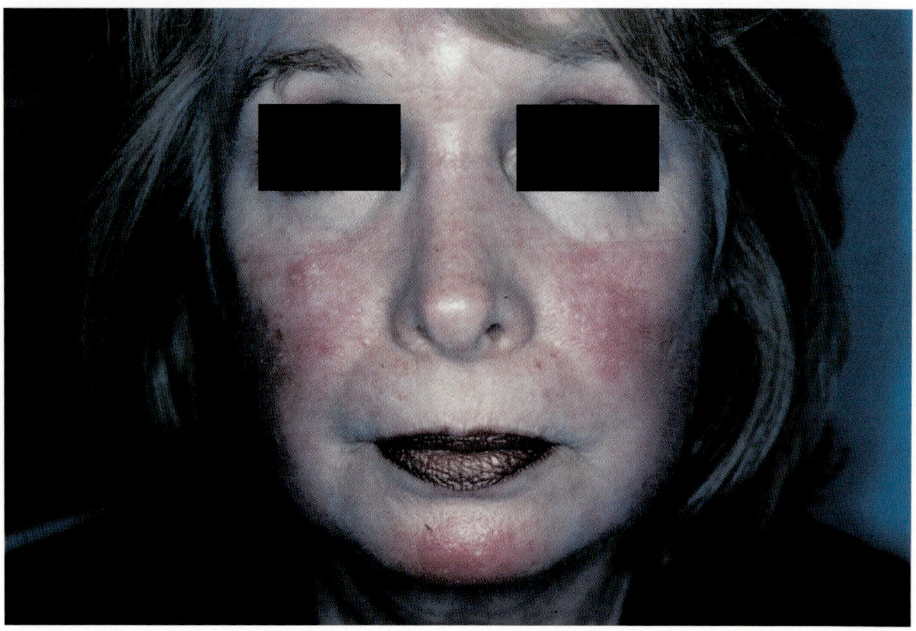

Figure 2.57. Persistent erythema 1 year after CO_2 laser resurfacing

The vulnerability of the resurfaced skin to the effects of ultraviolet light makes sun avoidance desirable until post-operative erythema has subsided.

Post-laser resurfacing erythema can be divided into focal and diffuse types. Focal bright erythema, especially when seen in the mandibular area, usually suggests the possibility of impending hypertrophic scarring. Immediate action is required to halt the process.

Focal persistent erythema also correlates with the appearance of hypopigmentation 6–12 months after the procedure in those areas. Diffuse focal erythema can be due to irritant or allergic contact dermatitis, and a careful search for a causal agent is helpful. Persistent diffuse erythema can eventuate in hyperpigmentation in darker-skinned individuals.

ACNE AND MILIA

After laser resurfacing, the skin temporarily becomes hypersebaceous, producing more sebum, with a consequent increased incidence of acne and milia (Figure 2.58).

Acne has been reported to occur in as many as 80% of patients who undergo laser resurfacing. Milia may be seen in up to 14% of treated patients. The clinical appearance is generally one of painless, small, white, dome-shaped elevations that most likely represent epidermal cysts resulting from occlusion of eccrine duct

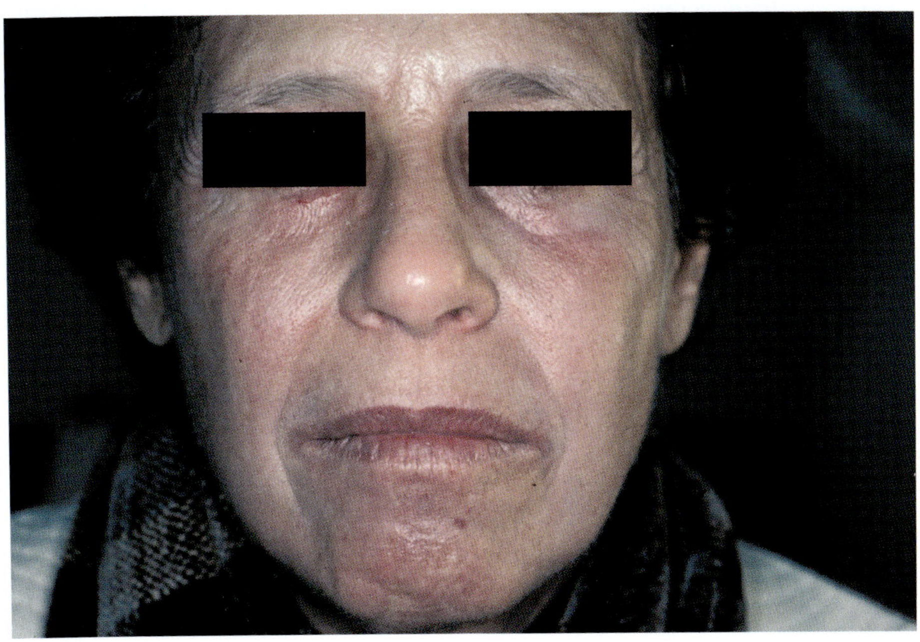

Figure 2.58. Milia beneath eyelids after CO_2 laser resurfacing

openings. These lesions usually become apparent between weeks 3 and 6 following the laser procedure, often lasting 2–4 weeks. Patients with a prior history of acne are at particular risk for its development after resurfacing. Milia may also be seen as a normal product of epidermal damage and repair. The milia that form after laser resurfacing are often superficial and usually resolve spontaneously. Treatment is usually not necessary for mild flares, since spontaneous resolution is commonly observed once the use of the occlusive ointments and dressings is discontinued.

PRURITUS

Pruritus occurs in up to 90% of the patients undergoing laser resurfacing.[15] It may occur as a result of the normal re-epithelialization and wound-healing process, or it may be associated with an infection or allergic process. Usually, the pruritus begins during the first week of re-epithelialization. Pruritis, when it occurs, tends to last for 2–4 weeks after laser resurfacing.

TEXTURAL CHANGES

Change in skin texture will inevitably occur after all resurfacing procedures. This result is usually desirable, as the skin is now smoother after laser treatment. Loss of skin translucency, a less desirable effect, may occur with deeper resurfacing.

ECTROPIAN

Ectropian of the lower eyelid is a rare, but potentially serious post-laser resurfacing complication.[17,19,20,50,51,55,56] Ectropian generally results from vertical shortening of the lower eyelid anterior lamella. Aggressive resurfacing of the lower eyelid increases the risk of ectropion. Lower eyelid laxity, and/or patients who have undergone previous lower lid blepharoplasty are at increased risk of forming ectropian.

CELLULITIS

Although unusual, cellulitis may be a complicating factor in the early post-operative period, and may be confused with erythema. Early institution of antibiotics rather than steroids is indicated.

PAIN

It is reasonable to expect pain and discomfort after laser resurfacing, as the wound created by lasers exposes tissue that is sensitive for almost 1 week after laser resurfacing.

The degree of pain and discomfort described as a burning sensation is variable. The single most reliable indicator of the existence and intensity of pain is the patient's own self-report. Although occlusive dressings may help to alleviate pain, the potential increased risk of infection may make this method less desirable.[49]

CONCLUSION

Complications may occur after both ablative and non-ablative treatments. In general, extensive scarring after ablative laser resurfacing results from either the poor technique and/or infection. Scarring after non-ablative treatments is rare and results from either the thermal effect or associated excessive cooling with these devices.

REFERENCES

1 Brody HJ. Chemical peeling. In: Baxter S, Brody HJ, eds. Chemical Peeling and Resurfacing. 2nd edn. St. Louis, MO: Mosby;1997:1–256.

2 Alt TH. The value of effective therapeutic and cosmetic dermabrasion. In: Epstein E, Epstein EJ, eds. Controversies in Dermatology. Philadelphia: WB Saunders; 1984:439–446.

3 Stanly RJ, Roenigk RK. Actinic cheilitis: treatment with carbon dioxide laser. Mayo Clin Proc 1988;63:230–235.

4 Fitzpatrick RE, Goldman MP. Carbon dioxide laser surgery. In: Goldman MP, Fitzpatrick RE, eds. Cutaneous Laser Surgery: The Art and Science of Selective Photothermolysis. St. Louis: Mosby; 1994:198–258.

5 Alster TS, Lewis AB. Dermatologic laser surgery: A review. Dermatol Surg 1996;22:797–805.

6 Gupta MA, Schork NJ, Ellis CN. Aging-related concerns and body image: Possible future implications for eating disorders. Int J Eat Disord 1993;14:481–486.

7 Gupta MA, Schrok NJ, Ellis CN. Psychosocial correlates of the treatment of photodamaged skin with topical retinoic acid: A prospective controlled study. J Am Acad Dermatol 1994;30:969–972.

8 Olsen EA, Katz HI, Levine N, et al. Tretinoin emollient cream: A new therapy for photodamaged skin. J Am Acad Dermatol 1992;26:215–224.

9 Pearlman SF. Late and mid-life astonishment: Disruptions to identity and self-esteem. Women Ther 1993;14:1–12.

10 Burks JW. Wire Brush Surgery: The Treatment of Certain Cosmetic Defects and Diseases of the Skin. Springfield, IL: Charles C Thomas: 1956.

11 Blau S, Rein CR. Dermabrasion of the acne pit. AMA Arch Derm Syphilol 1954;70:754–766.

12 Epstein ES. Dermabrasion. In: Epstein E, Epstein EJ, eds. Skin Surgery. 5th edn. Springfield, IL: Charles C Thomas; 1982:593–614.

13 Stuzin JM, Baker TJ, Gordon HL. Treatment of photoaging: Facial chemical peeling (phenol and trichloroacetic acid) and dermabrasion. Clin Plast Surg 1993;20:9–25.

14 Goldberg DJ. Laser surgery of the skin. Am Fam Physician 1989;40:109–116.

15 Bernstein LJ, Kauvar ANB, Grossman MC, Geronemus RG. The short- and long-term side effects of carbon dioxide laser resurfacing. Dermatol Surg 1997;23:519–525.

16 Waldorf HA, Kauvar AN, Geronemus RG. Skin resurfacing of fine to deep rhytides using a char-free CO_2 laser in 47 patients. Dermatol Surg 1995;21:940–946.

17 Nanni CA, Alster TS. Complications of carbon dioxide laser resurfacing. An evaluation of 500 patients. Dermatol Surg 1998;24:315–320.

18 Schwartz RJ, Burns AJ, Rohrich RJ, et al. Long-term assessment of CO_2 facial laser resurfacing: aesthetic results and complications. Plast Reconstr Surg 1999;103:592–601.

19 Alster TS. Side effects and complications of laser surgery. In: Alster TS, ed. Manual of Cutaneous Laser Techniques. 2nd edn. Philadelphia: Lippincott, Williams & Wilkins; 2000:175–187.

20 Alster TS. Cutaneous resurfacing with CO_2 and erbium:YAG lasers: preoperative, intraoperative, and postoperative considerations. Plast Reconstr Surg 1999;103:619–632.

21 Alster TS, Nanni CA, Williams CM. Comparison of four carbon dioxide resurfacing lasers: a clinical and histologic evaluation. Dermatol Surg 1999;25:153–159.

22 Phipps A. Skin healing. Probl Gen Surg 1989;6:235.

23 Lowe NJ, Lask G, Griffin ME. Laser skin resurfacing: pre and post treatment guidelines. Dermatol Surg 1995;21:1017–1019.

24 Fitzpatrick RE, Goldman MP, Satur NM, Tope WD. Pulsed carbon dioxide laser resurfacing of photoaged facial skin. Arch Dermatol 1996;132:395–402.

25 Lowe NJ, Lask G, Griffin ME, et al. Skin resurfacing with UltraPulse carbon dioxide laser: observations on 100 patients. Dermatol Surg 1995;21:1025–1029.

26 Alster TS, West TB. Resurfacing of atrophic facial scars with a high-energy, pulsed carbon dioxide laser. Dermatol Surg 1996;22:151–155.

27 Alster TS, Garg S. Treatment of facial rhytides with the UltraPulse high-energy carbon dioxide laser. Plast Reconstr Surg 1996;98:791–794.

28 Lask G, Keller G, Lowe NJ, et al. Laser skin resurfacing with the SilkTouch flashscanner for facial rhytides. Dermatol Surg 1995;21:1021–1024.

29 David LM, Sarne A, Unger WP. Rapid laser scanning for facial resurfacing. Dermatol Surg 1995;21:1031–1033.

30 Ho C, Nguyen Q, Lowe NJ, et al. Laser resurfacing in pigmented skin. Dermatol Surg 1995;21:1035–1037.

31 Weinstein C. Why I abandoned CO_2 laser resurfacing: The dilemma of evolving technologies. Aesthetic Surg J 1999;67.

32 Burns AJ. Erbium laser resurfacing: Current concepts. Plast Reconstr Surg 1999;103:617.

33 Laws RA, Finley EM, McCollough ML, Grabski WJ. Alabaster skin after carbon dioxide laser resurfacing with histologic correlation. Dermatol Surg 1998;24:633–636.

34 Weinstein C. Erbium laser resurfacing: Current concepts. Plast Reconstr Surg 1999;103:602–616.

35 Weinstein C, Roberts TL 3rd. Aesthetic skin resurfacing with the high-energy UltraPulse CO_2 laser. Clin Plast Surg 1997;24:379–405.

36 Olbricht SM, Stern RS, Tang SV, et al. Complications of cutaneous laser surgery. A survey. Arch Dermatol 1987;123:345–349.

37 Abergel RP, Meeker CA, Oikarinen H, et al. Retinoid modulation of connective tissue metabolism in keloid fibroblast cultures. Arch Dermatol 1985;121:632–635.

38 Jetten MA. Retinoids specifically enhance the number of epidermal growth factor receptors. Nature 1980;284:626–629.

39 Kenny MC, Shihh LM, Labereir U, et al. Modulation of rabbit keratinocyte production of collagen, sulphated glycosaminoglycans and fibronectin by retinol and retinoic acid. Biochem Biophys Acta 1986;889:156–162.

40 Alster TS. Side effects and complications of laser surgery. In: Alster TS, ed. Manual of Cutaneous Laser Techniques. Philadelphia: Lippincott-Raven; 1997:142–151.

41 Alster TS. Preoperative preparation for CO_2 laser resurfacing. In: Coleman WP, Lawrence N, eds. Skin Resurfacing, Baltimore: Williams & Wilkins; 1998:171–179.

42 Apfelberg D. Preoperative considerations in laser resurfacing. Int J Aesth Restor Surg 1997;5:21–28.

43 Dover J, Hruza G. Laser resurfacing. Semin Cutan Med Surg 1996;15:177–188.

44 Katz BE, MacFarlane DF. Atypical facial scarring after isotretinoin therapy in a patient with a previous dermabrasion. J Am Acad Dermatol 1994;30:852–853.

45 Munster AM. Immunologic response of trauma and burns: An overview. Am J Med 1989;75:142–145.

46 Yurt RW. In: Mandell GL, Bennett JE, Dolin R, eds. Mandell, Douglas and Bennett's Principles and Practice of Infectious Diseases. New York: Churchill Livingstone; 1995:2761–2765.

47 Alster TS, Nanni CA. Famciclovir prophylaxis of herpes simplex virus reactivation after laser skin resurfacing. Dermatol Surg 1999;25:242–246.

48 Monheit GD. Facial resurfacing may trigger the herpes simplex virus. Cosmetic Dermatol 1995;8:9–16.

49 Sriprachya-anunts S, Fitzpatrick RE, Goldman MP, Smith SR. Infections complicating pulsed carbon dioxide laser resurfacing for photoaged facial skin. Dermatol Surg 1997;23:527–535 [Discussion: 535–536].

50 Ratner D, Tse Y, Marchell N, et al. Cutaneous laser resurfacing. J Am Acad Dermatol 1999; 41:365–389.

51 Nanni CA. Postoperative management and complications of carbon dioxide laser resurfacing. In: Alster TS, Apfelberg DB, eds. Cosmetic Laser Surgery: A Practitioner's Guide. 2nd edn. New York, NY: Wiley-Liss; 1999:37–55.

52 Levy PM, Salomon D. Use of Biobrane after laser resurfacing. Dermatol Surg 1998;24:729–734.

53 Maloney BP, Millman B, Monheit G, McCollough EG. The etiology of prolonged erythema after chemical peel. Dermatol Surg 1998;24:337–341.

54 Lanzafame RJ, Naim JO, Rogers DW, et al. Comparisons of continuous-wave, chop-wave, and superpulsed laser wounds. Lasers Surg Med 1988;8:119–124.

55 Nanni CA. Handling complications of laser treatment. Dermatol Ther 2000;13:127–139.

56 Alster TS, Nanni CA. Complications of cutaneous laser resurfacing. In: Biesman B, ed. Carbon Dioxide Laser in Facial Aesthetic and Reconstructive Surgery. Baltimore: Williams & Wilkins; 1999:81–90.

57 Ruiz-Esparza J, Gomez JMB, De La Torre OLG, et al. Erythema after laser skin resurfacing. Dermatol Surg 1998;24:31–34.

58 Goodman GJ. Carbon dioxide laser resurfacing. Dermatol Surg 1998;24:665–672.

59 Trelles MA, Mordon S, Svaavand LO, et al. The origin and role of erythema after carbon dioxide laser resurfacing: a clinical and histological study. Dermatol Surg 1998;24:25–29.

60 Massey R, Jones D, Diamond J, et al. The importance of patient selection in CO_2 laser skin resurfacing. Cosmetic Dermatol 1997;10:9–14.

3 COMPLICATIONS IN LASER TREATMENT OF TATTOOS AND PIGMENTED LESIONS

KEY POINTS

(1) Q-switched laser treatment of both tattoos and pigmented lesions has a low incidence of complications
(2) Transient hypopigmentation after Q-switched laser treatment of tattoos and pigmented lesions is common and generally resolves
(3) Transient hyperpigmentation after Q-switched laser treatment of tattoos and pigmented lesions is common in darker skin types and generally resolves
(4) Scarring when it occurs after Q-switched laser treatment of tattoos and pigmented lesions is generally of the atrophic variety

TATTOOS

Decorative human tattooing is an ancient art form, the origins of which can be traced back as far as the Stone (12 000 BC) and Bronze (8000 BC) Ages.[1] Archeologists have found crude tattoos on the skin of mummies dating from 4000 BC.[2] Evidence suggests that ornamental tattooing was practiced in a large variety of geographic locations and by widely differing cultures.

A consistent theme throughout studies involving tattooed persons is the quest for a symbolic display of significant personal identity.[3] Studies have shown that the average age for acquiring a professional tattoo is 18 years, whereas amateur tattoos, most often self-inflicted, are seen on average at 14 years of age.[4]

Chemical and Photophysical Analysis of Tattoo Pigments

In the past, tattoo coloring agents were inorganic pigments, such as titanium dioxide (white), cadmium sulfide (yellow), chromic oxide (green), cadmium selenide (red),

red cinnabar (red), ferric oxide (brown-red), and carbon (black). For dark blue amateur tattoos, commercially available ink is still often used.

Professional tattoos have a variety of different colors and consist of a variety of pigments. Black is the most commonly used tattoo ink. This is followed by shades of blue, green, red, yellow, and orange. Additional colors found in professional tattoos are various shades of pink, brown, purple, and white. Usually, neither the tattoo artist nor the tattooed person have any information about the compounds placed within the tattooed skin. Because tattoo compounds, in comparison with cosmetics, are not generally controlled, the origin and chemical structure of these coloring agents are usually not known.

Tattoos having similar colors may contain completely different pigments and, therefore, exhibit a different absorption behavior. In addition, electron microscopic analysis of tattoo pigment shows a variety of shapes such as needles, platelets, cubes, bars, and a number of irregular shapes. The diameters of these pigments can vary from about 20 nm to 900 nm. With such variability in color and particle size, Q-switched laser treatment of tattoos can lead to a tremendous variability in clinical response.

Skin Reactions to Tattoos

Although artists use numerous different pigments of unknown purity and composition, these pigments are, in general, histologically unreactive. Pigments used for tattooing are usually well tolerated by the skin. Nevertheless, adverse reactions have been noted. These include allergic reactions,[5–8] pseudolymphoma,[9–11] systemic sarcoidosis,[12,13] and granulomatous or lichenoid reactions.[14,15]

In addition, several malignant lesions have occurred in tattoos (possibly coincidental), including basal cell carcinoma,[16] squamous cell carcinoma,[17] and malignant melanomas.[18,19] In one case, an evolution to B-cell lymphoma from pseudolymphoma has been reported.[20] A sarcoidal reaction in a tattoo can be an isolated finding or it can represent a cutaneous sign of systemic disease. Occasionally, localization of various skin diseases, such as lichen planus and psoriasis, has been reported within tattoos.[21]

Allergic reactions can be induced by a variety of commonly used tattoo pigments. These include mercury, chromium, and cobalt ions. Cadmium sulfide and cadmium selenide are mainly responsible for phototoxic reactions.

The most commonly reported allergic reactions are those seen in red tattoos containing mercury compounds. Most of these cases involve allergic eczematous dermatitis.[7,22–25]

Histology of Tattoos

At 24 hours, freshly tattooed skin shows an intense inflammatory reaction, with histologic and ultrastructural evidence of extensive damage to the epidermis and papillary dermis. Ink particles are found concentrated in keratinocytes and inflammatory cells within large membrane-bound phagosomes or free in the cytoplasm.

At 1 month, necrotic and inflammatory cells have disappeared and the basement membrane at the dermal–epidermal junction has re-formed. This limits further pigment loss through transepidermal elimination. Ink-containing cells are found concentrated along the dermal–epidermal junction.

Biopsies obtained from tattoos at 1, 3, and 40 years post-tattooing show ink particles distributed throughout the upper dermis. Most particles are found within the boundary of a cell membrane. Cells containing ink aggregates are found in the dermis surrounded by a matrix of collagen and elastic fibers. Most of the tattoo ink found in the dermis is concentrated in a single cell type. Ultrastructurally, the cells appear to be fibroblasts, although tattoo pigment has been found free within the dermis and contained in perivascular mast cells and macrophages.[26] In time, pigment deposits are seen deeper in the dermis, in contrast with the typical upper dermal deposits seen in new tattoos. Tattoo pigments have also been found in regional lymph nodes.

Motivation for Tattoo Removal

Tattoos are often applied impulsively,[27] and for a variety of reasons. Tattoos are usually applied for fashion, because of peer pressure, rebellion, or romance. Of tattooed individuals, 28% voice remorse within one month of tattoo application.[28] More than 80% of the tattoos are present on exposed body locations, such as shoulders and arms. The most common tattoos feature designs of animals, names and/or initials, crosses, or other self-designed marks.

Requests for tattoo removal appear to be increasing, presumably because of both effective laser therapy and an increasing incidence of tattoo application and subsequent dissatisfaction with the placed tattoos. In time, many tattooed individuals find their tattoos lead to considerable personal unhappiness, and impose significant psychological and social burdens.

Non-laser Tattoo Removal

The search for a successful means of removing or concealing tattoos is as old as the art of tattooing itself. Regardless of the initial reasons for acquiring tattoos, at some point many people regret their decision and seek methods of tattoo removal. Unfortunately, most non-laser methods of tattoo removal have disadvantages, such as incomplete pigment removal, non-selective tissue destruction, and unsatisfactory cosmetic results (e.g. atrophic and hypertrophic scarring).

Historically, crude methods of tattoo removal have involved the topical application of caustic chemicals, such as salicylic acid, trichloracetic acid, phenol, sulfuric acid, tannic acid, and zinc chloride. Physical modalities of tattoo removal have included salabrasion, cryosurgery, dermabrasion, electrocoagulation, and the use of an infrared coagulator.[29] The use of sodium chloride to remove tattoos dates back to ancient times, when in AD 543, Atius, a Greek physician, first used salt for the removal of tattoos. Although there are numerous reports describing the use of salabrasion to remove tattoos, the results, in general, have been unsatisfactory, with a high incidence of residual pigmentation and post-operative scarring.[30,31]

Cryosurgical tattoo removal has also been reported. Many treatments are necessary and the results are generally unsatisfactory with residual pigmentation and scarring noted in a significant number of treated patients.[32,33] Conventional dermabrasion has also been used to remove tattoos. In its simplest form, tattoo pigment is brushed away under visual control, with further loss of pigment noted in the post-operative tissue slough followed by healing by secondary intention.[34] Post-operative complications, such as incomplete pigment removal, pigment disturbances, and scarring are also frequently noted as a result of this procedure.[35,36]

Thermal cautery by means of various electrical devices has also been reported. Regardless of the method used, these devices are associated with inadequate pigment removal and a high incidence of post-operative scarring. In 1979, the infrared coagulator was developed. This device is capable of delivering intense, non-coherent, multispectral light energy. A tungsten halogen light provides the energy source, with most energy in the near infrared range, at 900–960 nm. Pre-set pulse durations are used in an attempt to deliver a controlled cutaneous thermal injury. Unfortunately, the use of this device is also associated with incomplete pigment removal and a high incidence of post-operative scarring.[37–39]

Intense pulsed light sources have recently been introduced for the treatment of tattoos. These devices use a powerful flashlamp, that generates intense, polychromatic, visible pulsed light at variable pulsewidths and intervals. With the placement of cut-off filters, specific wavelengths are selected that can target a variety of skin disorders. Unfortunately, these devices show little wavelength specificity for tattoo ink and produce non-specific tissue thermal damage. Once again, these techniques are often associated with incomplete pigment removal and hypertrophic scarring.

Finally, conventional surgical methods have been used to treat tattoos; however, their use is limited to the removal of small tattoos.[40] Larger tattoos have been managed by means of serial excisions, flaps or grafts; however, the results of these procedures in most instances provide a suboptimal cosmetic outcome.[41,42]

PIGMENTED LESIONS

A variety of epidermal and dermal pigmented lesions occur in the skin. Some pigmented lesions are congenital, most are acquired later in life. The difficulties in removing such lesions generally relates to their etiology and depth of pigment.

LASERS IN THE TREATMENT OF TATTOOS AND PIGMENTED LESIONS

Laser technology, through the process of selective photothermolysis,[43] can lead to improvement in a variety of pigmentary abnormalities in the skin. Properly chosen wavelengths of light used with appropriate pulse durations can selectively alter pigment cells and disrupt exogenous (tattoo) and endogenous pigment in a manner that leaves the adjacent skin intact.

Ruby Laser

The first laser ever used on man, the non-Q-switched ruby laser, has an emission wavelength of 694 nm. This wavelength is well absorbed by melanin leading to selective destruction of melanin-containing cells. Goldman and colleagues used the normal-mode ruby laser with a pulse duration in the microsecond range.[44–47] Destruction of melanin-containing cells was achieved. However, clinical outcomes with these early ruby lasers were variable. Superficial pigmented lesions responded best; deeper lesions were only partially removed. Complications, such as hypopigmentation and skin textural changes, often depended on the delivered laser fluence.[44–47]

Argon Laser

In 1979, Apfelberg first reported the use of the argon laser (488–514 nm) to remove tattoos. His work renewed interest in evaluating the role of laser treatment of pigmented lesions and tattoos. Although effective on a variety of pigmented lesions, the response with this laser was quite variable.[48,49] Argon laser emission is well absorbed by melanin. However, the argon laser's short wavelength does not penetrate very deeply into the dermis. Unfortunately, in the treatment of pigmented lesions, the 488–514 nm wavelength is also well absorbed by hemoglobin. This may lead to undesired thermal damage to the surrounding structures. Finally, the argon laser's emitted pulse duration, generally 20–50 milliseconds or more, distributes the thermal damage far beyond the targeted cells. Because of all these factors, argon laser-induced non-specific heat absorption results in diffuse tissue necrosis. This is the likely cause of the high incidence of scarring noted with the use of this laser.

Carbon Dioxide Laser

In 1978, the continuous wave carbon dioxide (CO_2) laser was first successfully used for tattoo removal. CO_2 lasers emit energy at 10 600 nm in the infrared region. The primary chromophore for CO_2 lasers is tissue water. This water undergoes instantaneous vaporization on exposure to laser energy. CO_2 lasers produce varying degrees of residual dermal damage related to energy and pulse duration. Unfortunately, variation of the depth of ink placement results in a thermal wound of varying depth after laser treatment. The CO_2 laser removes tattoo pigment by means of a thermal tissue coagulative effect in a way similar to that seen with the argon laser. No specific effects on the tattoo ink particles are seen using this modality. CO_2 laser treatment of tattoos often causes prolonged healing and the development of thick hypertrophic scars (Figures 3.1–3.20).[50]

Complications such as pigmentation changes, persistent tattoo pigmentation, and the occurrence of atrophic and hypertrophic scars, are to be expected from the thermal effects of this laser.

Erbium:Yttrium-Aluminum-Garnet Laser

In contrast to CO_2 lasers, whose mechanism of action involves tissue coagulation, Er:YAG lasers (2940 nm) are capable of precise tissue ablation with limited residual thermal effects in the dermis.

Clinical and histologic studies suggest that Er:YAG lasers can mimic the tissue effects of dermabrasion, albeit with a far greater degree of accuracy and control. Dermal effects are also seen with this laser. This dermal effect may result in

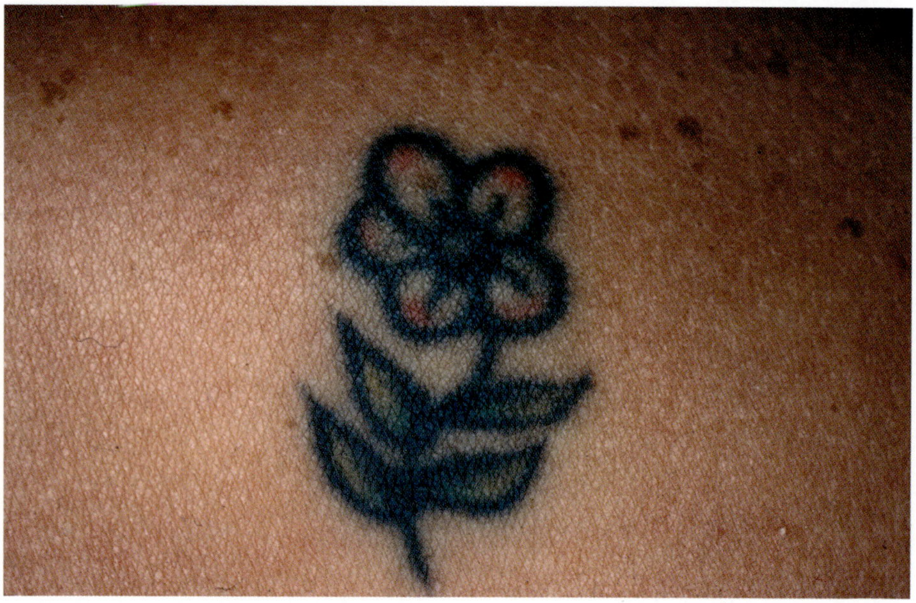

Figure 3.1. Tattoo before CO_2 laser treatment

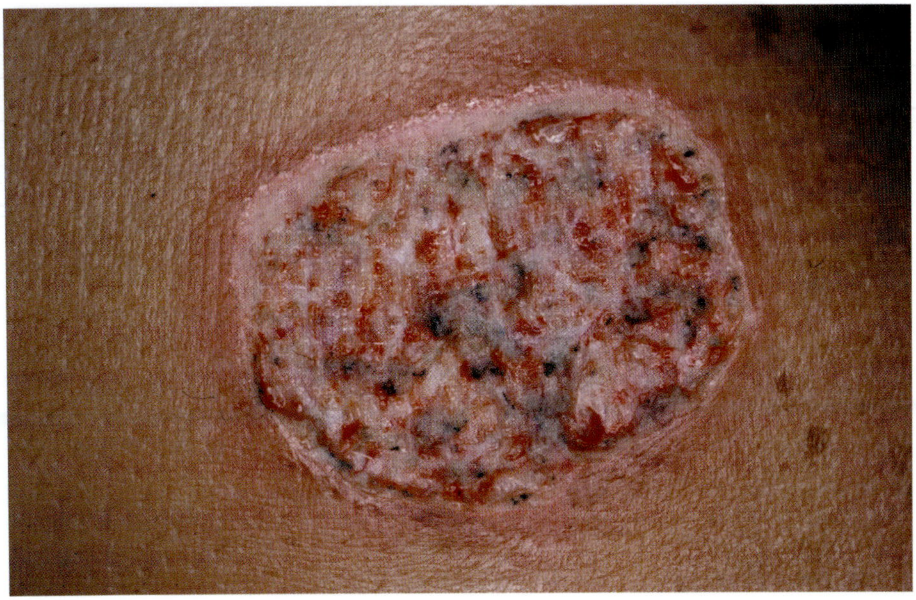

Figure 3.2. Tattoo immediately after CO_2 laser treatment

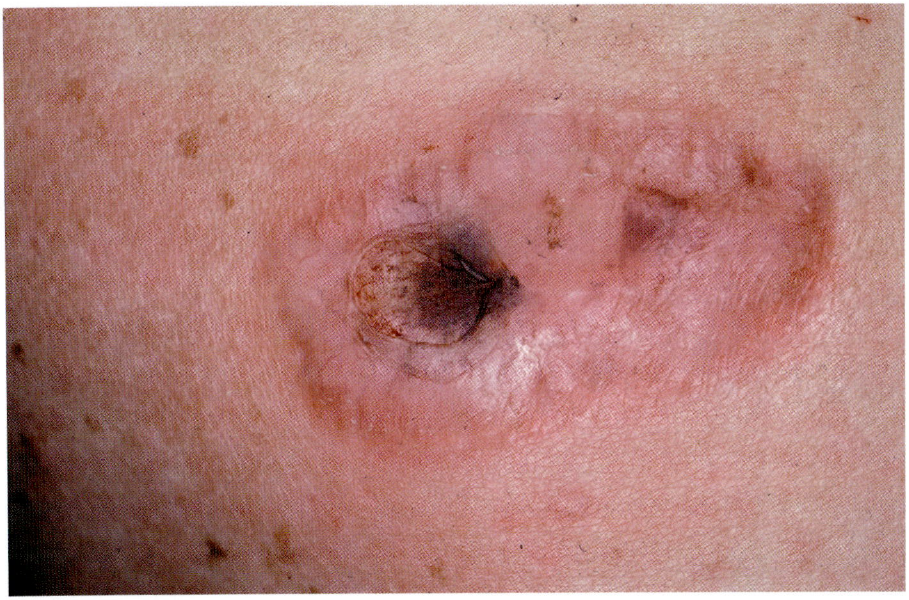

Figure 3.3. Early hypertrophic scar 6 weeks after CO_2 laser treatment of tattoo

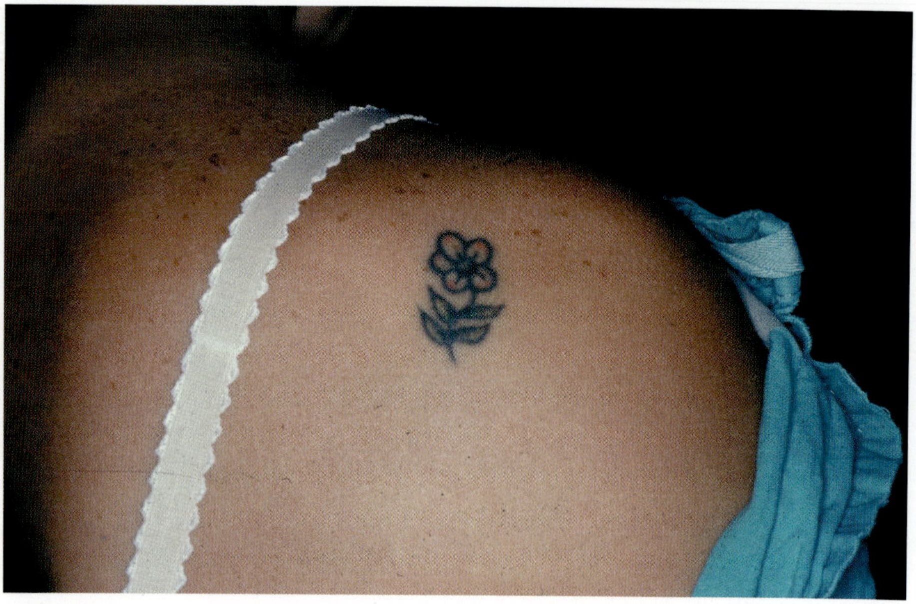

Figure 3.4. Tattoo before CO_2 laser treatment

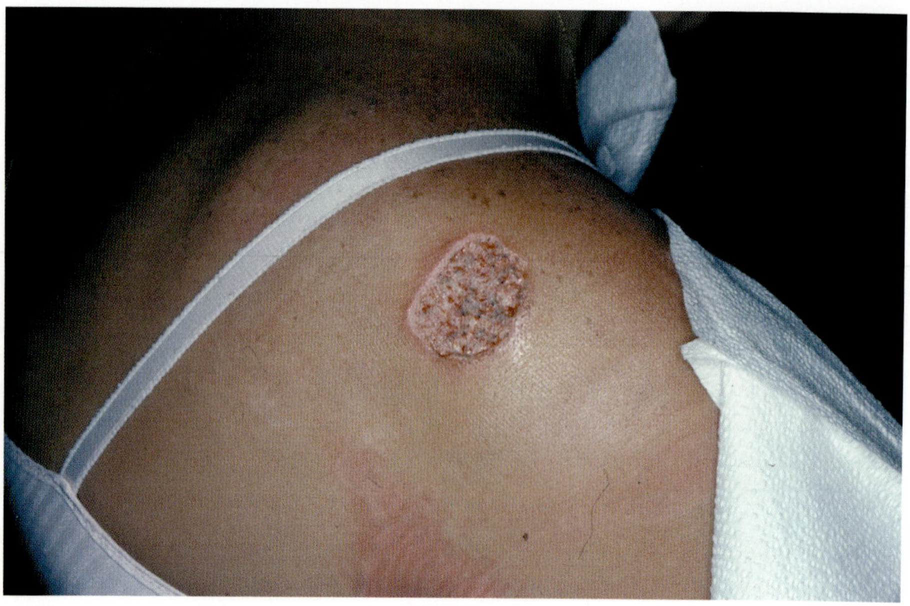

Figure 3.5. Tattoo immediately after CO_2 laser treatment

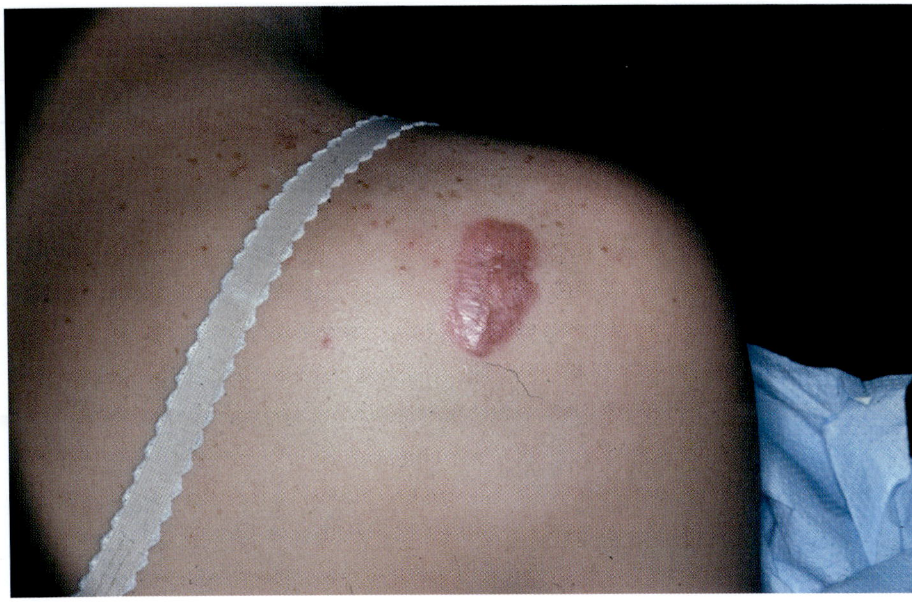

Figure 3.6. Hypertrophic scar 2 months after CO_2 laser treatment of tattoo

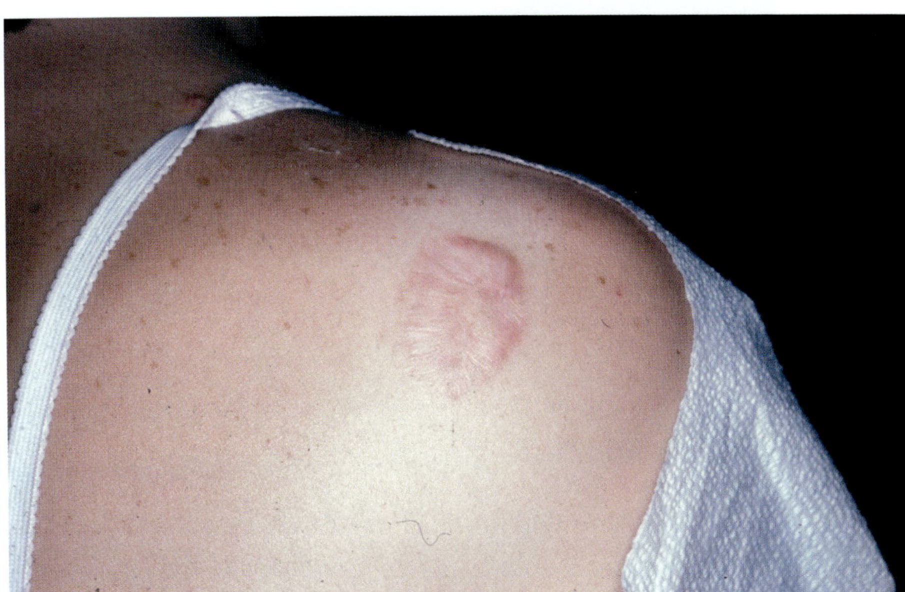

Figure 3.7. Hypertrophic scar 6 months after CO_2 laser treatment of tattoo

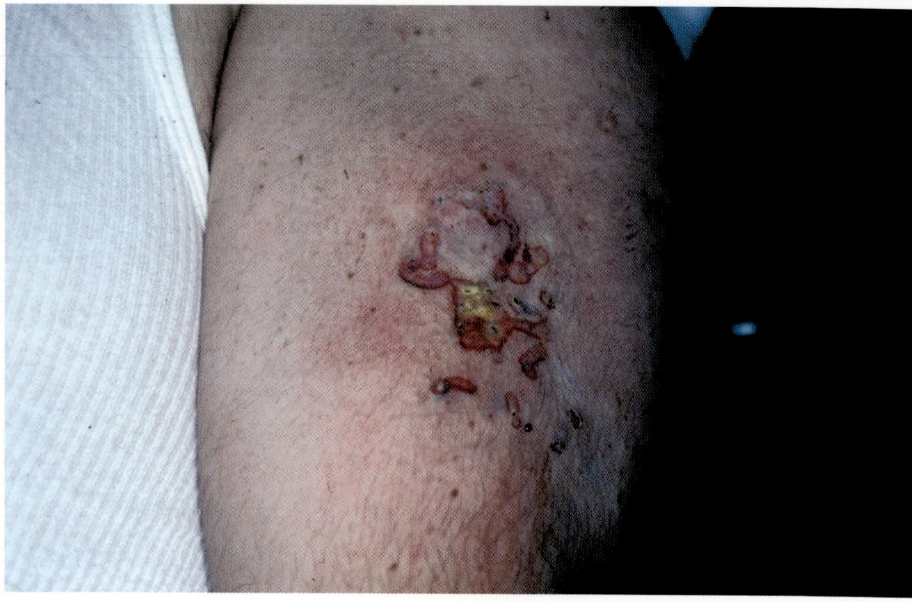

Figure 3.8. Four weeks after CO_2 laser treatment of tattoo

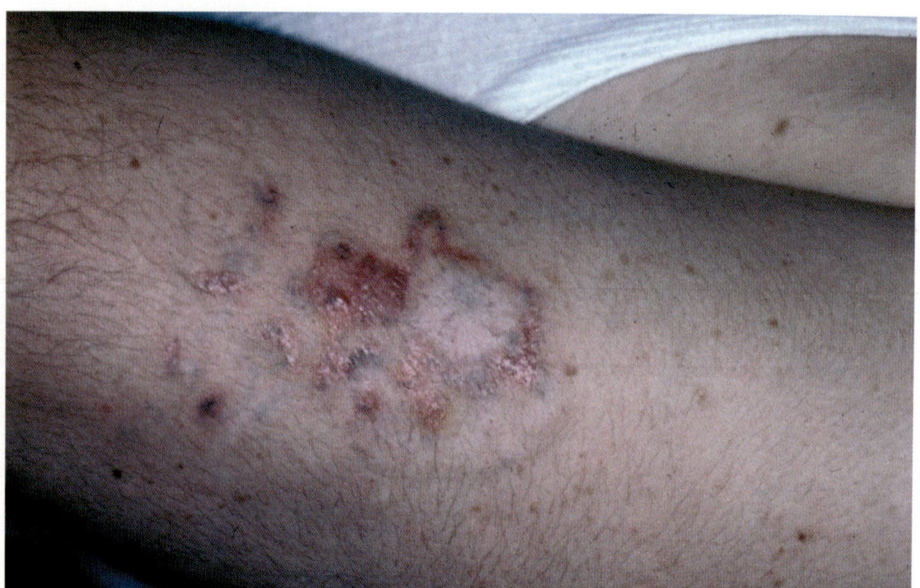

Figure 3.9. Slow healing and early hypertrophic scar 2 months after CO_2 laser treatment of tattoo

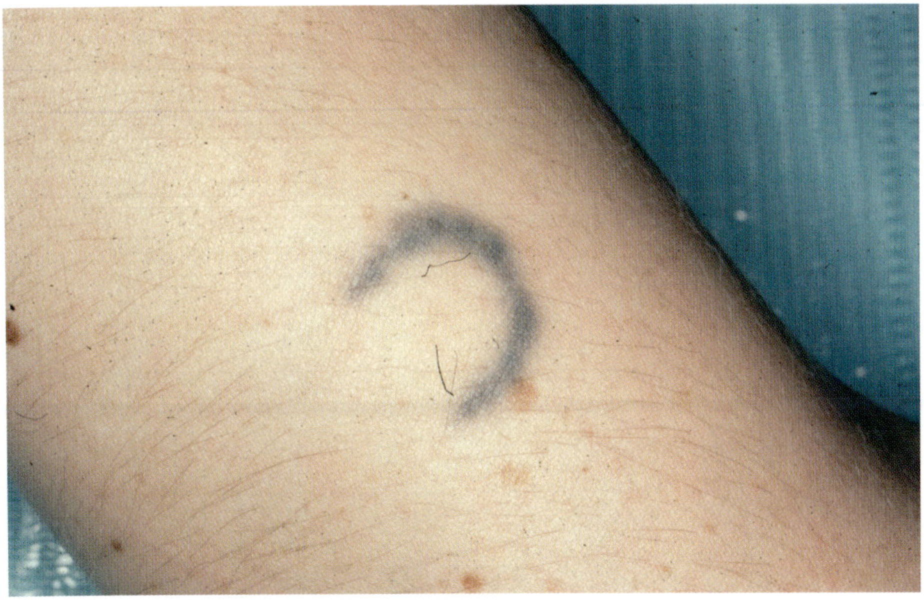

Figure 3.10. Tattoo before CO_2 laser treatment

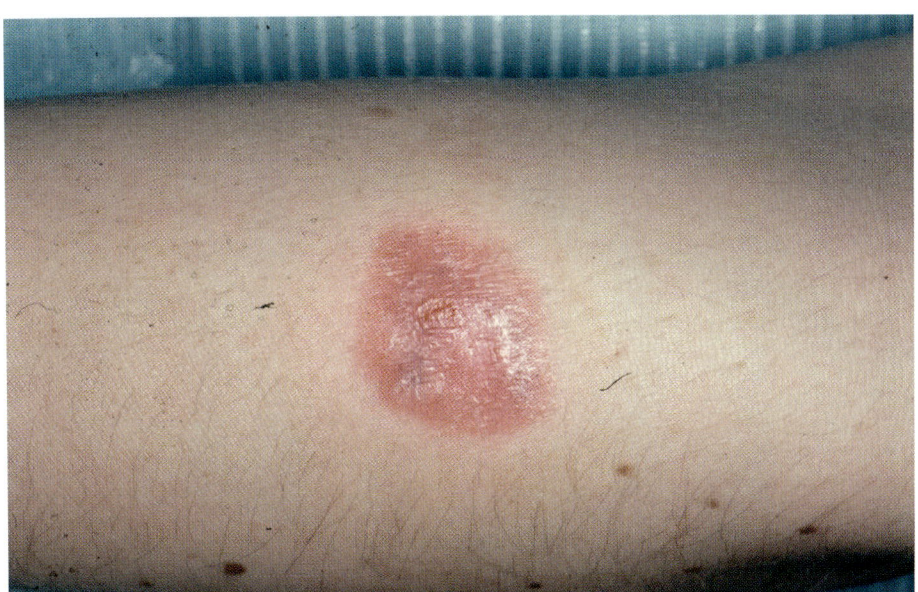

Figure 3.11. Early hypertrophic scar 8 weeks after CO_2 laser treatment of tattoo

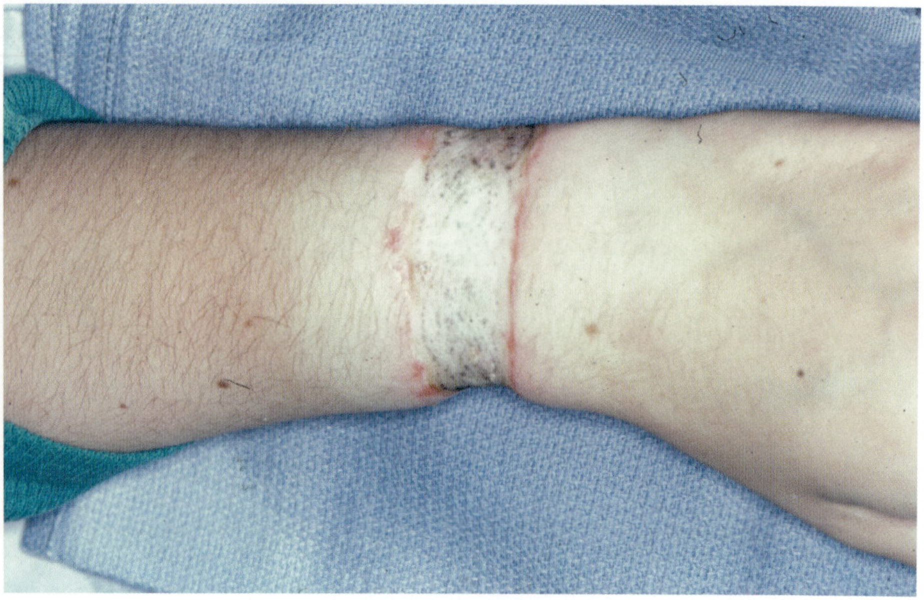

Figure 3.12. Tattoo immediately after CO_2 laser treatment

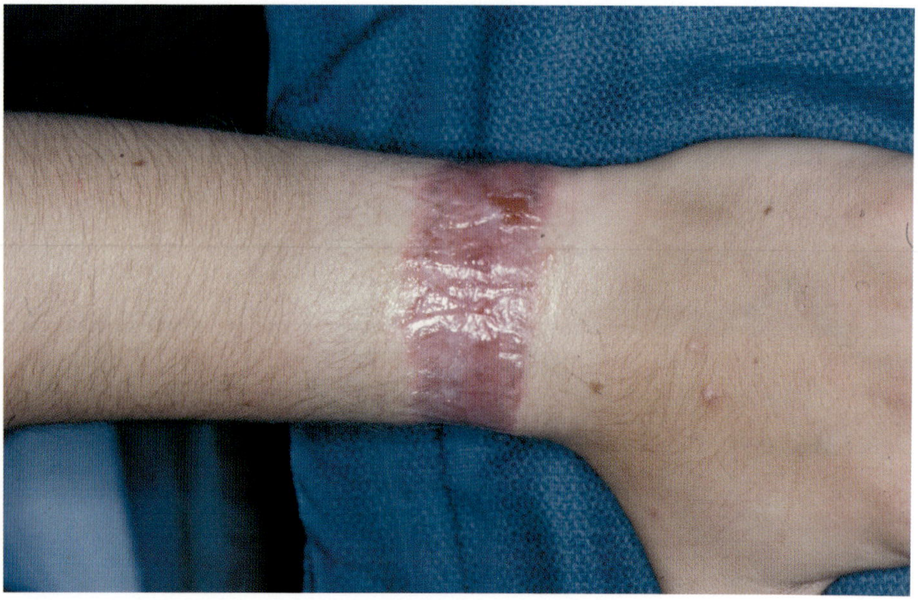

Figure 3.13. Tattoo 1 month after CO_2 laser treatment

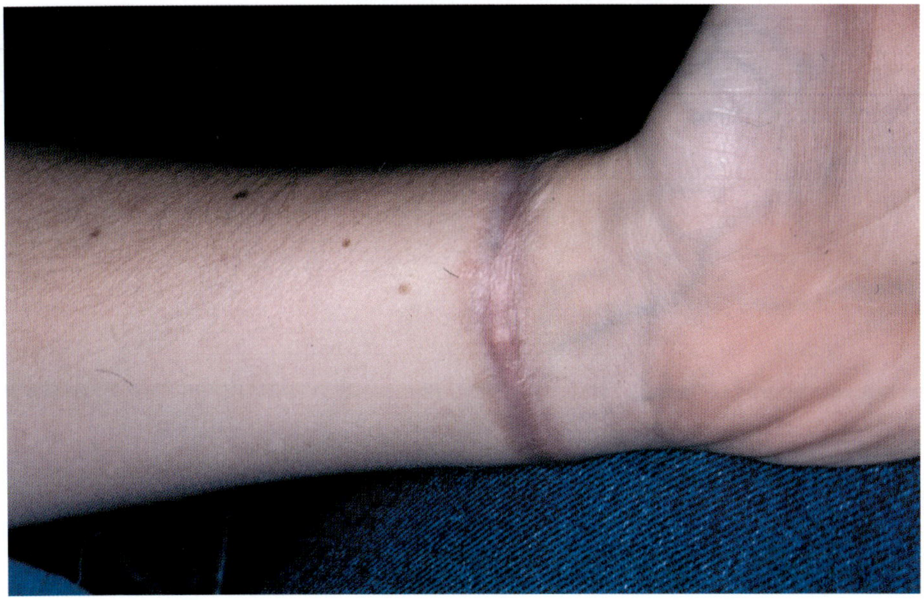

Figure 3.14. Hypertrophic scar 2 months after CO_2 laser treatment of tattoo

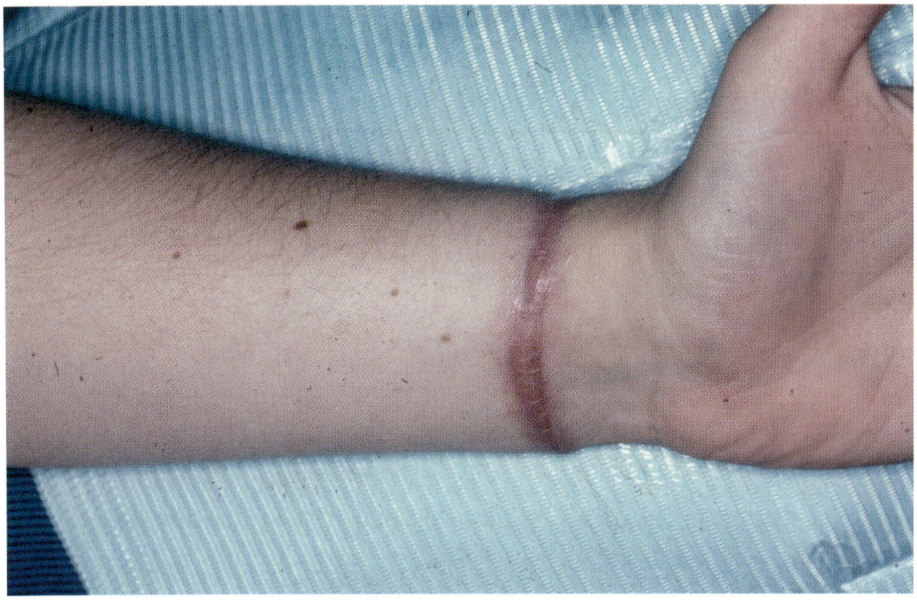

Figure 3.15. Hypertrophic scar 3 months after CO_2 laser treatment of tattoo

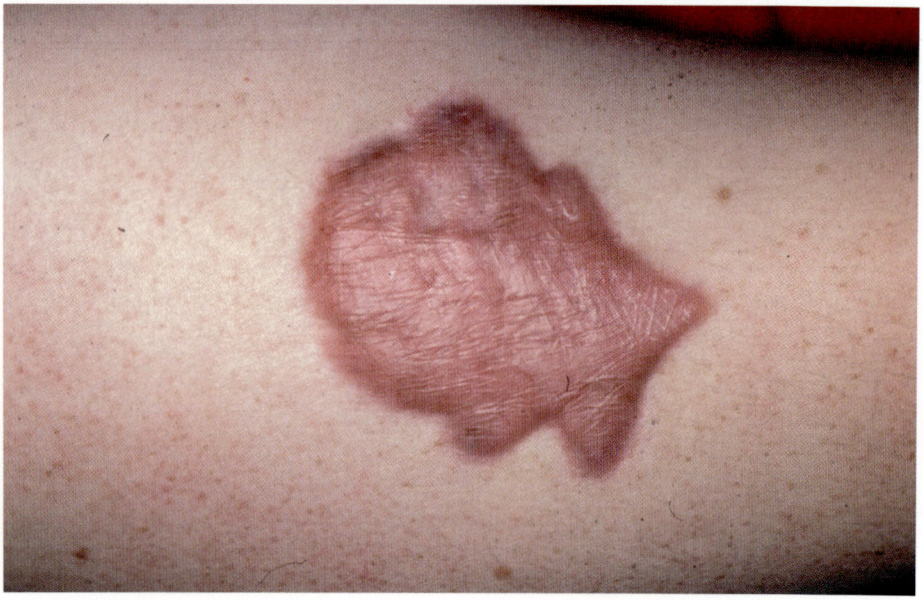

Figure 3.16. Hypertrophic scar 6 months after CO_2 laser treatment of tattoo

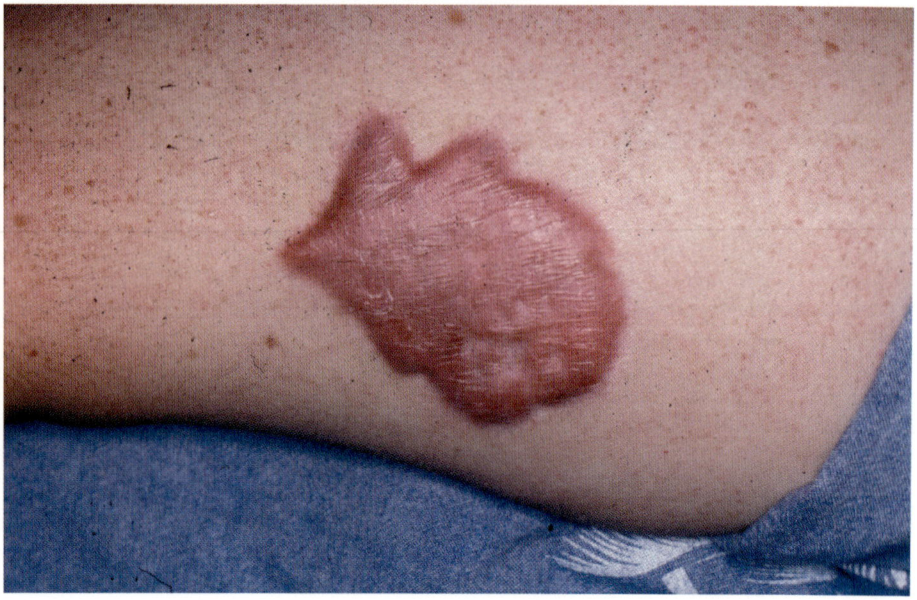

Figure 3.17. Hypertrophic scar 9 months after CO_2 laser treatment of tattoo

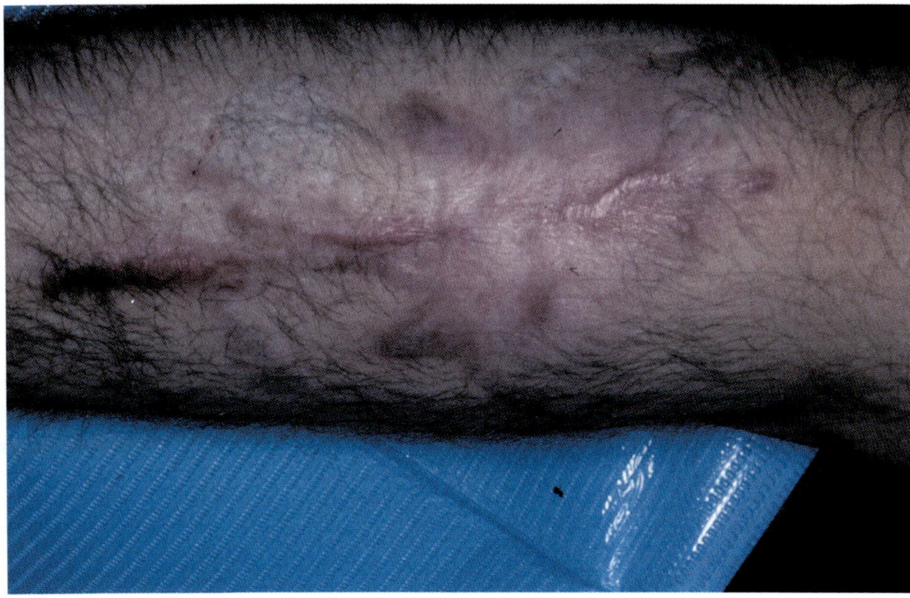

Figure 3.18. Hypertrophic scar 6 months after CO_2 laser treatment of tattoo

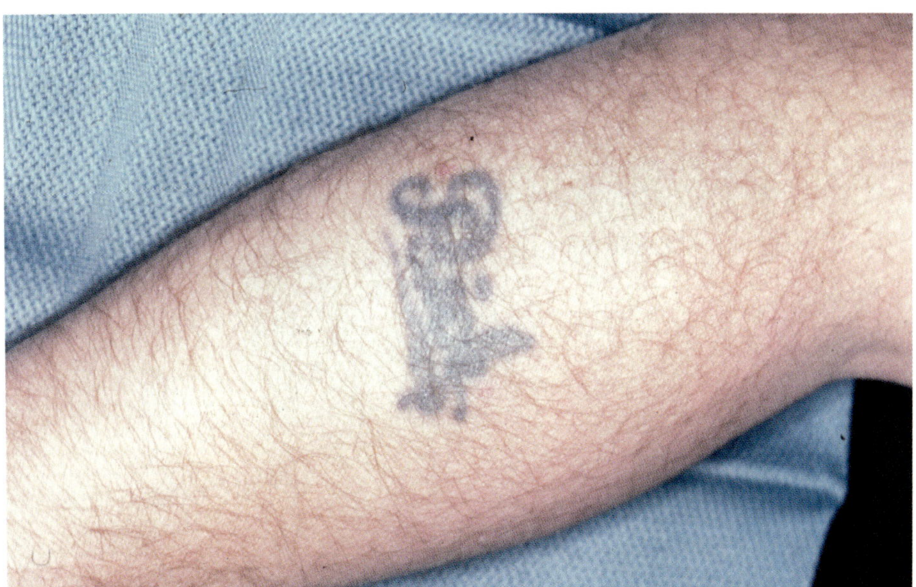

Figure 3.19. Tattoo before CO_2 laser treatment

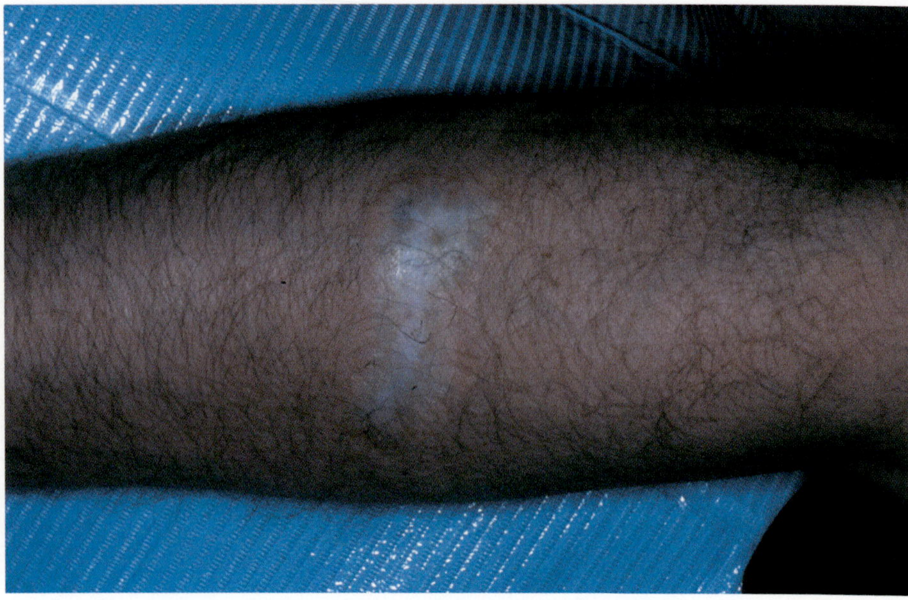

Figure 3.20. Atrophic scar 6 months after CO_2 laser treatment

post-operative textural changes and scarring (Figures 3.21 and 3.22). Despite this problem, Er:YAG and CO_2 lasers are quite useful for the treatment of cosmetic tattoos containing iron or titanium oxide.

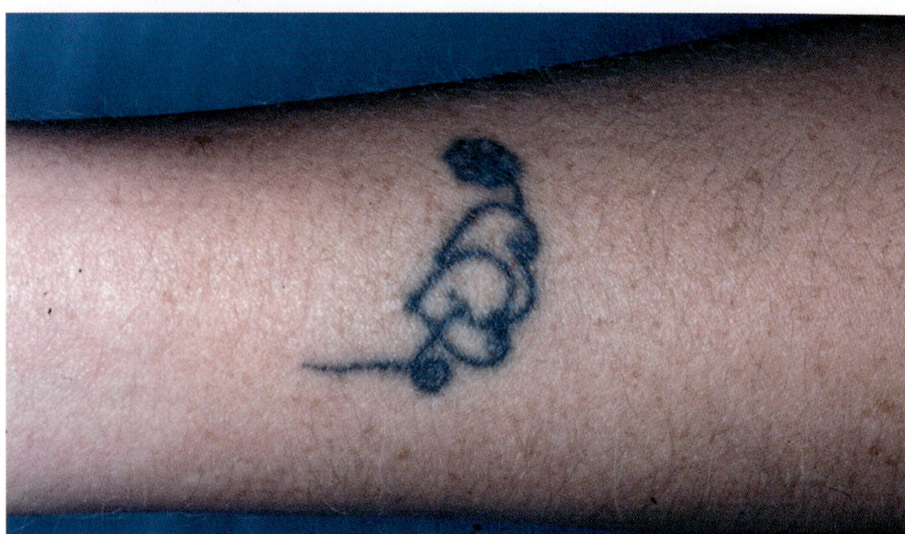

Figure 3.21. Tattoo before Er:YAG laser treatment

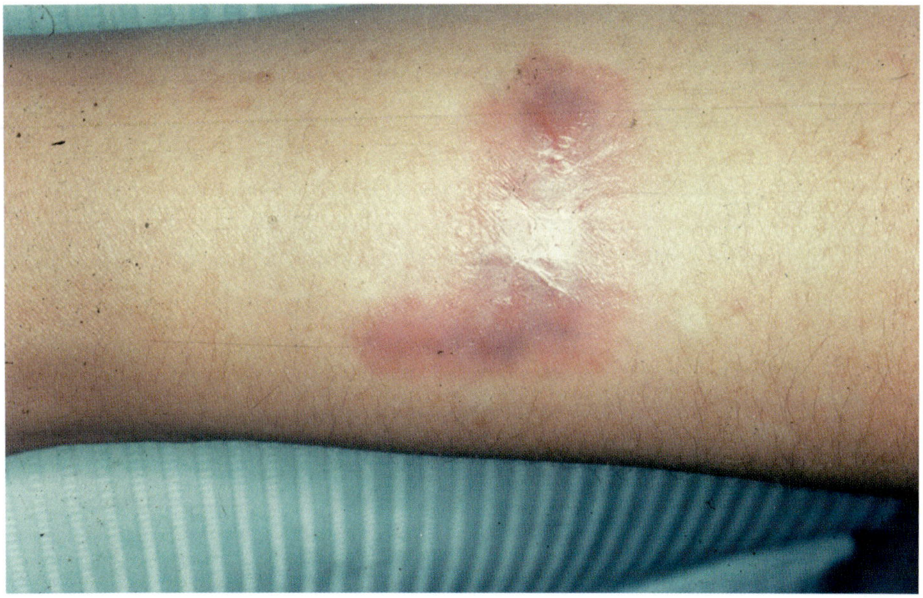

Figure 3.22. Atrophic scar 6 months after Er:YAG laser treatment

When the concept of selective photothermolysis is applied to the treatment of pigmented lesions and tattoos,[43] selective destruction of melanin and/or tattoo ink can be accomplished by choosing an appropriate pigment-absorbing wavelength. Reflectance spectrographic data of tattoo ink colors has been used to choose the best wavelength to treat an individual tattoo pigment. Black tattoo pigment absorbs all wavelengths and is a competing chromophore with melanin pigmentation in the epidermis. Absorption of blue and green tattoo ink appears concentrated from 625 nm to 755 nm. Red tattoo pigment absorbs energy poorly above 550 nm. Many tattoo inks are color mixtures and can be difficult to classify as a single pigment. Pigmented lesions and tattoos respond best to nanosecond pulses delivered by Q-switched lasers.[51]

Q-switched Laser

Mechanism of Action

The mechanism behind Q-switched laser melanosome pigment destruction is unknown. It most likely represents a submicroscopic, mechanical form of damage mediated through an extreme temperature gradient generated within heated melanosomes.[52] These changes cause rapid thermal expansion, local vaporization, and generation of acoustic waves that damage the nucleus and eventually destroy the pigment-laden cells. A nearly identical photomechanical mechanism appears to occur in laser removal of tattoos. As with melanosomes, tattoos consist of insoluble, submicrometer-sized pigmented particles that are phagocytosed by dermal cells.[53] Treatment with short-pulsed lasers results in both fragmentation of tattoo particles and selective death of pigment-containing cells.[54] The released pigment is then removed through transepidermal elimination, phagocytosis by dermal macrophages, or elimination through lymphatic drainage. Other mechanisms of clearance include pyrolytic chemical alteration of the pigment particles and fibrosis, which alters the dermal scattering coefficient, resulting in obscuring of the deeper pigment.[54]

ALLERGIC REACTIONS TO TATTOO PIGMENT AFTER LASER TREATMENT

The most serious complication reported after tattoo treatment with Q-switched lasers, is the occurrence of a localized as well as systemic allergic reaction.[55] Most of these patients never experienced any problem with their tattoo prior to treatment with a Q-switched laser. Allergic reactions to metal salts used in tattoos can occur with many different tattoo pigments. The different colors used in tattoos are often derived from either chromium oxide, cobalt, or cadmium sulfide. All of these substances can cause swelling, erythema, and pruritus in tattooed individuals.[56] Cadmium sulfide can also be phototoxic.[56] In addition, manganese found in purple tattoos has been shown to cause granulomatous reactions in certain patients.[57,58]

Generally, red tattoo pigment is due to cinnabar, which is a mercury derivative and can produce pruritis, swelling, eczematous, granulomatous, and sarcoidal reactions. Frequently, this allergic reaction, which occurs at the site of the red tattoo area, can occur several years after a tattoo has been quiescent. There have been reports of a generalized eczematous eruption after laceration of the tattoo, in a patient who was mercury-sensitive.[59] This can also occur after laser treatment.

Biopsy specimens obtained from these tattoo-induced cutaneous allergic reactions show acanthosis with or without spongiosis and an inflammatory cell infiltrate consisting of lymphocytes, macrophages, and scattered plasma cells and eosinophils. Foreign body giant cells, and in some instances, pseudolymphomatous reactions have been noted.[60]

Q-switched laser-induced extracellular fragmented and mobilized pigments are likely recognized by the patient's immune system as a foreign antigen, potentially triggering an allergic response, initiating a localized as well as potentially generalized allergic reaction.

Systemic allergic reactions are more prevalent in patients exhibiting a localized allergic reaction at the tattoo site. Therefore, if a patient exhibits a cutaneous reaction within the tattoo,[61–63] Q-switched laser treatment is not advised.

In those cases where cutaneous allergy is a concern, Er:YAG and/or high energy, pulsed CO_2 lasers can be used to de-epithelialize the tattoo, promoting transepidermal elimination of the ink.[64] Unfortunately, however, multiple treatments are required, and the risk for dyspigmentation and scarring is increased.

TATTOO INK DARKENING

The mechanism by which tattoos may darken after laser treatment is not completely understood. One factor may be the laser-induced reduction of metallic compounds used in certain dyes. Potential offenders are ferric oxide and titanium dioxide (TiO_2).

Tattoos containing ferric oxide, a brown-red ingredient widely used in red, pink, and flesh-colored tattoos, has been reported to result in a black discoloration when treated with the Q-switched ruby laser. The mechanism is thought to involve the reduction of ferric oxide, which is rust-colored, to ferrous oxide, which is jet black.[65]

A similar phenomenon may be involved in white and other iron-free inks that contain titanium (Figures 3.23–3.25). Titanium dioxide is an increasingly popular white ink used to enhance the brilliance of green, blue, yellow, flesh-colored, and purple tattoos.[66] It has been identified in tattoos of almost any color.[67] In untreated tattoos, titanium is in the TiO_2 form, which is bright white. High-intensity laser irradiation has been shown to result in the reduction of Ti^{4+} to Ti^{3+}, which is responsible for the blue color.[68]

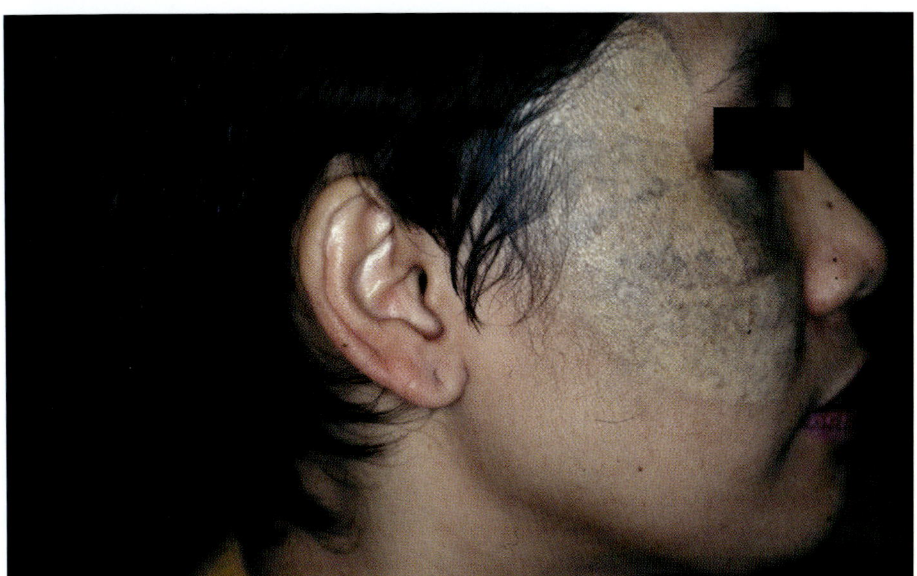

Figure 3.23. Nevus of Ota with overlying titanium dioxide cosmetic tattoo

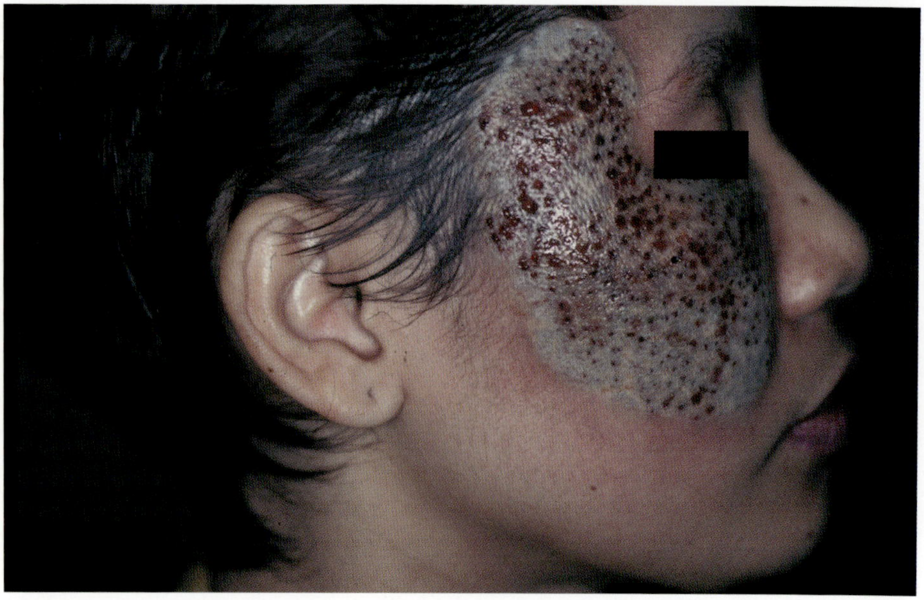

Figure 3.24. Immediate darkening of titanium dioxide tattooed nevus of Ota after Q-switched laser treatment

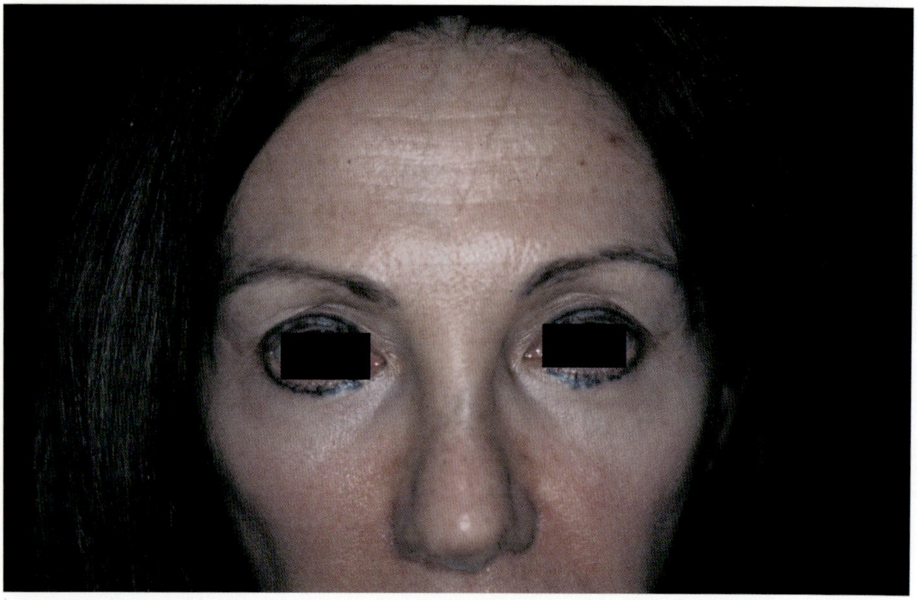

Figure 3.25. Cosmetic tattoo on lower eyelids. No immediate darkening after Q-switched laser treatment

A study of tattoo ink gels containing TiO_2 and iron oxide,[69] found that laser-induced changes were both wavelength- and pulse duration-dependent. Investigators were unable to induce tattoo ink darkening in tattoos with delivered pulse durations greater than 1 millisecond. These data suggest that a threshold power density is required for tattoo ink darkening.

Blackened tattoo pigment, generally, but not always, can be removed with successive laser treatments.[70] Laser treatment of these tattoos must be approached with extreme caution. If one recognizes the possibility of the presence of iron or titanium oxides, a single pulse can be performed as a test site. If the tattoo darkens one might consider using another modality (e.g. pulsed CO_2 or Er:YAG lasers) or abandon attempts at removal.

PIGMENTARY CHANGES

Pigmentary changes after laser treatment of tattoos or pigmented lesions are partially a wavelength-dependent phenomenon. The postulated Q-switched laser mechanism of injury to the melanized cells is a photothermal and photoacoustic effect. This results in disruption of melanosomes with a secondary lethal injury to the melanocytes. This preferential injury to melanized cells may lead to transient hypopigmentation followed by re-pigmentation.[71,72]

Hypopigmentation

The Q-switched, frequency doubled, 532 nm laser invariably produces temporary hypopigmentation that resolves readily. This rapid resolution probably occurs because of the limited depth of penetration of this short wavelength.[73] Prolonged post laser-induced de-pigmentation is rare. The 694 nm and 755 nm Q-switched laser wavelengths have a similar incidence of temporary hypopigmentation, because of their high melanin specificity (Figures 3.26–3.31).

However, the Q-switched ruby laser (694 nm) may also induce long-term hypopigmentation. The 1064 nm Q-switched Neodymium:YAG (Nd:YAG) laser wavelength is least injurious to melanocytes, and is, therefore, the wavelength of choice for dark-skinned individuals undergoing Q-switched laser tattoo removal treatment.[74–76]

Hyperpigmentation

Unlike laser-induced hypopigmentation, hyperpigmentation is more related to the patient's skin type. Darker skin is more likely to hyperpigment no matter which wavelength is used.[77] This increased pigmentation can be caused by deposition of either

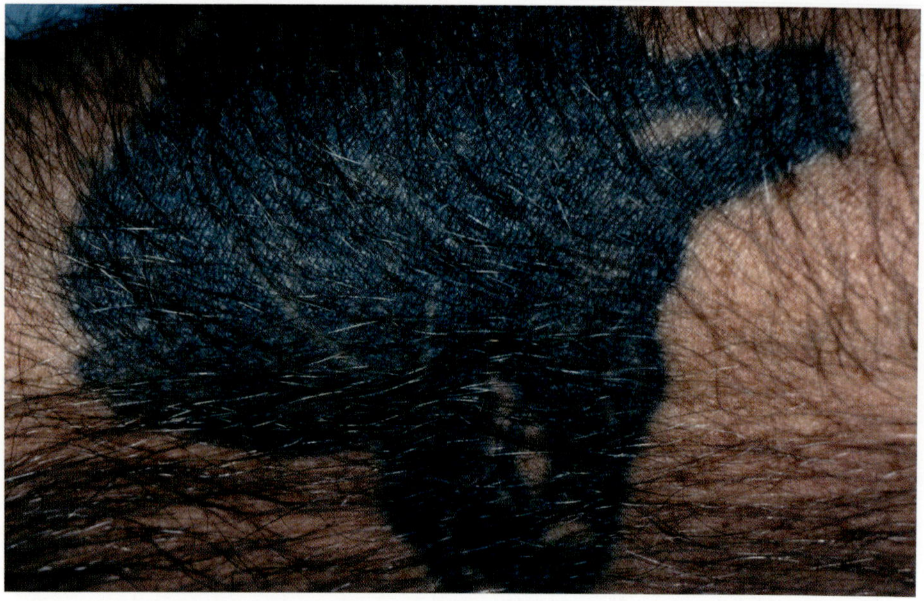

Figure 3.26. Tattoo before Q-switched laser treatment

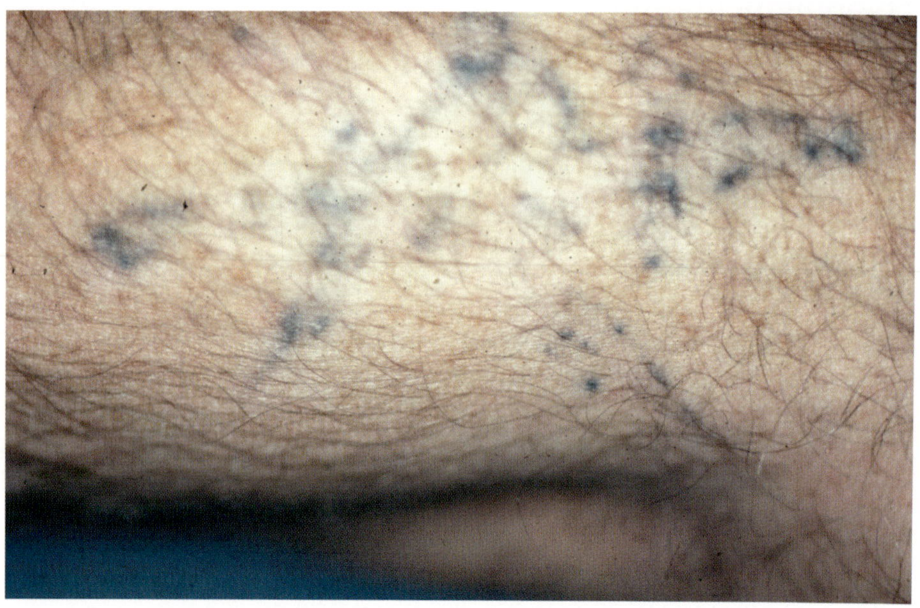

Figure 3.27. Early hypopigmentation 2 months after Q-switched laser treatment

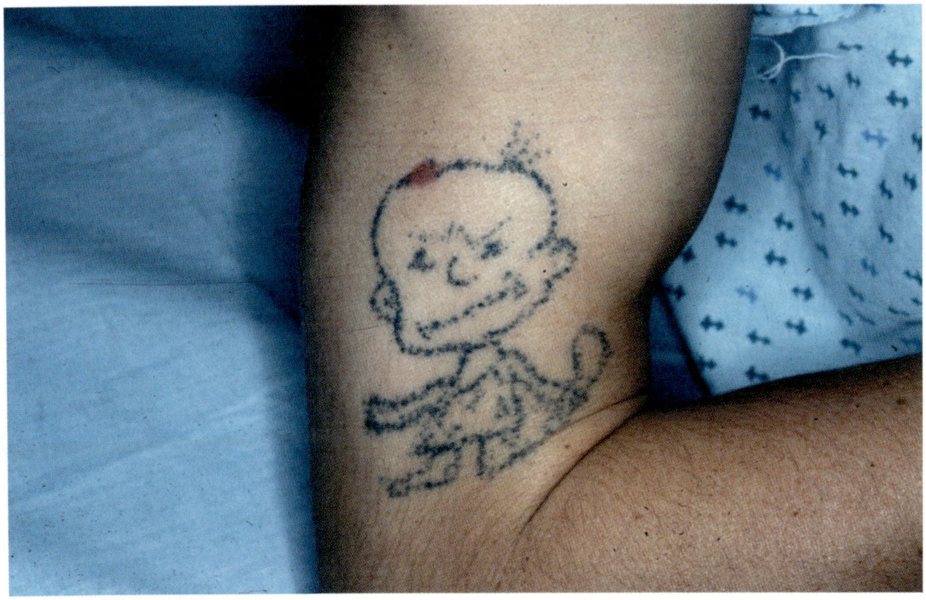

Figure 3.28. Tattoo with small scar after test spot with CO_2 laser and before Q-switched laser treatment

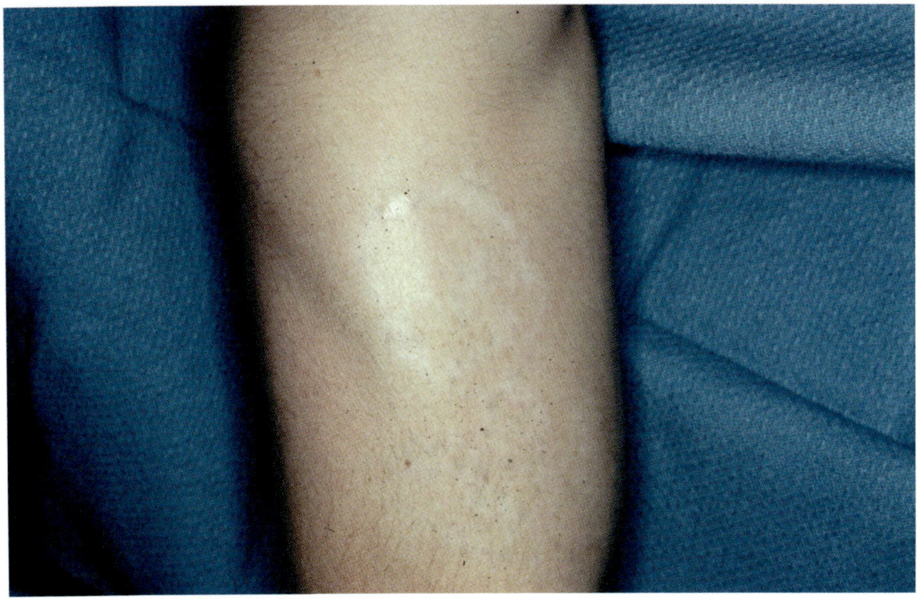

Figure 3.29. Hypopigmentation 3 months after Q-switched laser treatment

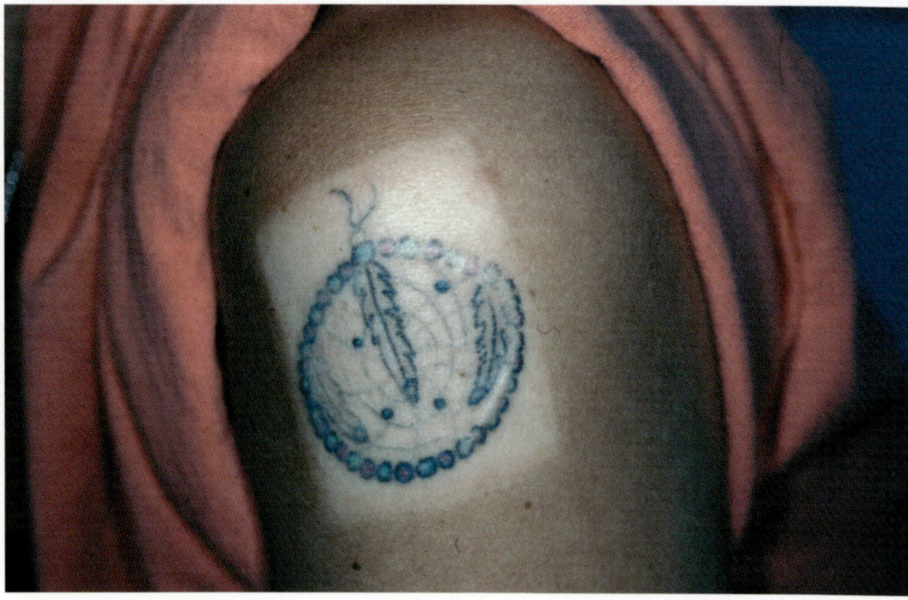

Figure 3.30. Tattoo after two superficial treatments with CO_2 laser and before Q-switched laser treatment

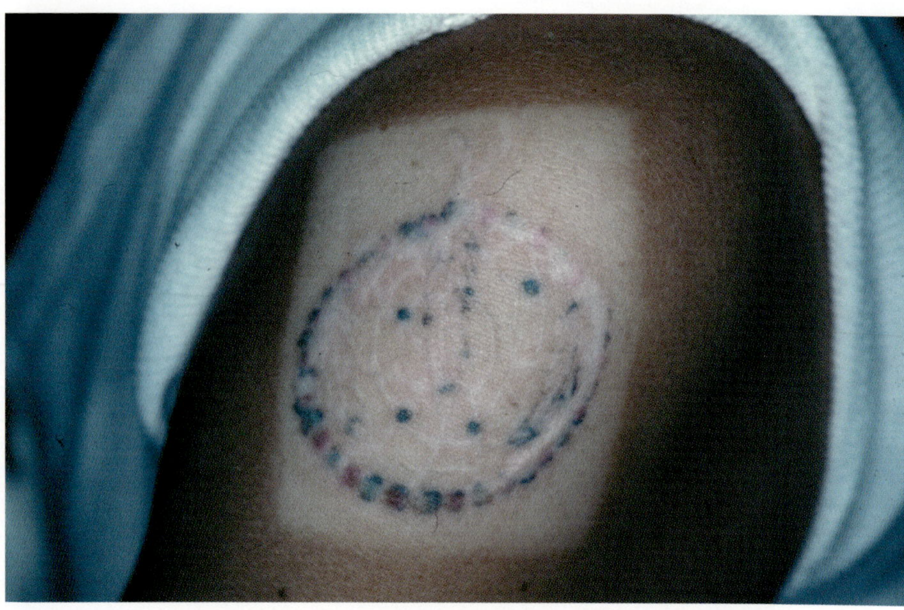

Figure 3.31. Areas of permanent hypopigmentation from CO_2 laser and temporary hypopigmentation induced by Q-switched laser

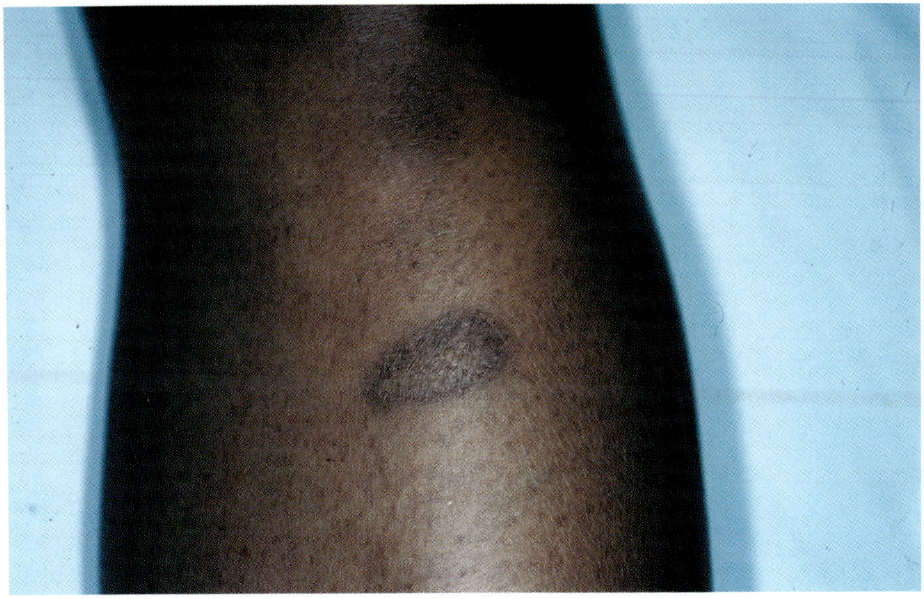

Figure 3.32. Post-inflammatory hyperpigmentation induced by Q-switched Nd:YAG laser treatment of tattoo

melanin or hemosiderin. Q-switched laser-induced epidermal hyperpigmentation may be related to transiently increased melanin formation. These observations, of apparent melanocyte stimulation, have also been seen in guinea pigs after Q-switched laser irradiation.[71,72]

Patients with Fitzpatrick skin type III or greater, and those with a tendency to hyperpigment after superficial skin injuries, are at greater risk for Q-switched laser-induced hyperpigmentation (Figure 3.32). While higher delivered laser fluences may be more successful in tattoo pigment removal, the risk of adverse effects is also greater.

SCARRING/TEXTURAL CHANGES

Textural changes and scarring rarely occur after Q-switched laser treatment of pigmented lesions and tattoos. Despite the extent of histologic dermal vacuolization seen immediately after Q-switched laser treatment, visible microscopic changes in collagen are limited to within a few micrometers of the treatment area. The absence of disruption or necrosis of collagen suggest that vacuolation causes reversible deformation of collagen without significantly altering the dermal architecture. Without significant tissue destruction, the stimulus to healing with fibrosis is minimized. Tissue injury is rarely enough to initiate uncontrolled reparative mechanisms, such as keloid or hypertrophic scar formation. However, transient textural changes (fine cigarette paper-like wrinkling, mild erythema, or a waxy, shiny surface), as well as hypertrophic and atrophic scarring have been noted when higher fluences are used. The incidence of any form of scarring has been reported to be less than 0.5% (Figures 3.33–3.38).[78]

In some instances, the original placement of a tattoo can also produce minor scarring. This may not be easily visible when the ink is in place. However, Q-switched laser removal of the ink may make those textural changes more noticeable.

Textural changes associated with the healing response may also be seen after multiple treatments. Larger laser handpiece spot sizes do tend to minimize epidermal damage and are associated with fewer textural changes.[79] Pruritus can also be significant in the healing phase and topical corticosteroids may be helpful in minimizing local trauma from scratching.

Double tattoos (one tattoo superimposed above another tattoo) should also be treated with caution because they may be associated with an increased risk of scarring. Because of the high density of pigment in double tattoos, laser energy is strongly absorbed.[80] Such laser absorption may produce heat so intense that even the surrounding dermis is thermally damaged, with subsequent scarring.

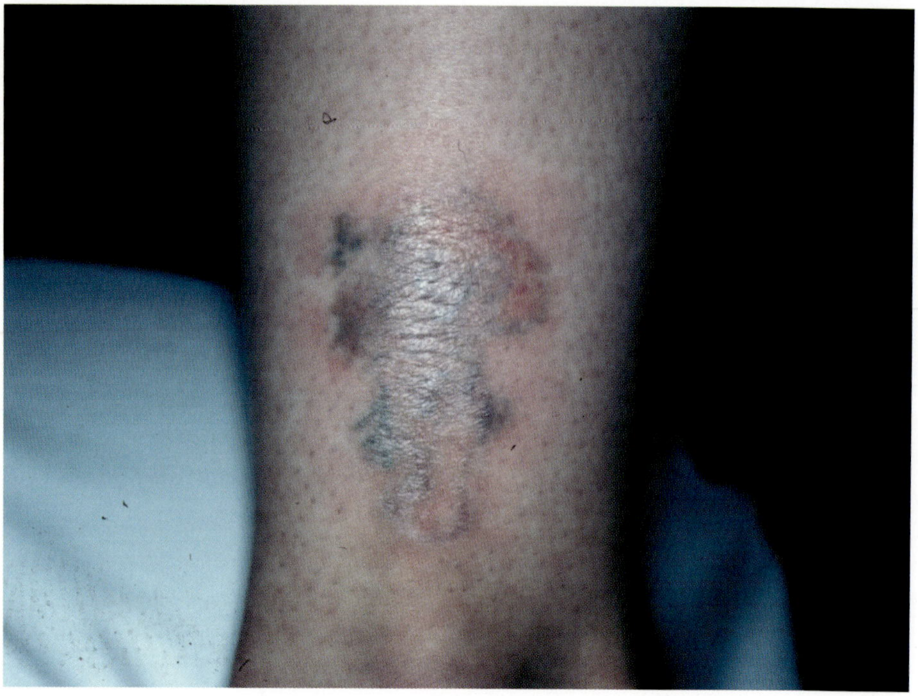

Figure 3.33. Q-switched ruby induced hypopigmentation and early atrophy

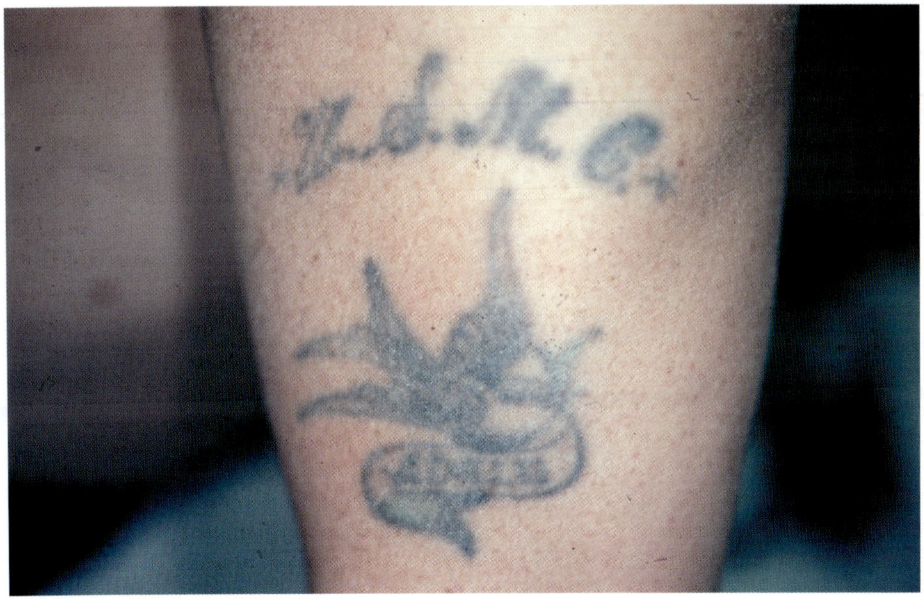

Figure 3.34. Tattoo before Q-switched ruby laser treatment

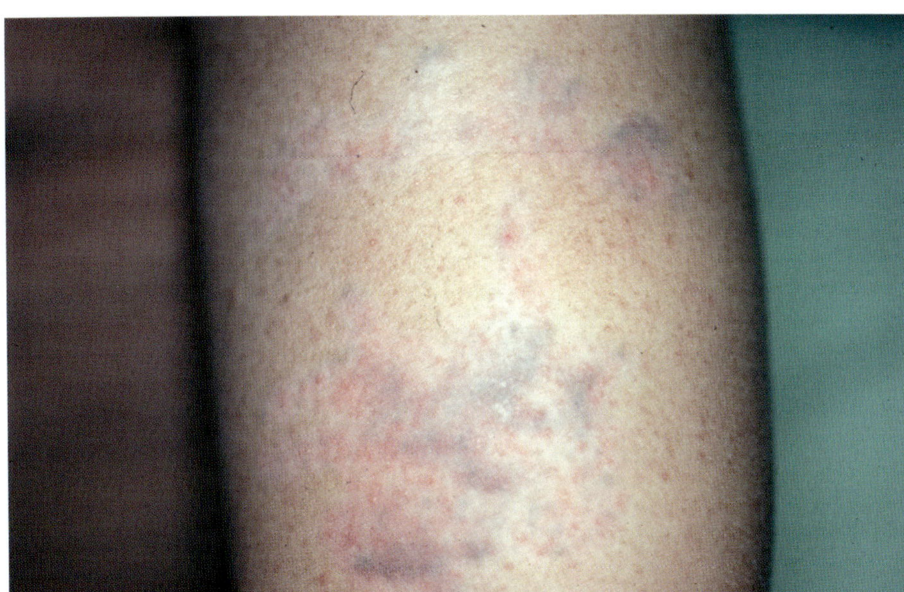

Figure 3.35. Mild atrophy induced by 10 Q-switched ruby laser treatments

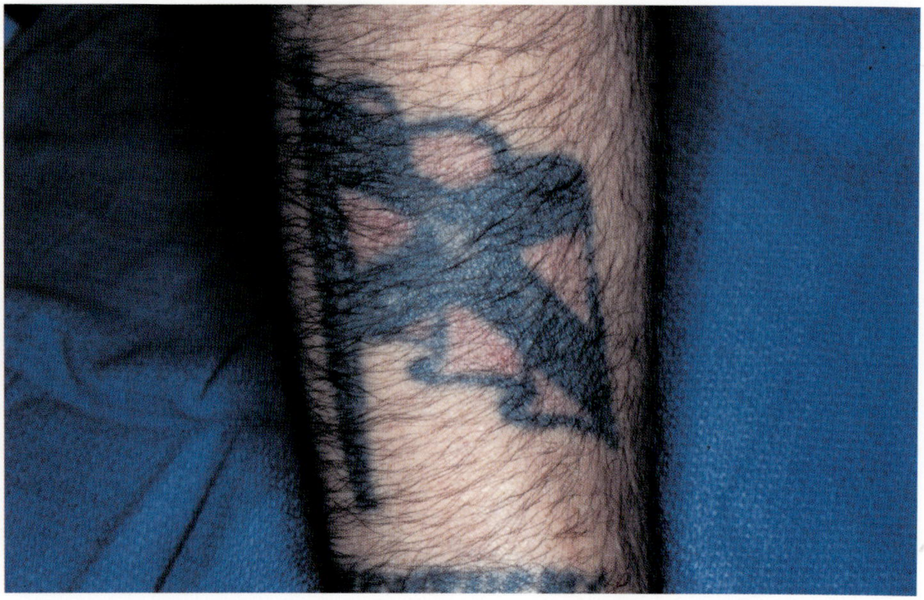

Figure 3.36. Tattoo before treatment with Q-switched Nd:YAG laser treatment

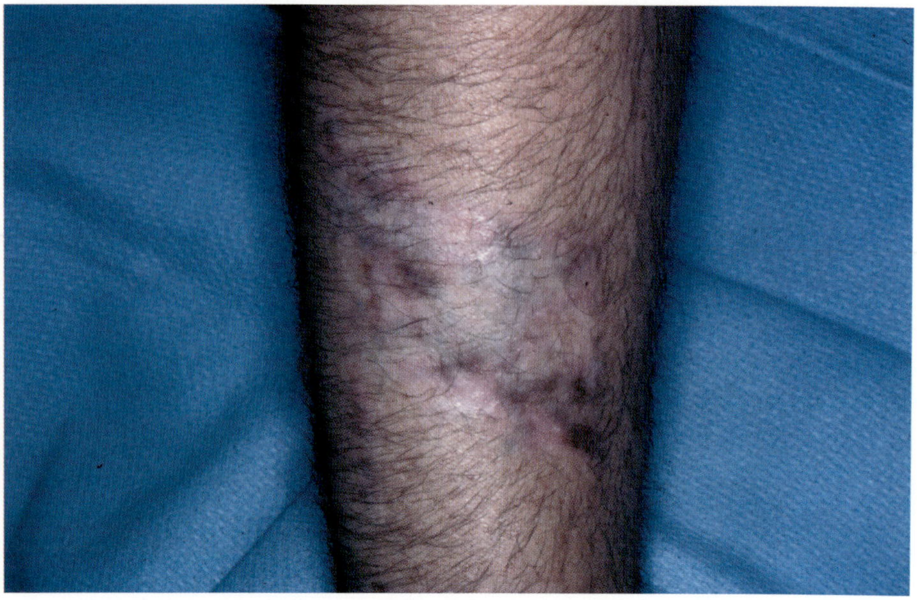

Figure 3.37. Atrophy of skin after 15 Q-switched Nd:YAG laser treatments

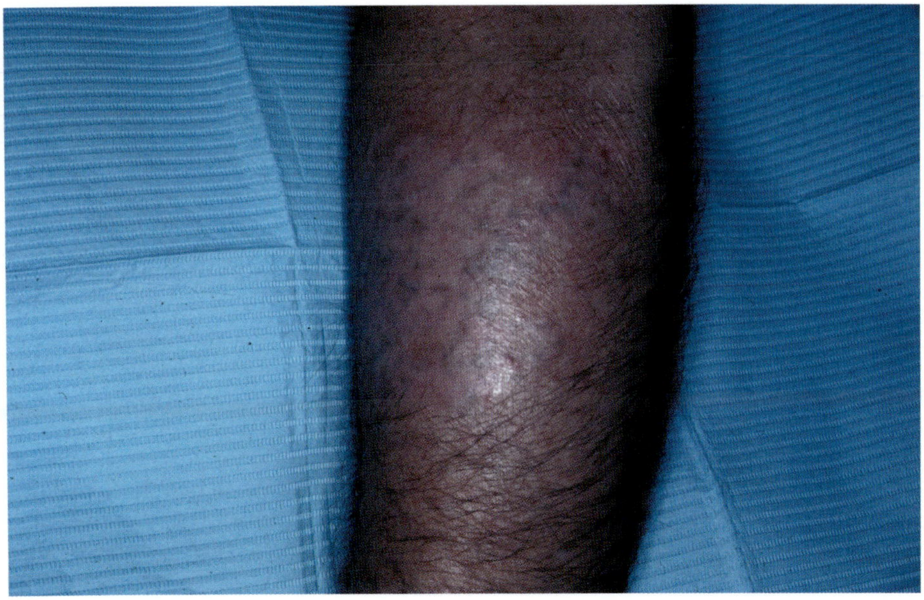

Figure 3.38. Persistence of atrophy 6 months after 15 Q-switched Nd:YAG laser treatments

PRURITUS

Post-treatment pruritus occurs in approximately 25% of Q-switched laser-treated patients. The onset is variable, occurring immediately post-treatment, after 24 hours, after 2–3 days, and in some cases up to 14 days later. In each case, pruritus usually resolves within 2–3 days of the onset. Excessive scratching secondary to the pruritis may lead to scarring.[81]

TREATMENT COMPLICATIONS OF TRAUMATIC TATTOOS

Traumatic tattoos, unlike most professional and amateur tattoos, involve the skin implantation of asphalt, gravel, earth, and/or vegetative matter. Occasionally, traumatic tattoos may involve the deposition of combustible materials, such as gunpowder.[82]

Q-switched laser treatment of traumatic tattoos suspected of containing gunpowder should be carefully undertaken (Figure 3.39). A careful history regarding the potential content of a traumatic tattoo must be elicited. A test treatment should

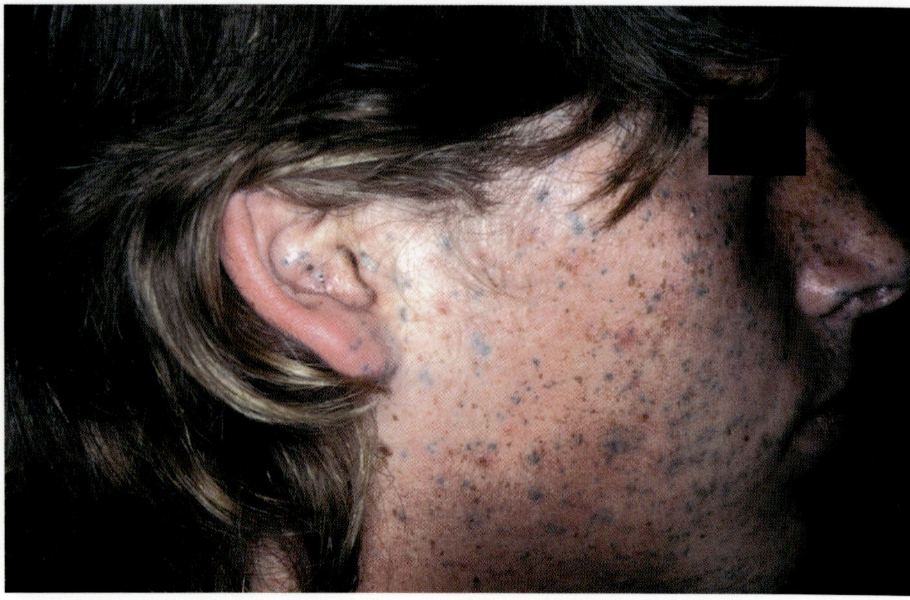

Figure 3.39. Traumatic tattoo of face prior to Q-switched ruby laser treatment

be considered and treatment must not be started if an abnormal reaction with sparking, transepidermal pitting, and/or the smell of burned sulfur occurs in the area of skin being tested.[83–85]

PIGMENTED LESIONS

Melanosomal disruption, after laser treatment of pigmented lesions, will usually lead to the cellular death of either the melanocyte producing the melanosome, the keratinocyte containing them, or the melanophages trying to remove them.[71,72,86–88] Post-treatment pigmentary changes can occur much in the same manner as after the treatment of tattoos. However, these changes are usually of a lesser degree (Figures 3.40–3.48).

Finally, localized chrysiasis was induced in a patient receiving parenteral gold therapy who underwent treatment with a Q-switched ruby laser for post-inflammatory hyperpigmentation. This effect is probably due to a physiochemical alteration of the dermal gold deposits by the laser. It resembles the darkening or blackening effect on flesh-colored tattoos containing ferric oxide.[89]

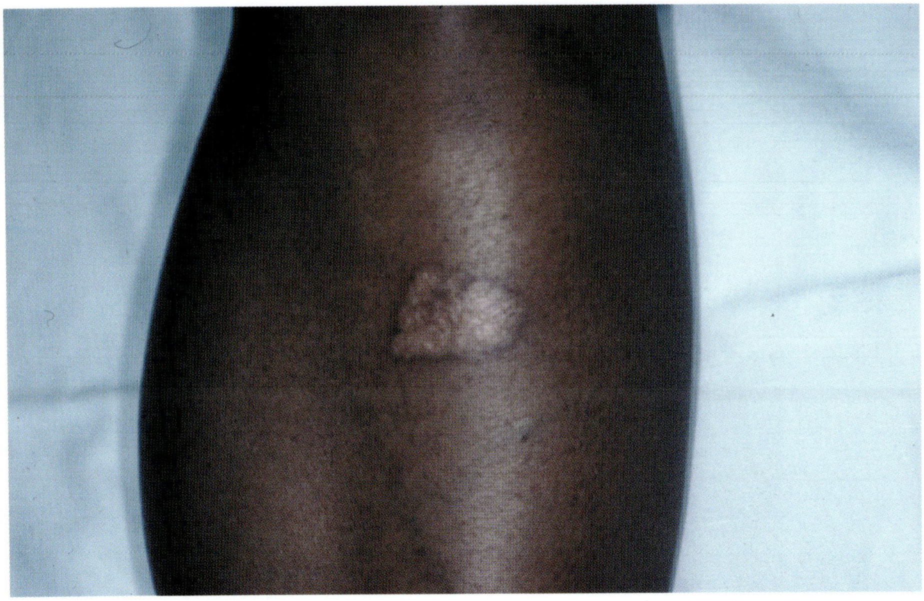

Figure 3.40. Hypopigmentation of skin after Q-switched laser treatment of post-inflammatory hyperpigmentation

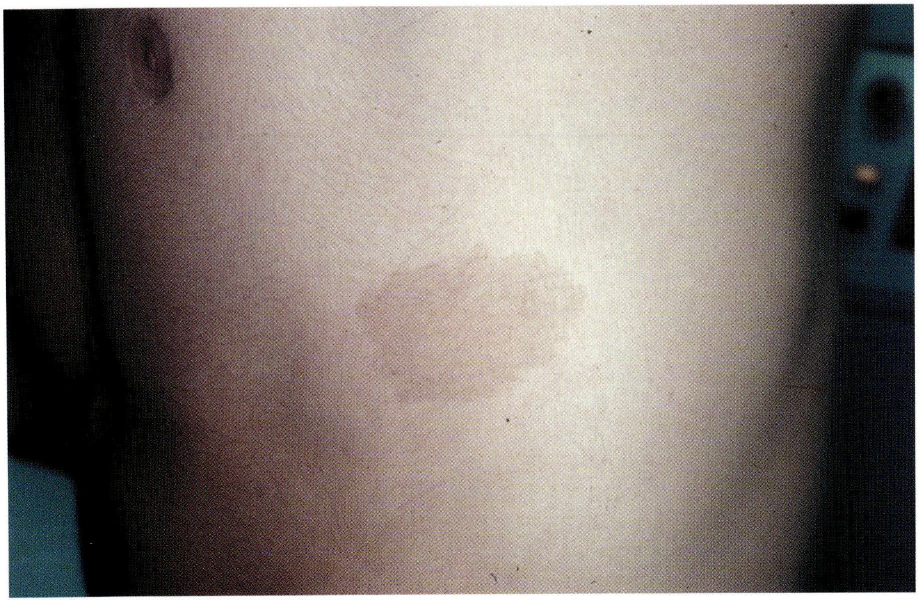

Figure 3.41. Café-au-lait macule before Q-switched Nd:YAG laser treatment

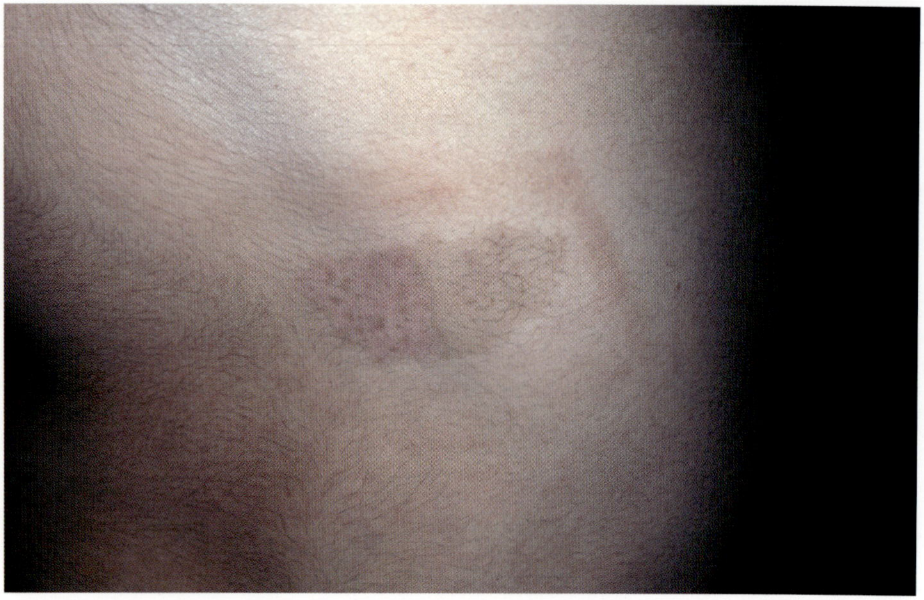

Figure 3.42. Areas of both hyper- and hypopigmentation 4 months after Q-switched Nd:YAG laser treatment

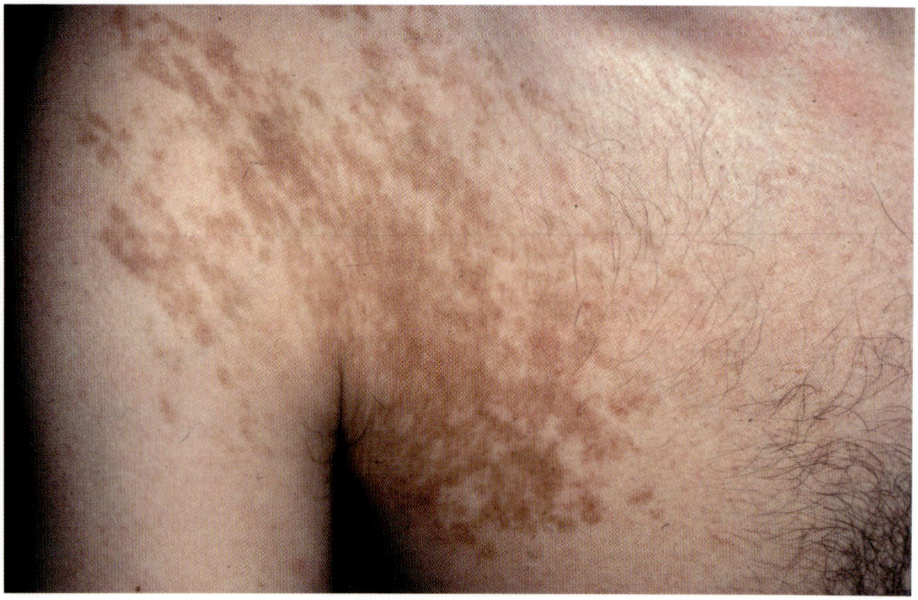

Figure 3.43. Becker's nevus before Q-switched ruby laser treatment

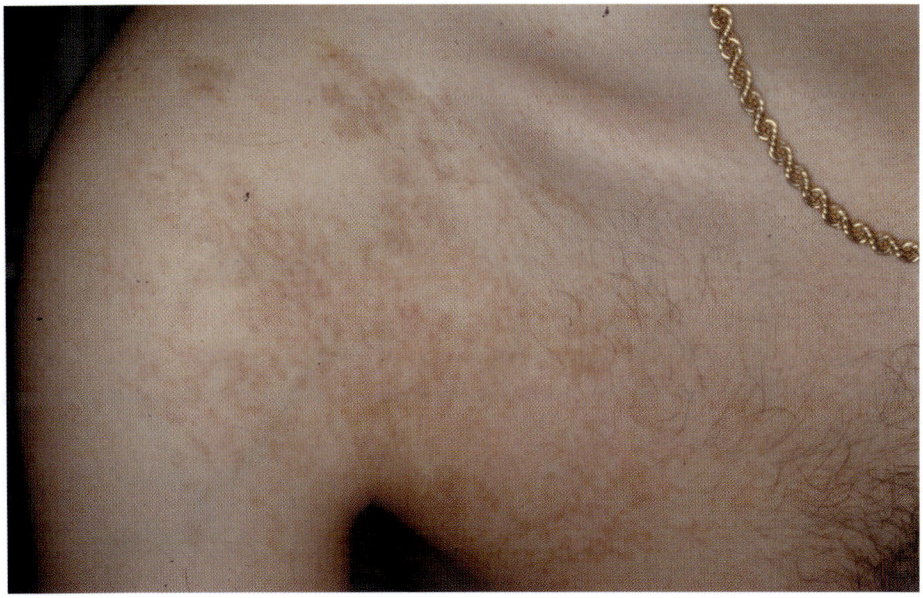

Figure 3.44. Some clearing on chest noted. Mild hypopigmentation also seen

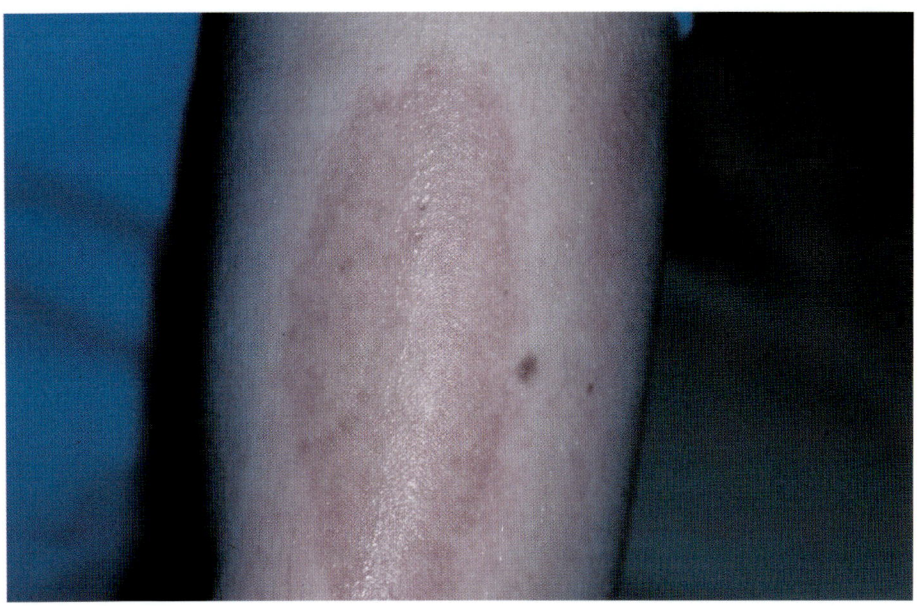

Figure 3.45. Erythema and hypopigmentation noted 4 months after Q-switched ruby laser treatment of café-au-lait macule

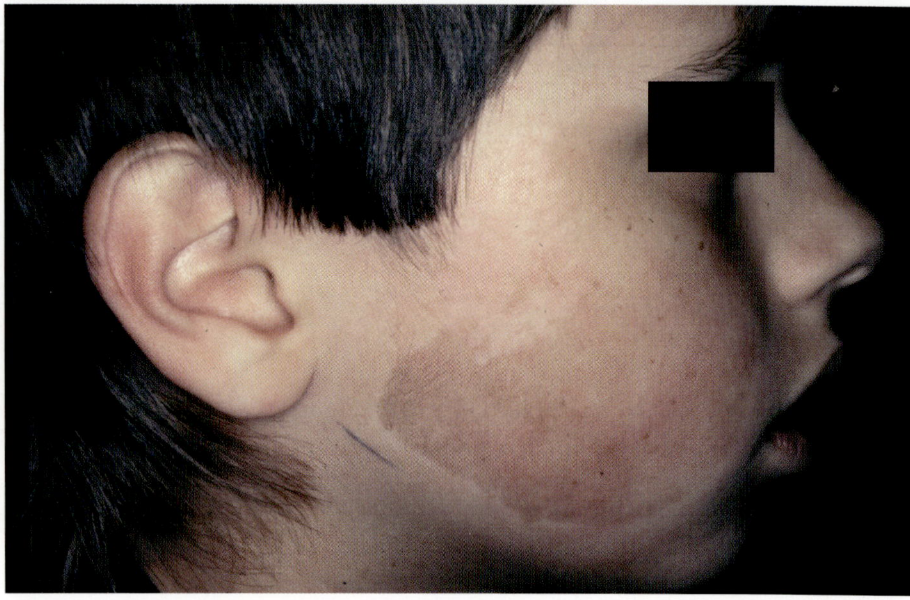

Figure 3.46. Becker's nevus on right cheek before treatment with Q-switched ruby laser

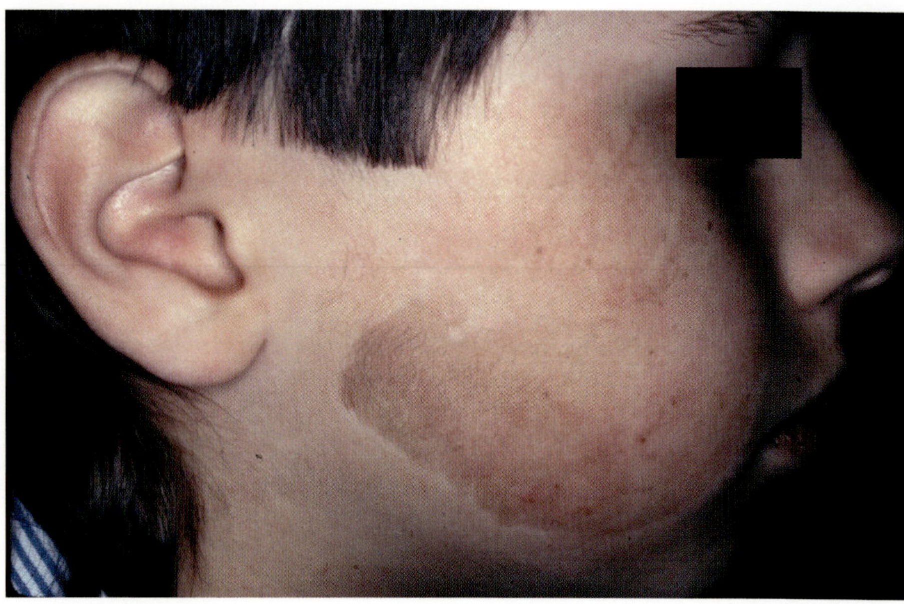

Figure 3.47. Mild hyerpigmentation noted at lateral portion of cheek after treatment with Q-switched ruby laser

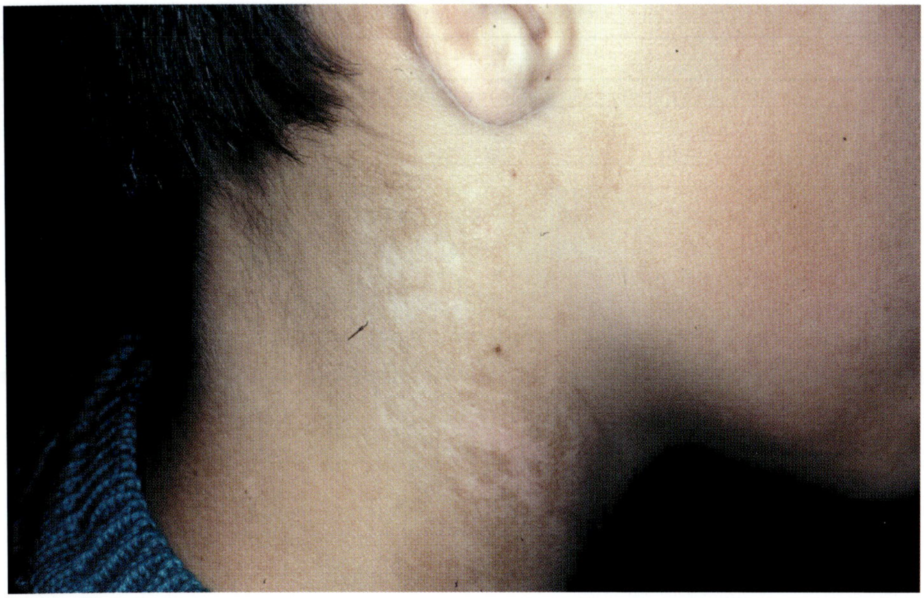

Figure 3.48. Hypopigmentation at site of Q-switched laser treatment of café-au-lait macule

CONCLUSION

Q-switched laser treatment of tattoos and pigmented lesions is in general very safe. Transient hypo- or hyperpigmentation, although common, generally resolves with time. Atrophic and hypertrophic scars, although rare, can occur. Special attention must be paid to those tattoos that contain ferric oxide, titanium dioxide, or gunpowder.

REFERENCES

1 Grumet GW. Psychodynamic implications of tattoos. Am J Orthopsychiatry 1983;53:482–492.
2 Scutt R, Gotch C. Art, Sex and Symbol: The Mystery of Tattooing. South Brunswick, NJ: AS Barnes; 1974.
3 Goldstein N. Psychological implications of tattoos. J Dermatol Surg Oncol 1979;5:883–888.
4 Scutt RWB. The chemical removal of tattoos. Br J Plast Surg 1972;25:189–194.
5 Goldberg HM. Tattoo allergy. Plast Reconstr Surg 1998;98:1315–1316.
6 Sulzberger MB. Tattoo dermatitis. AMA Arch Derm Syphilol 1937;36:1265.
7 Baumler W, Eibler ET, Hohenleutner U, et al. Q-switch laser and tattoo pigments: First results of the chemical and photophysical analysis of 41 compounds. Lasers Surg Med 2000;26:13–21.
8 Caron GA. Tattoo reactions. Arch Dermatol 1968;97:589.
9 Nilles M, Eckert F. Pseudolymphoma following tattooing. Hautarzt 1990;41:236–238.

10 Zinberg M, Heilman E, Glickman F. Cutaneous pseudolymphoma resulting from a tattoo. J Dermatol Surg Oncol 1982;8:955–958.
11 Blumenthal G, Okun MR, Ponitch JA. Pseudolymphomatous reactions to tattoos. Report of three cases. J Am Acad Dermatol 1982;6:485–488.
12 Jones MS, Malony ME, Helm KF. Systemic sarcoidosis presenting in the black dye of a tattoo. Cutis 1997;59:113–115.
13 Sowden JM, Cartwright PH, Smith AG, et al. Sarcoidosis presenting with a granulomatous reaction confined to red tattoos. Clin Exp Dermatol 1992;17:446–448.
14 Hindson C, Foulds I, Cotterill J. Laser therapy of lichenoid red tattoo reaction. Br J Dermatol 1992;133:665–666.
15 Clarke J, Black MM. Lichenoid tattoo reactions. Br J Dermatol 1979;100:451–454.
16 Wiener DA, Scher RK. Basal cell carcinoma arising in a tattoo. Cutis 1987;39:125–126.
17 McQuarrie D. Squamous cell carcinoma arising in a tattoo. Minn Med 1996;49:799–801.
18 Kircik L, Armus S, van den Broek H. Malignant melanoma in a tattoo. Int J Dermatol 1993;32:297–298.
19 Soroush V, Gurevitch AW, Peng SK. Malignant melanoma in a tattoo: a case report and review of the literature. Cutis 1997;59:111–112.
20 Saungueza OP, Yadav S, White CR Jr, et al. Evolution of B-cell lymphoma from pseudo lymphoma. A multidisciplinary approach using histology, immunohistochemistry, and Southern blot analysis. Am J Dermatopathol 1992;14:408–413.
21 Goldstein AP. Histologic reaction in tattoos. J Dermatol Surg Oncol 1979;5:896.
22 Goldstein N. Complications from tattoos. J Dermatol Surg Oncol 1979;5:869–878.
23 Hamberger E. Tattooing as psychic defence mechanism. Int J Soc Psychiatry 1966;12:60.
24 Tazelaar DJ. Hypersensitivity to chromium in a light-blue tattoo. Dermatologica 1970;141:282–287.
25 Tindball JP, Smith JG Jr. Unusual reactions in yellow tattoos. Microscopic studies on histologic sections. South Med J 1962;55:792.
26 Taylor CR, Gange RW, Dover JS, et al. Treatment of tattoos by Q-switched ruby laser: a dose-response study. Arch Dermatol 1990;126:893–899.
27 Dupont C. Decorative tattoos: an analysis of 100 cases. Acta Derm Venereol (Stockh) 1994;74:236.
28 Verma S, Lanigan SW. Reasons for requesting laser removal of unwanted tattoos. Br J Dermatol 1999;140:483–485.
29 Goldstein N, Penoff J, Price N, et al. Techniques of removal of tattoos. J Dermatol Surg Oncol 1979;5:901–910.
30 DeCoste SD, Anderson RR. Comparison of Q-switched ruby and Q-switched Nd:YAG laser treatment of tattoos. Lasers Surg Med (Suppl) 1991;3:64.
31 Strong AMM, Jackson IT. The removal of amateur tattoos by salabrasion. Br J Dermatol 1979;101:693–696.
32 Colver GB, Dawber RPR. Tattoo removal using a liquid nitrogen cryospray. Clin Exp Dermatol 1984;9:364–366.
33 Dvir E, Hirshowitz B. Tattoo removal by cryosurgery. Plast Reconstr Surg 1980;66:373–379.
34 Boo-Chai K. The decorative tattoo: Its removal by dermabrasion. Plast Reconstr Surg 1963;32:559–563.
35 Clabaugh WA. Removal of tattoos by superficial dermabrasion. Arch Dermatol 1968;98:515–521.
36 Clabaugh WA. Tattoo removal by superficial dermabrasion. Plast Reconstr Surg 1975;55:401–405.
37 Colver GB, Jones RL, Cherry GW, Dawber RP, Ryan TJ. Precise dermal damage with an infrared coagulator. Br J Dermatol 1986;114:603–608.
38 Groot DW, Arlette JP, Johnston PA. Comparison of the infrared coagulator and the carbon dioxide laser in removal of decorative tattoos. J Am Acad Dermatol 1986;15:518–522.
39 Venning VA, Colver GB, Millard PR, Ryan TJ. Tattoo removal using infrared coagulation: a dose comparison. Br J Dermatol 1987;117:99–105.

40 Penoff JH. The office treatment of tattoos: a simple and effective method. Plast Reconstr Surg 1987;79:186–191.

41 Buncke HJ Jr, Conway H. Surgery of decorative and traumatic tattoos. Plast Reconstr Surg 1957;20:67–77.

42 Wheeler ES, Miller TA. Tattoo removal by split thickness tangential excision. West J Med 1976;124:272–275.

43 Anderson RR, Parrish JA. Selective photothermolysis: Precise microsurgery by selective absorption of pulsed radiation. Science 1983;220:524.

44 Goldman L, Blaney DJ, Kindel DJ Jr, Franke EK. Effect of the laser beam on the skin. J Invest Dermatol 1963;40:121–122.

45 Goldman L, Ingelman JM, Richfield DF. Impact of the laser on nevi and melanosomes. Arch Dermatol 1964;90:71–75.

46 Goldman L, Wilson RG, Hornby P, et al. Radiation from a Q-switched ruby laser: Effect of repeated impacts of power output of 10 megawatts on a tattoo of man. J Invest Dermatol 1965;44:69.

47 Goldman L, Rockwell RJ, Meyer R, et al. Laser treatment of tattoos: A preliminary survey of three years clinical experience. JAMA 1967;201:841.

48 Apfelberg DB, Maser MR, Lash H. Argon laser treatment of decorative tattoos. Br J Plast Surg 1979;32:141–144.

49 Apfelberg DB, Rivers J, Masers MR, Lash H. Update on laser usage in the treatment of decorative tattoos. Lasers Surg Med 1982;2:169–177.

50 Reid R, Muller S. Tattoo removal by CO_2 laser dermabrasion. Plast Reconstr Surg 1980;65:717.

51 Goldman MP, Fitzpatrick RE. Tattoo Removal in Cutaneous Laser Surgery. St. Louis, MO: Mosby: 1999.

52 Ara G, Anderson RR, Mandell KG, et al. Irradiation of pigmented melanoma cell with high intensity pulsed radiation generates acoustic waves and kills cells. Lasers Surg Med 1990;**10**:52–59.

53 Ort RJ. Tattoos and their treatments. Med Surg Dermatol 1998;5:265–269.

54 Taylor CR, Anderson RR, Gange RW, et al. Light and electron microscopic analysis of tattoo treated by Q-switched ruby laser. J Invest Dermatol 1991;97:131–136.

55 Bailin PL, Ratz JR, Levine HL. Removal of tattoos by CO_2 laser. J Dermatol Surg Oncol 1980;6:997–1001.

56 Fisher AA. Contact Dermatitis. Philadelphia: Lea & Febiger; 1986:713–714.

57 Schwartz RA, Mathias EG, Miller CH, et al. Granulomatous reaction to purple tattoo pigment. Contact Dermatitis 1987;16:199–202.

58 Ravits HG. Allergic tattoo granuloma. Arch Dermatol 1962;86:287–289.

59 Biro L, Klein WP. Unusual complications of mercurial (cinnabar) tattoo. Arch Dermatol 1967;96(2):165–167.

60 Kyanko NE, Pontasch MJ, Brodell RT. Red tattoo reactions: Treatment with carbon dioxide laser. J Dermatol Surg Oncol 1989;15:652–656.

61 Bjornberg A. Allergic reaction to cobalt in light blue tattoo markings. Acta Venereol (Stockh) 1961;41:259.

62 Bjornberg A. Reaction to light in yellow tattoos from cadmium sulphide. Arch Dermatol 1963;88:267–271.

63 Lowenthal LA. Reactions in green tattoos. Arch Dermatol 1973;107:101.

64 Kaufman R, Hibst R. Pulsed erbium:YAG laser ablation in cutaneous surgery. Lasers Surg Med 1996;19:324–330.

65 Anderson RR, Geronemus R, Kilmer SL, et al. Cosmetic tattoo ink darkening: a complication of Q-switched and pulsed-laser treatment. Arch Dermatol 1993;129:1010–1014.

66 Lehmann G, Pierchalla P. Tattooing dyes [in German]. Dermatosen Beruf Umwelt 1988;36:152–156.

67 Slater DN, Durrant TE. Tattoos: Light and transmission electron microscopic studies with X-ray microanalysis. Clin Exp Dermatol 1984;9:167–173.

68 Torimoto T, Fox R III, Fox M. Photoelectric electrochemical doping of TiO_2 particles and the effect of charged carrier density on the photocatalytic activity of microporous semiconductor electrode film. J Electrochem Soc 1996;143:3712–3717.

69 Tope W, Tsoukas M, Farinelli W, Anderson RR. Tattoo ink darkening: The effect of wave length, fluence and pulse duration. Lasers Surg Med 1994;15:364 [abstract].

70 Zelickson BD, Mehregan DA, Zarrin AA, et al. Clinical, histologic, ultrastructural evaluation of tattoos treated with three laser system. Lasers Surg Med 1994;15:364–372.

71 Dover JS, Margolis RJ, Polla LL, et al. Pigmented guinea pig skin irradiated with Q-switched ruby laser pulses. Morphologic and histologic findings. Arch Dermatol 1989;125:43–49.

72 Polla LL, Margolis RJ, Dover JS, et al. Melanomas are a primary target of Q-switched ruby laser irradiation in guinea pig skin. J Invest Dermatol 1987;89:281–286.

73 Kilmer SL, Casparian JM, Wimberly JM, et al. Hazards of Q-switched lasers. Lasers Surg Med Suppl 1993;5:56.

74 Grevelink JM, Casparian JM, Gonzalez E, et al. Undesirable effects associated with the treatment of tattoos and pigmented lesions with Q-switched lasers at 1064 nm and 694 nm. The MGH clinical experience. Lasers Surg Med Suppl 1993;5:55.

75 Kilmer SL, Anderson RR. Clinical use of the Q-switched ruby laser and the Q-switched Nd:YAG (1064 nm and 532 nm) lasers for treatment of tattoos. J Dermatol Surg Oncol 1993;19:330–338.

76 Kilmer SL, Lee MS, Grevelink JM, Flotte TO, Anderson RR. The Q-switched Nd:YAG laser (1064 nm) effectively treats tattoos: A controlled, dose response study. Arch Dermatol 1993;129:971–978.

77 Kilmer SL, Garden JM. Laser treatment of pigmented lesions and tattoos. Seminars in Cutaneous Med Surg 2000;4:232–244.

78 Levine PC, Anderson RR. Q-switched ruby laser treatment of pigmented lesions and tattoos. Clinical Dermatol 1995;13(1):75–79.

79 Kilmer SL, Farinelli W, Tearney G, et al. Use of a large spot size for the treatment of tattoos enhances clinical efficacy and decreases potential side effects. Lasers Surg Med Suppl 1994;6:5.

80 Alora MB, Arndt KA, Taylor CR. Scarring following Q-switched laser treatment of 'Double Tattoos'. Arch Dermatol 2000;136:269–270.

81 Ferguson JE, August PJ. Evaluation of the Nd:YAG laser for the treatment of amateur and professional tattoos. Br J Dermatol 1996;135:586–591.

82 Taylor CR. Laser ignition of traumatically embedded firework debris. Lasers Surg Med 1998;22:157–158.

83 Fusade T, Toubel G, Grognard G, Mazer JM. Treatment of gunpowder traumatic tattoo by Q-switched Nd:YAG laser: An unusual adverse effect. Dermatol Surg 2000;26:1057–1059.

84 Taylor CR, Gange RW, Dover JS, et al. Treatment of tattoos by Q-switched ruby laser. A dose response study. Arch Dermatol 1990;126:893–899.

85 Apfelberg DB, Manchester GH. Decorative and traumatic tattoo biophysics and removal. Clin Plast Surg 1987;14:243–251.

86 Hruza GJ, Dover JS, Flotte TJ, Goetschkes M, Watanabe S, Anderson RR. Q-switched ruby laser radiation of normal human skin. Histological and ultrastructural findings. Arch Dermatol 1991;127:1799–1805.

87 Hruza GJ, Margolis RJ, Watanabe S, et al. Selective photothermolysis of pigmented cells by Q-switched Nd:YAG laser pulses at 1064, 532, 355 nm wave lengths. J Invest Dermatol 1987;88:496.

88 Murphy GF, Shepard RS, Paul BS, et al. Organelle specific injury to melanin-containing cells in human skin by pulsed laser irradiation. Lab Invest 1987;49:680.

89 Yun PL, Arndt KA, Anderson RR. Q-switched laser-induced chrysiasis treated with long-pulsed laser. Arch Dermatol 2002;138:1012–1014.

4 COMPLICATIONS IN LASER TREATMENT OF UNWANTED HAIR

KEY POINTS

(1) Laser treatment of unwanted hair has a low incidence of complications
(2) Transient hypopigmentation after laser treatment of unwanted hair is common and generally resolves
(3) Transient hyperpigmentation after laser treatment of unwanted hair is common and generally resolves
(4) Although laser hair removal, and the resultant injury to the hair follicle must be performed over many sessions, there is no evidence of any mutagenic or carcinogenic potential

INTRODUCTION

Melanin, in the form of eumelanin, is the major cutaneous chromophore used as a target for hair removal lasers and light sources. Most individuals demonstrate greater melanin density in their hair as compared to their epidermis such that the absorption coefficient of the hair shaft and bulb is roughly 2 to 6 times that of the epidermis.[1] Optimally, one would want no absorption by any skin components except the targeted pigmented hair. Unfortunately, such a situation does not exist. The advantage of choosing melanin as a hair absorbing target is that it is already present in both the hair follicle and shaft. However, this choice of chromophore also has disadvantages. One disadvantage is that not all hair has melanin. White hair has no melanin; blonde or red hair has poorly absorbing pheomelanin. More importantly, in terms of complications, melanin is found not only in the hair follicle, but in the epidermis as well. Light must initially pass through the epidermis in order to get to the deeper hair follicle and is therefore potentially absorbed first in the epidermis. This may have several consequences. Absorption of light in the epidermis results in possible adverse effects, such as vesiculation, crusting, burns, and dyspigmentation. Finally, the more the laser light is absorbed in the epidermis, the less is that light available for damaging the follicle. As a result, higher fluences are required for effectiveness, and higher fluences can lead to more adverse effects.

The incidence of cutaneous adverse effects, after laser hair removal, is both patient- and wavelength-dependent.[2] Patients with darker colored skin, especially Fitzpatrick skin types V and VI, are more likely to experience cutaneous adverse effects related to the abundance of melanin in their epidermis. It should be noted that such complications are not limited to patients with genetically determined dark skin. This may also be seen in patients with darker skin due to other reasons, such as suntanning and lentiginous photoaging. A constitutionally higher reactivity to a variety of trauma in these darker skin types may be the reason for this observed effect (Figures 4.1–4.7).

Factors that could theoretically impact on the incidence of adverse effects include utilized wavelength, fluence, and pulse duration. A laser with a longer wavelength and longer pulse duration is less likely to be absorbed by epidermal melanin. This may have some advantages and disadvantages as are described below.

Although the circulation of blood undoubtedly considerably aids the dissipation of heat from the skin after laser hair removal,[3] it is unlikely that blood flow would significantly affect the peak temperatures recorded at the depth of hair follicles. More likely, any complication associated with laser depilation is mainly a direct result of the presence of melanin within the epidermis and the consequent localized

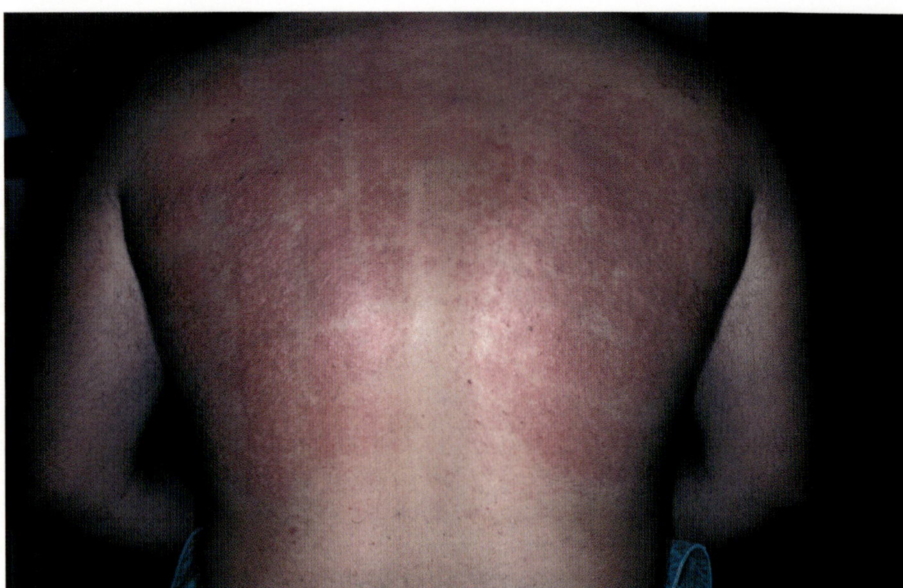

Figure 4.1. Early blistering immediately after alexandrite laser treatment

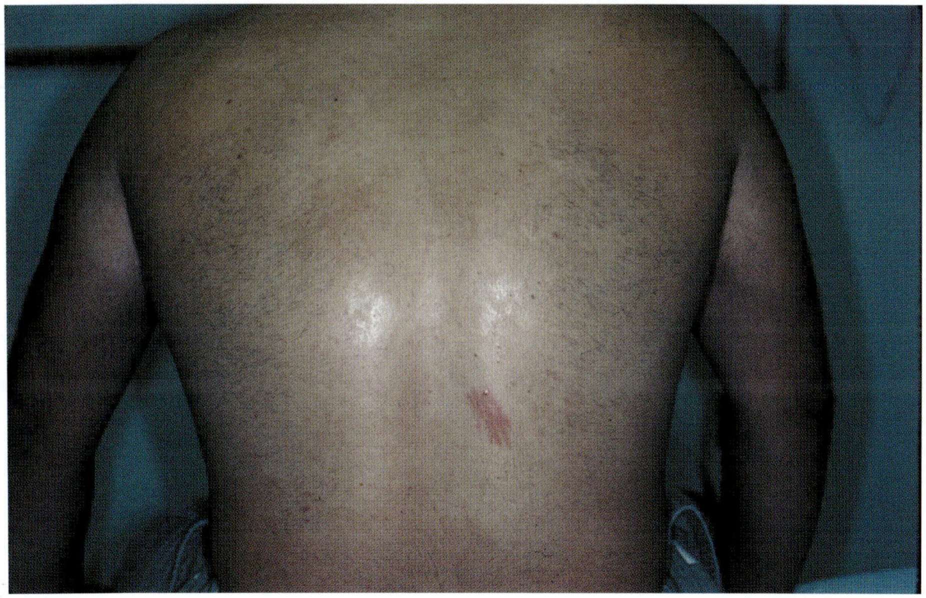

Figure 4.2. Back and shoulder hair before ruby laser hair removal

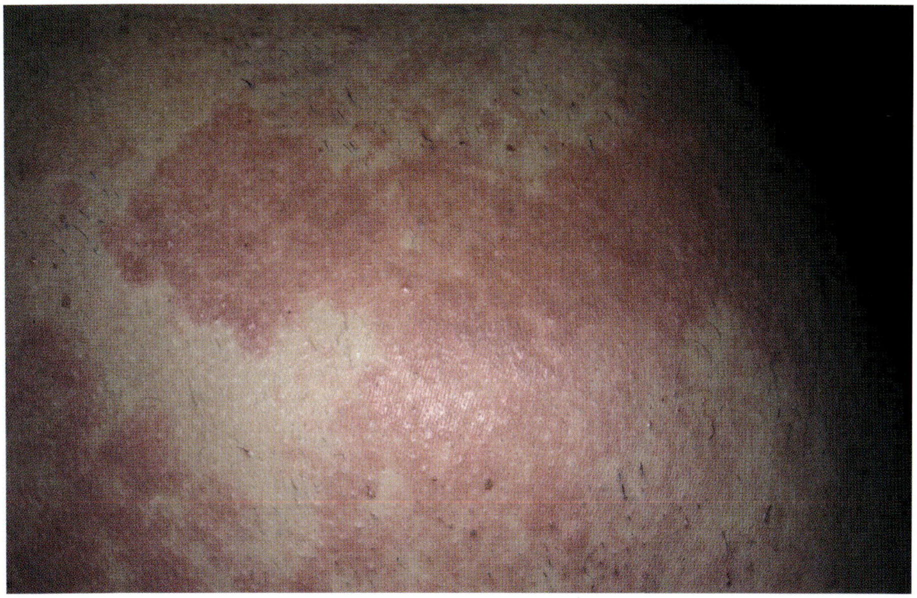

Figure 4.3. Extensive urticarial reaction immediately after ruby laser treatment

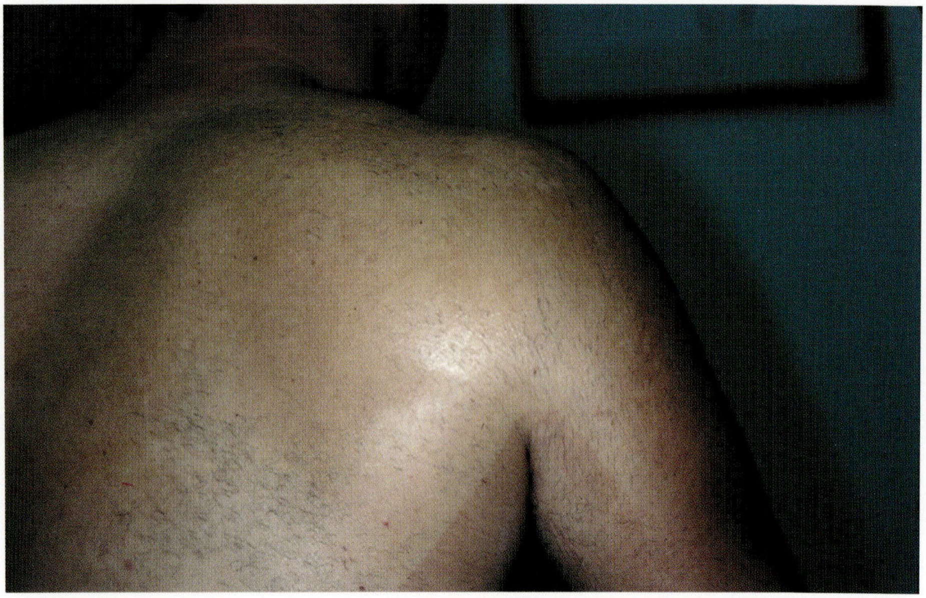

Figure 4.4. Shoulder and back hair prior to alexandrite laser hair removal

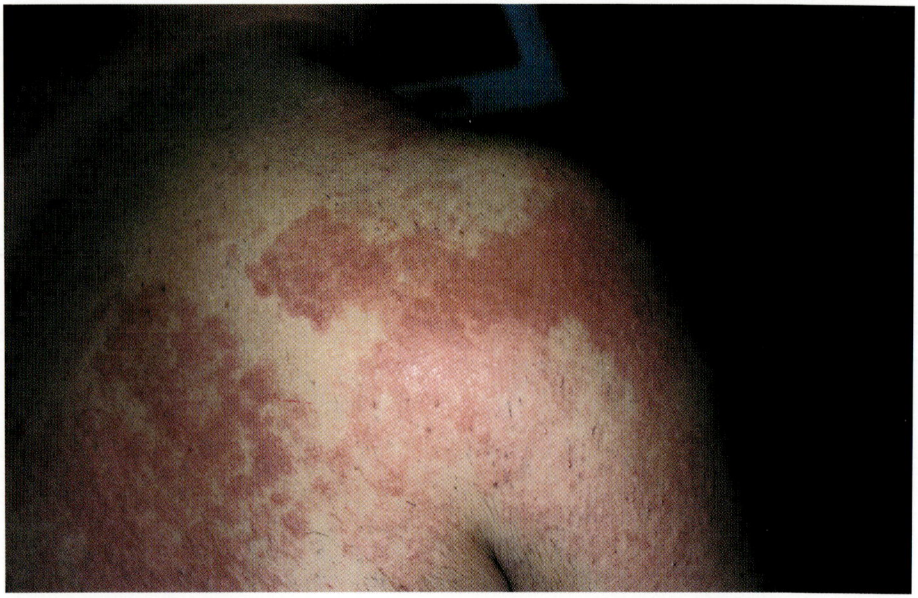

Figure 4.5. Urticarial and early blister formation 4 hours after treatment with the alexandrite laser

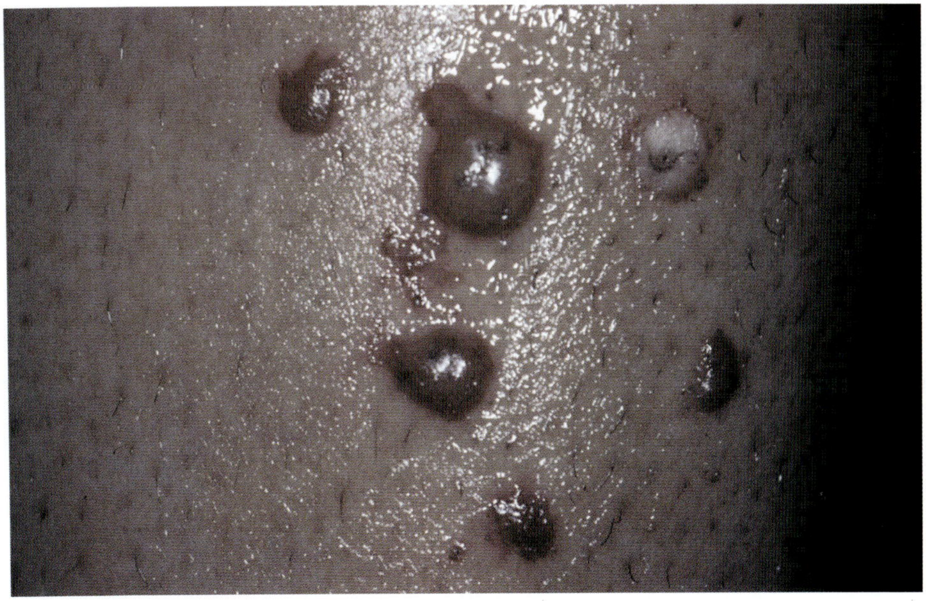

Figure 4.6. Blisters induced by diode laser hair removal

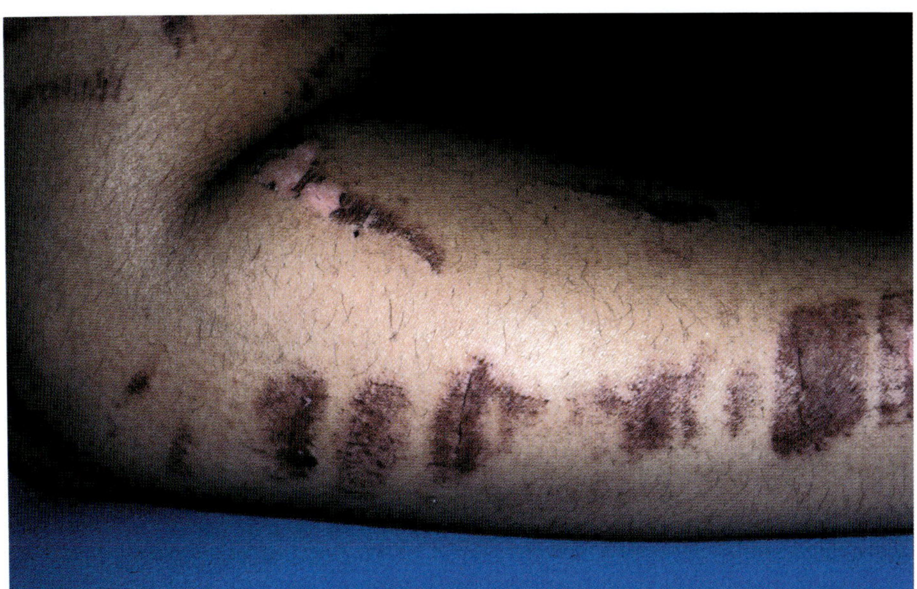

Figure 4.7. Blisters becoming crusted 6 days after intense pulsed light hair removal

production of heat. This is in agreement with the common observation that side effects are more prevalent in patients with darker skin. In addition, one sees in darker skin ultrastructural findings of damage to the keratinocyte-containing melanosomes in such treated patients.[4]

PIGMENTARY CHANGES

There is a remarkable variation in the reported incidence of post-operative pigmentary changes after laser hair removal. Unfortunately, these studies have not been carried out under standardized conditions. Different laser parameters have been used; the follow-up period has varied from 90 days to 2 years; the pre-operative skin characteristics were not standardized (hair color, skin pigmentation, anatomical region); and the majority of studies estimate the incidences of side effects by subjective clinical evaluations.

In one study,[5] skin reflectance measurements were documented by the presence of sub-clinical post-operative pigmentary changes. These changes generally depended on the degree of pre-treatment pigmentation. The post-operative reflectance-determined skin pigmentation differed from the pre-operative skin pigmentation in 47 out of 51 treated areas; yet clinically visible pigmentary changes were only seen in 6 of the treated areas. No linear dose–response relationship was observed. However, this may be due to non-homogenicity in the treated patients' skin characteristics (hair color and density, collagen density).

In general, light-pigmented skin types potentially experience more post-operative sub-clinical hyperpigmentation. Darker-pigmented skin types experience more post-operative sub-clinical hypopigmentation. This finding is in accordance with the notion that laser light in dark-pigmented skin types is strongly absorbed by epidermal melanin. This absorption leads to the damage of melanocytes.[6] In contrast, thermal effects in light-pigmented skin may provoke post-inflammatory hyperpigmentation.

Hypopigmentation

Hypopigmentation, although generally transient, can be unpleasant for the cosmetic laser hair removal patient. This loss of pigment may last for many months. Transient post-treatment hypopigmentation occurs in 10–17% of treated patients.[7–9] The exact etiology of post-laser hair removal-induced hypopigmentation is unclear. This hypopigmentation may be related to the destruction of melanocytes, suppression of melanogenesis, or the redistribution of melanin in the keratinocytes.

Most patients experience some degree of xerosis in laser-treated areas. This peeling after laser hair removal may result in a hypopigmented, spotted look to the skin. Loss of freckles or pigmented lesions is not uncommon and can result in a persistent geographic loss of pigment.

Recent research has shown that the number of melanocytes with tyrosinase activity (the first enzyme in the synthesis pathway of melanin) decreases dramatically immediately after laser treatment.[10] Yet, the absolute number of S-100 positive melanocytes remains constant. In addition, there appears to be no definite alteration in the distribution of melanosomes in the keratinocytes after treatment. It is therefore likely that the hypopigmentation seen after laser treatment is related to the suppression of melanin synthesis, rather than a change in the number of melanocytes in the basal layer of the epidermis. The mechanism of tyrosinase block is unknown. It could be due to the effect of heat, as tyrosinase enzymatic activity is normally suppressed by high temperatures. It could also be due to the mechanical disruption of melanosomes following laser irridiation. The sub-disruptive damage sustained by the patient's melanocytes may lead to a reparative process, which causes a delaying halt in tyrosinase activity. This is all consistent with the general clinical finding of reversibility of skin hypopigmentation after laser-assisted hair removal.[10,11] This observation is generally true for all degrees of epidermal pigmentation and fluences used. However, in those circumstances where melanocytes in the periglandular and perifollicular areas are destroyed or significantly disabled, the mechanisms of trauma-induced pigmentary changes may be different. Permanent loss of pigment is very rare (Figures 4.8–4.14).

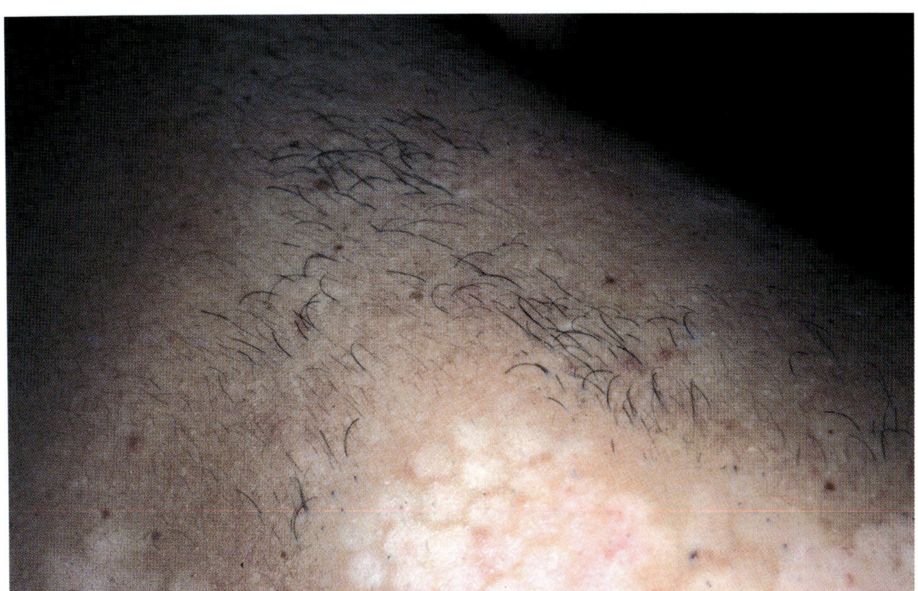

Figure 4.8. Hypopigmentation in ruby laser-treated areas 1 month after treatment

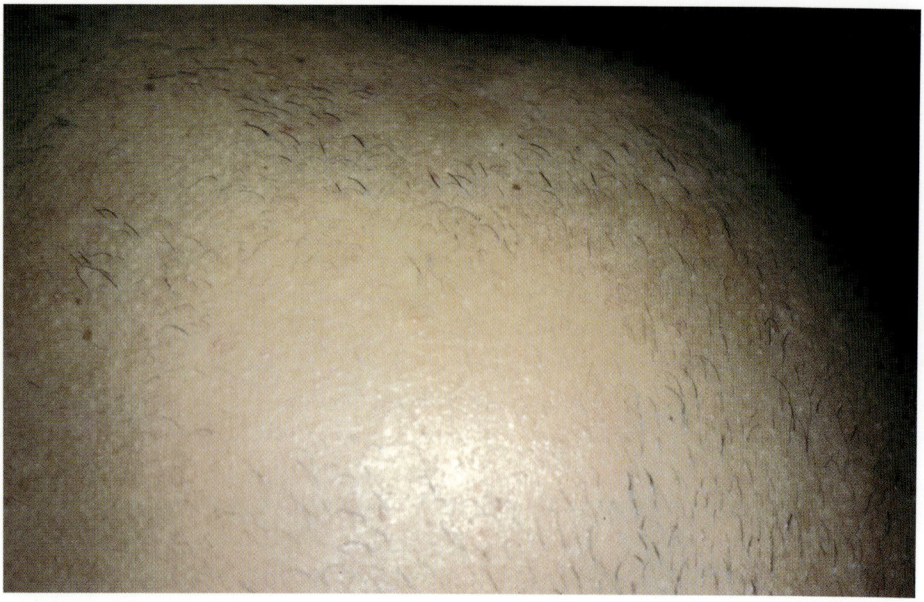

Figure 4.9. Patient in Figure 4.8 hypopigmentation is almost resolved at 6 months

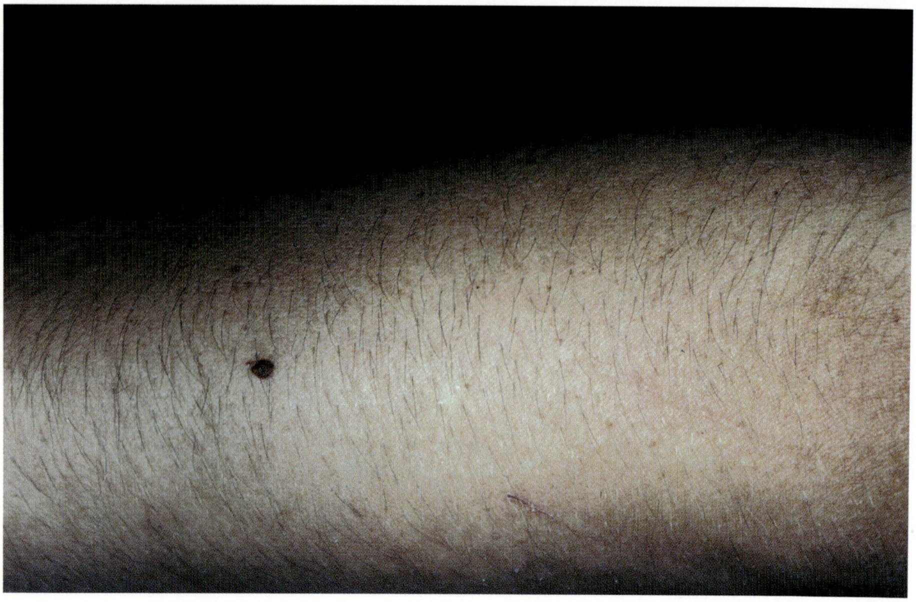

Figure 4.10. Unwanted hair in a recently tanned Fitzpatrick skin type III individual

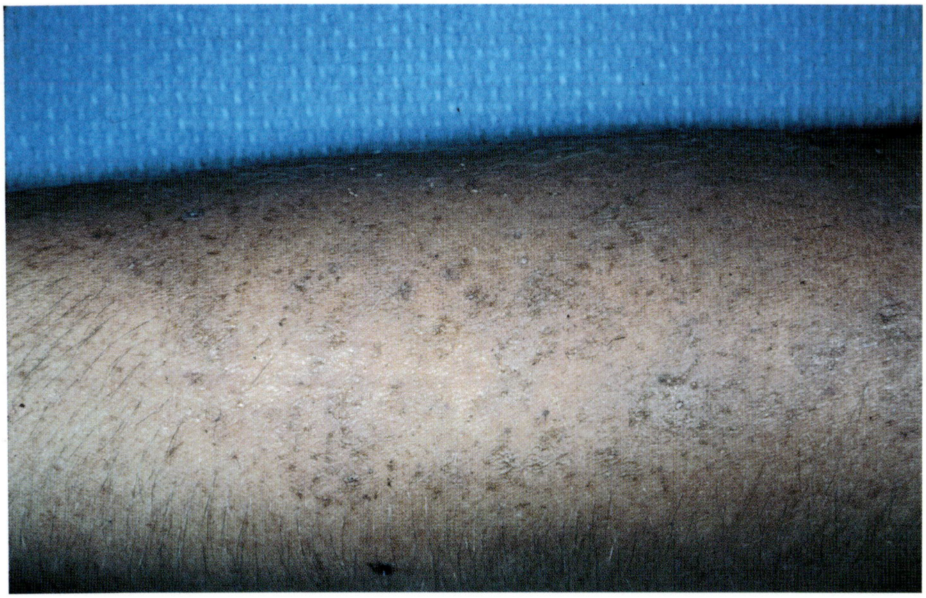

Figure 4.11. Patient in Figure 4.10 immediately after treatment with alexandrite laser

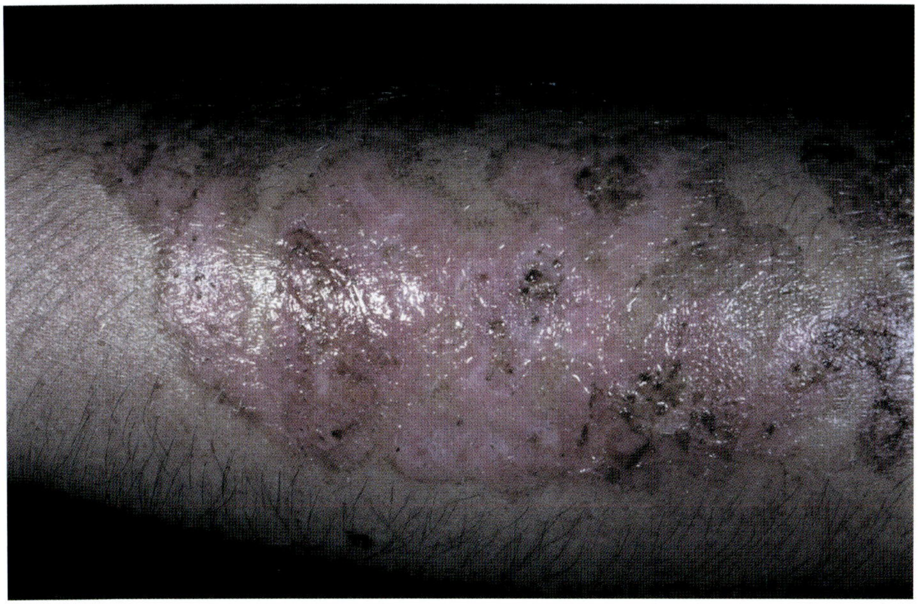

Figure 4.12. Patient in Figure 4.10 3 days after treatment with alexandrite laser

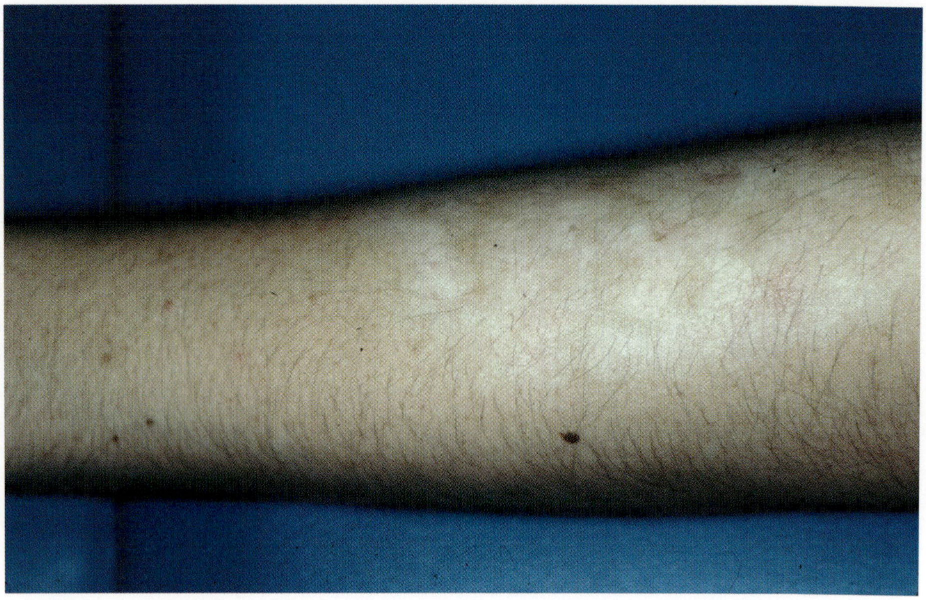

Figure 4.13. Patient in Figure 4.10 3 months after treatment with alexandrite laser

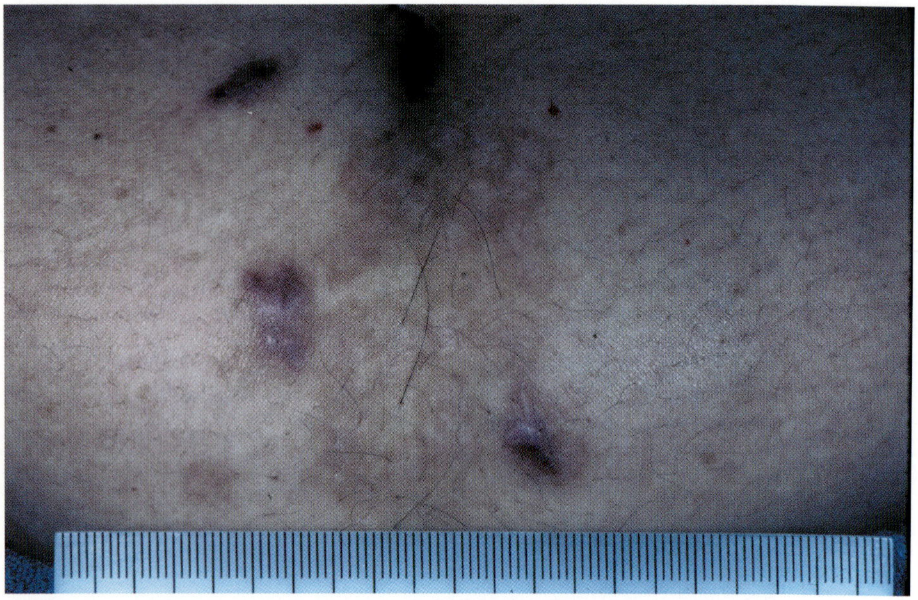

Figure 4.14. Hypertropic scarring, hypo- and hyperpigmentation 6 months after treatment with alexandrite laser

Hyperpigmentation

The exact pathogenesis of post-treatment hyperpigmentation is also obscure. Hyperpigmentation of the skin after most cutaneous skin injuries is related to melanocytic stimulation. In addition, arachidonic acid metabolites and histamine, which are found in increased amounts in inflamed skin, are thought to play a key role in post-injury pigmentary changes. Transient post-treatment hyperpigmentation occurs in 14–25% of laser hair removal patients.[7–9]

The causes of hyperpigmentation include delayed tanning, epidermal injury, or an immediate pigment-darkening phenomenon resulting from photooxidation of preexisting melanin. This darkening is usually transient, lasting only 3–4 weeks and resolving spontaneously without sequelae.[12,13]

A potentially more serious hyperpigmentation resulting from epidermolysis and blistering can occur at an energy threshold higher than those associated with immediate pigment darkening. Although immediate pigment darkening always resolves, this second type of hyperpigmentation has the potential for permanent dyschromia, both in very dark-skinned individuals and darkly tanned individuals (Figures 4.15–4.29).

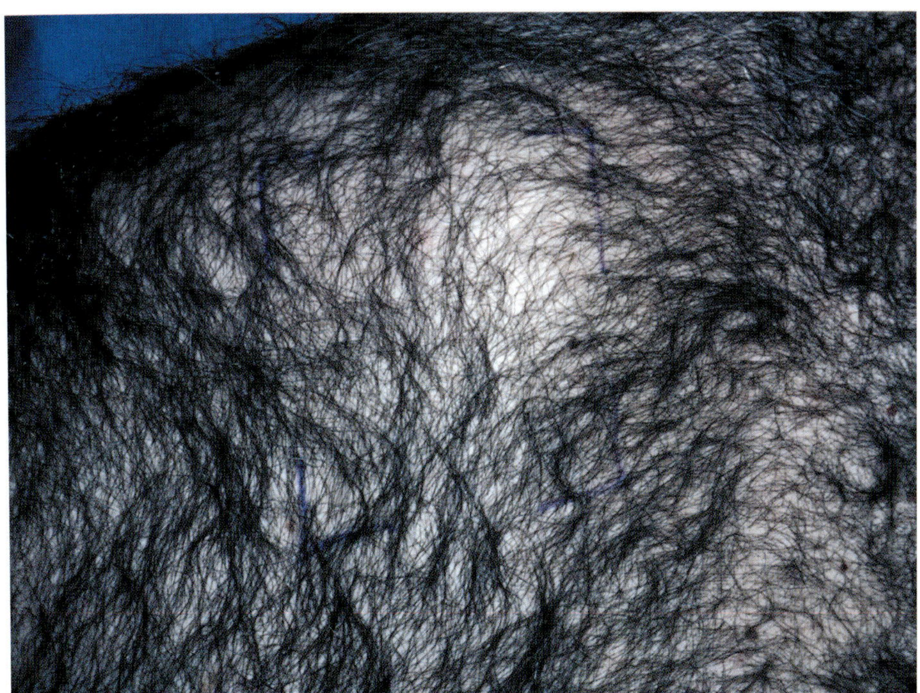

Figure 4.15. Unwanted trunk hair before intense pulsed light treatment

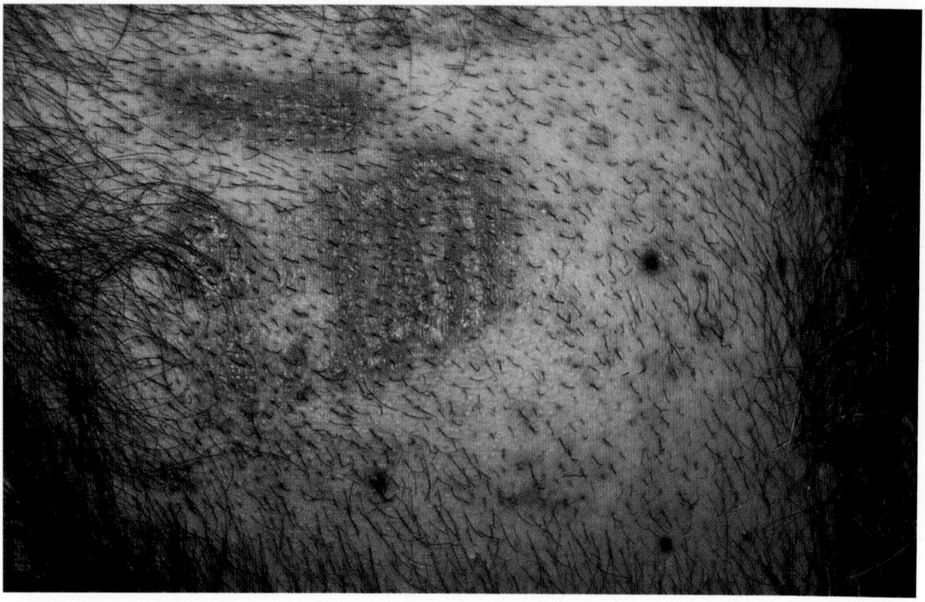

Figure 4.16. Crusting 5 days after intense pulsed light hair removal

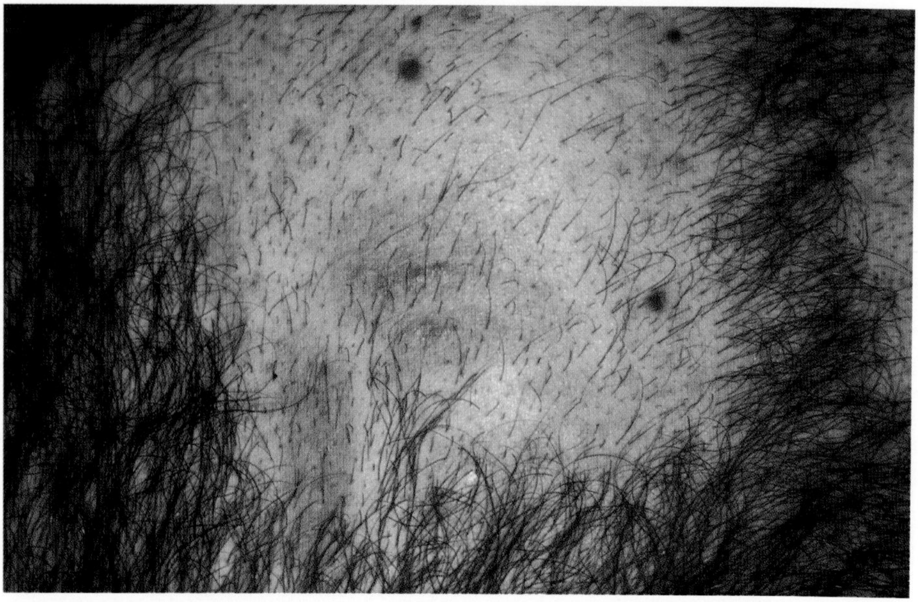

Figure 4.17. Post-inflammatory hyperpigmentation 1 month after treatment with an intense pulsed light

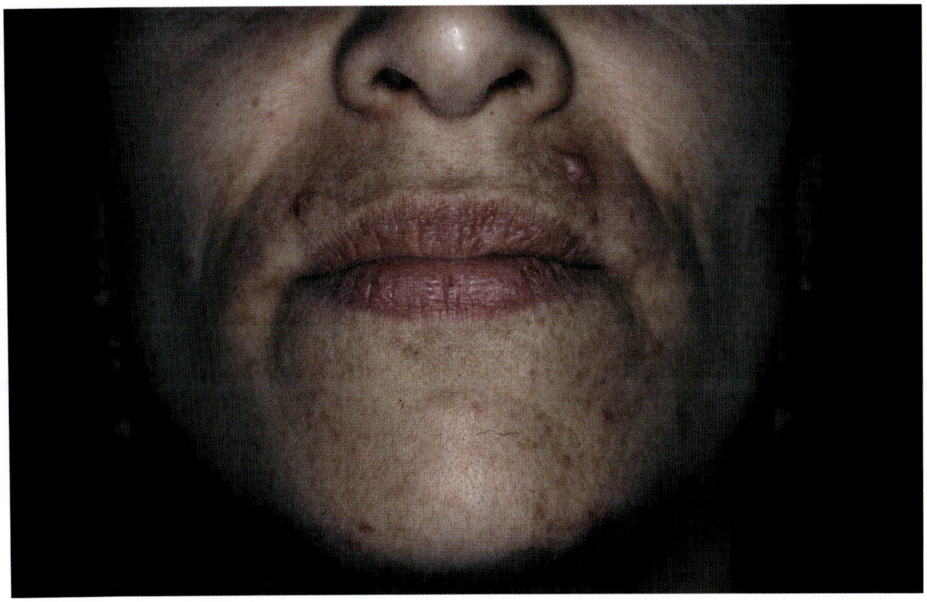

Figure 4.18. Post-inflammatory hyperpigmentation and scarring after ruby laser hair removal

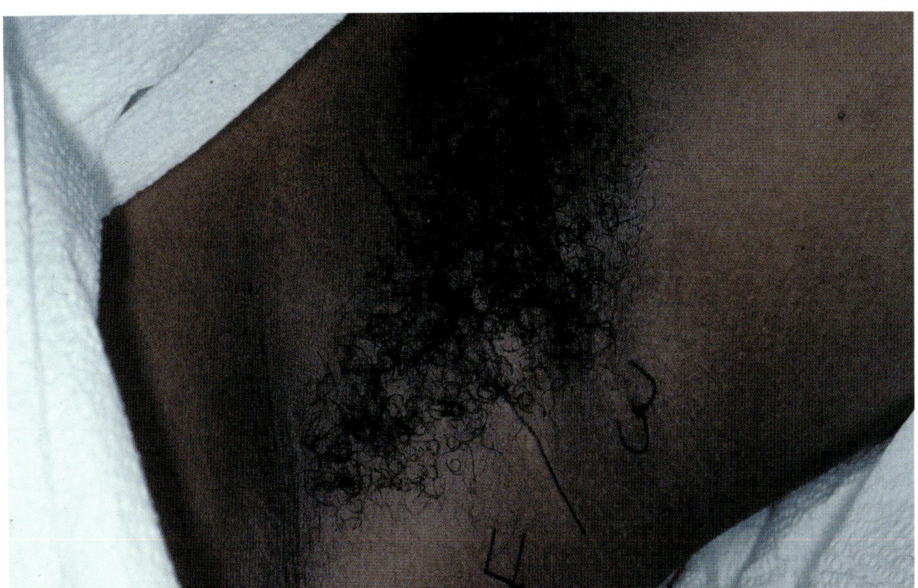

Figure 4.19. Fitzpatrick skin type VI before treatment with alexandrite laser

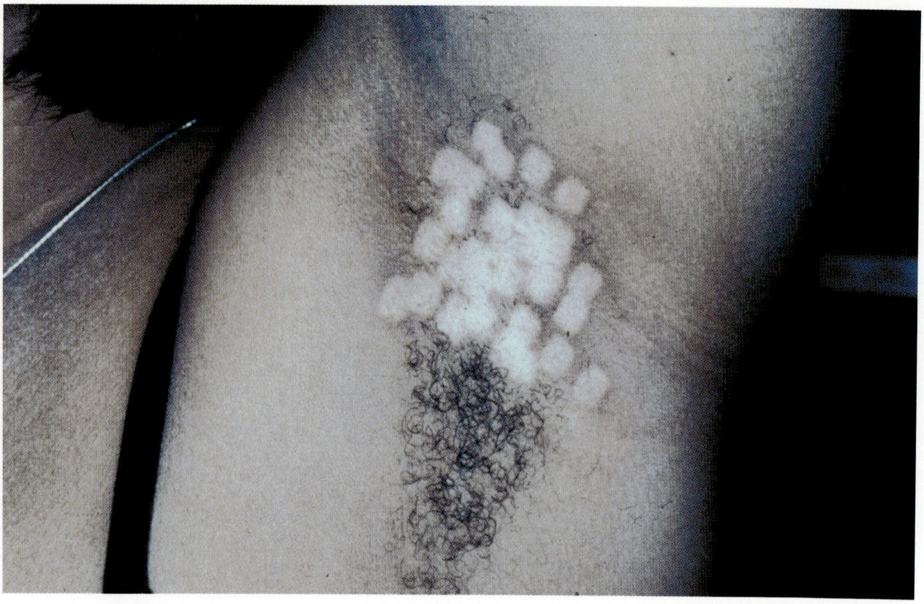

Figure 4.20. Immediately after treatment with alexandrite laser

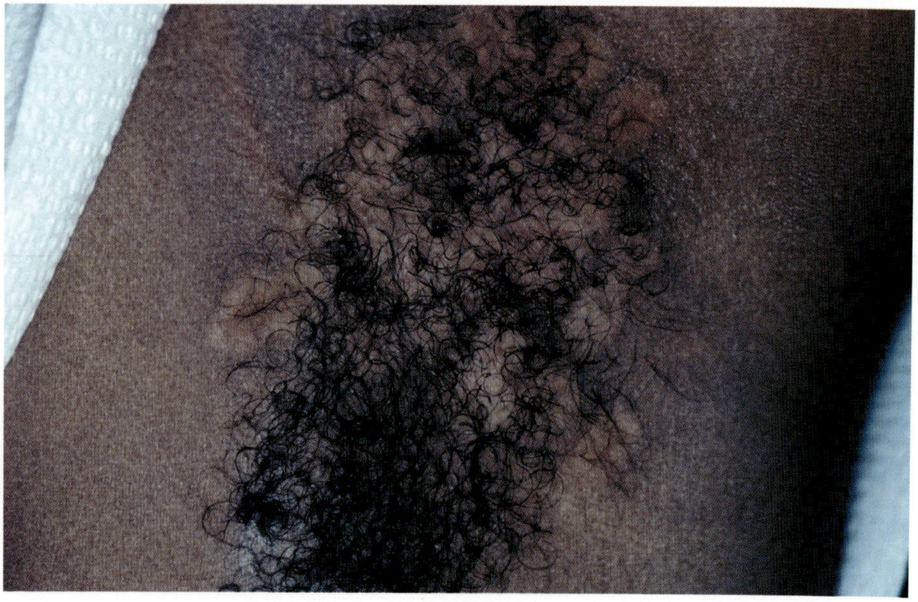

Figure 4.21. Post-inflammatory hyper- and hypopigmentation 6 months after treatment

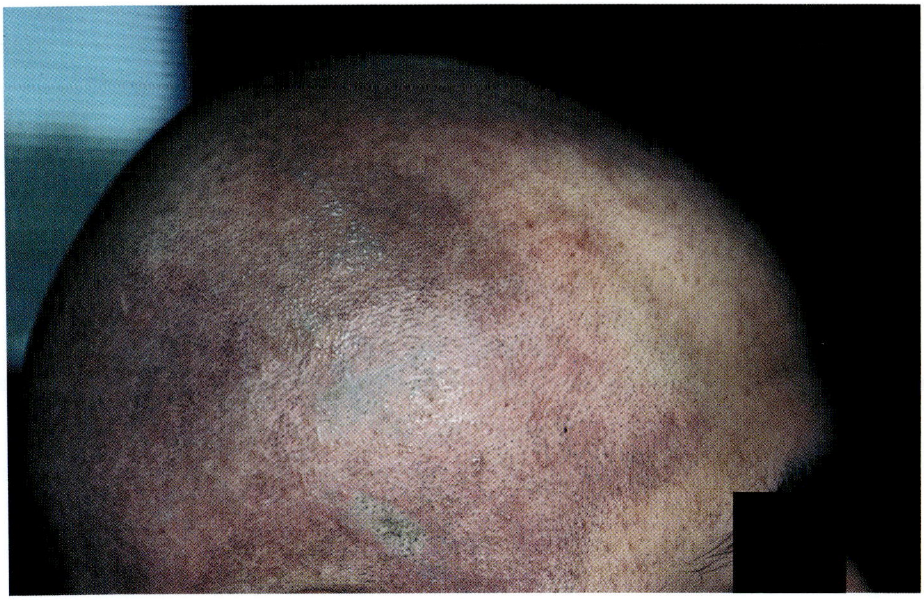

Figure 4.22. Immediately after intense pulsed light treatment for scalp hair

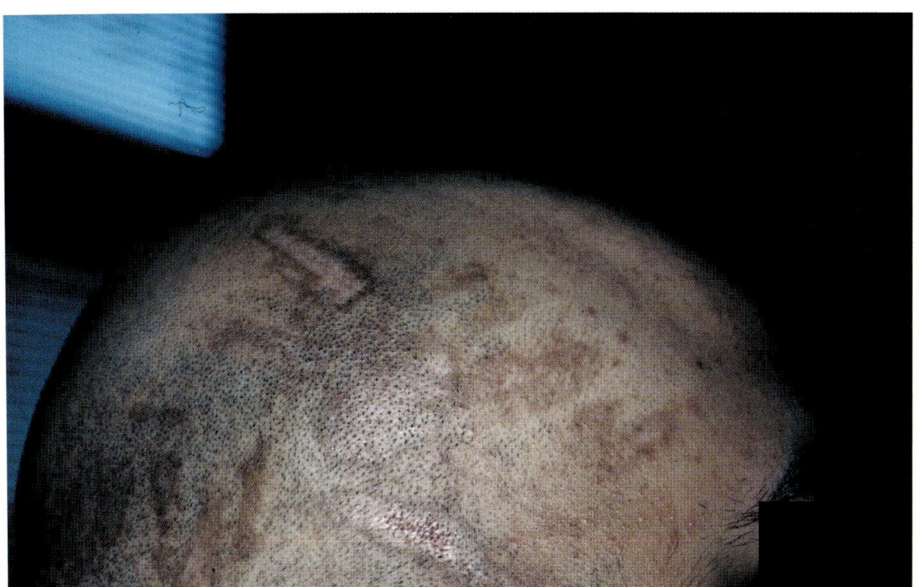

Figure 4.23. Post-inflammatory hyperpigmentation 6 months after intense pulsed light treatment

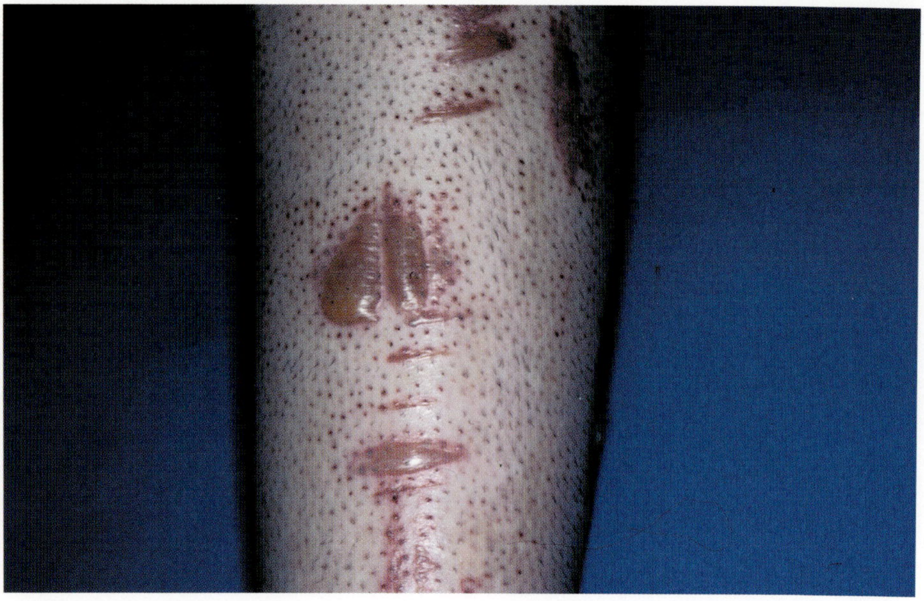

Figure 4.24. Blistering induced by intense pulsed light hair removal

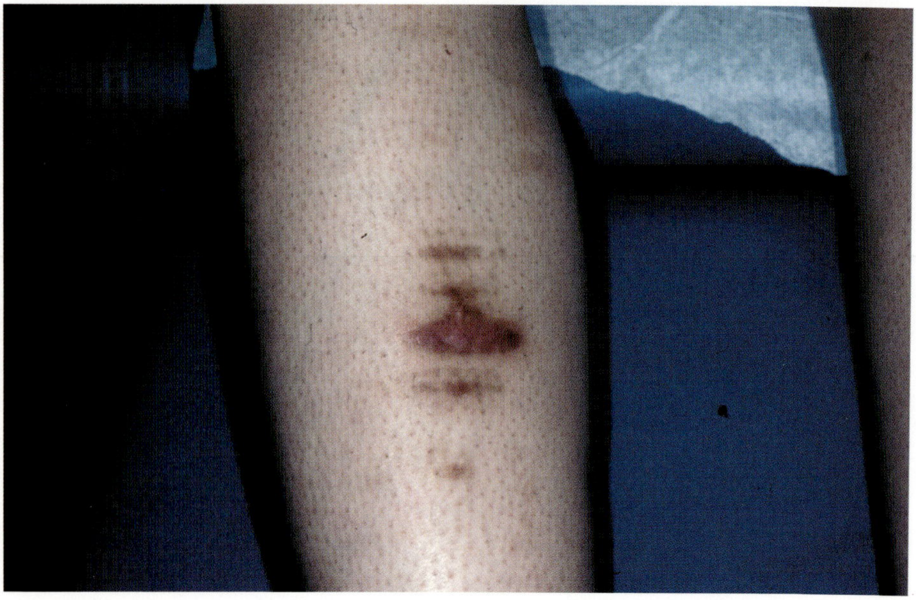

Figure 4.25. Hyperpigmentation and scars 6 months after treatment of patient in Figure 4.24

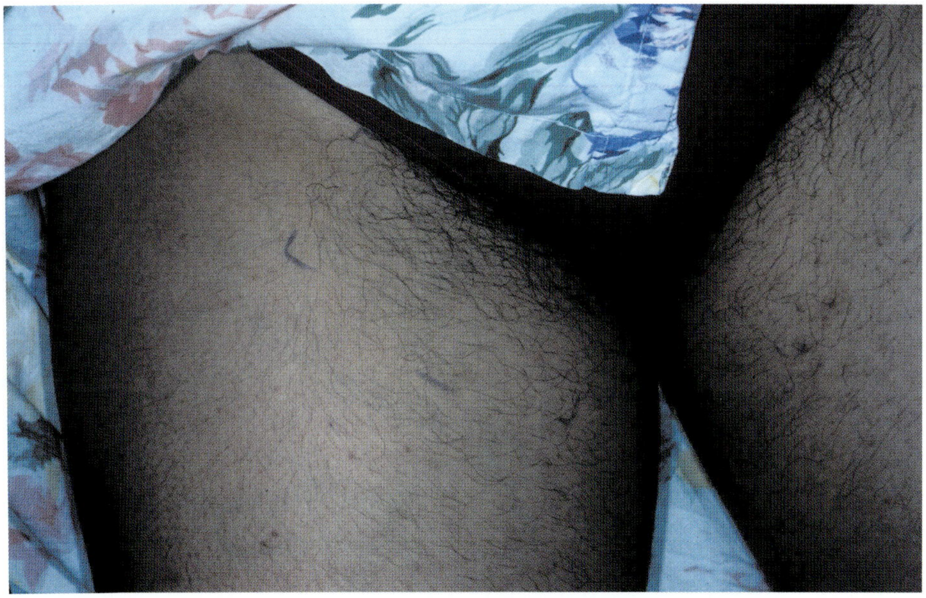

Figure 4.26. Unwanted hair on thigh in Fitzptatrick skin type IV individual

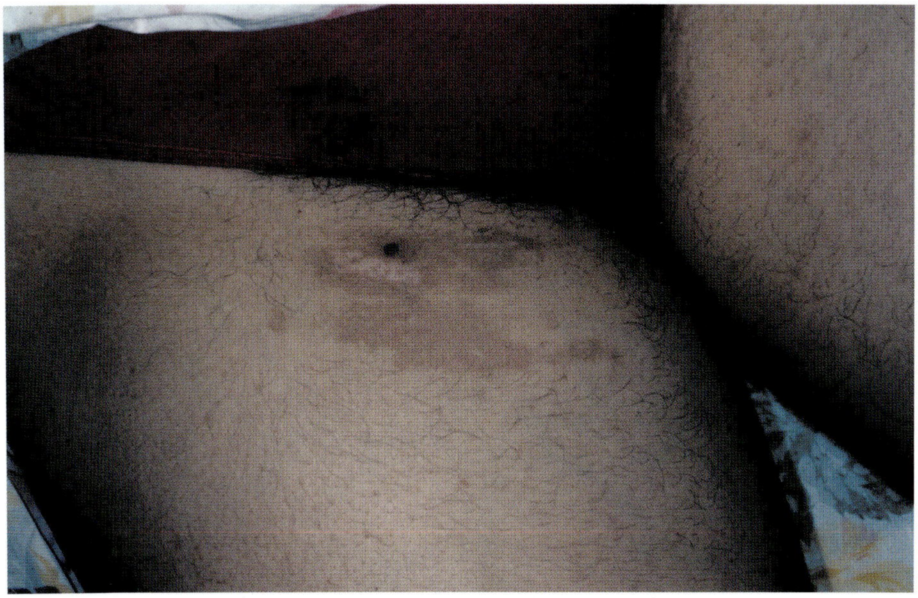

Figure 4.27. Post-inflammatory hyperpigmentation, confirmed by biopsy, 3 months after treatment

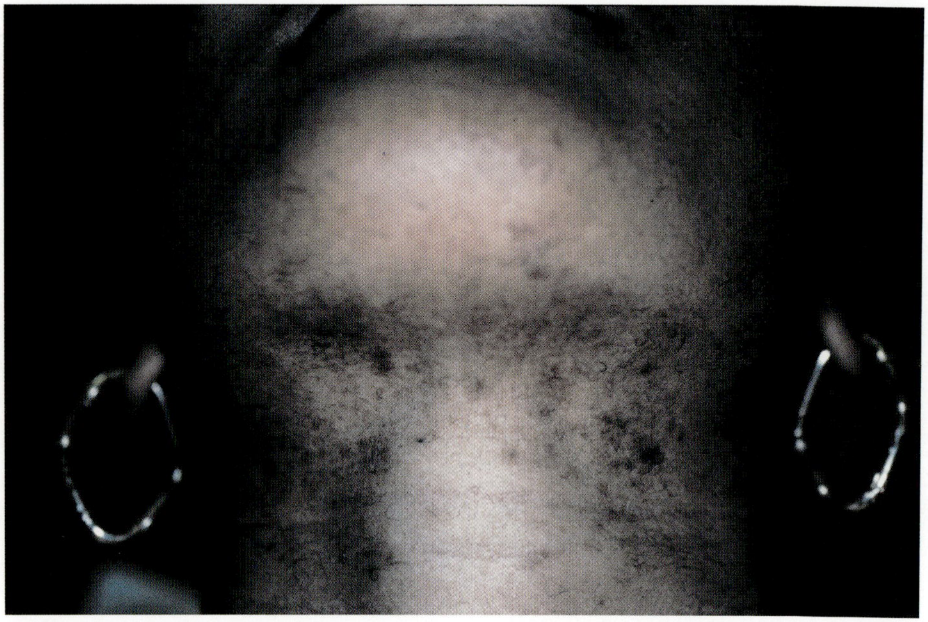

Figure 4.28. Hyperpigmentation seen 3 months after laser hair removal

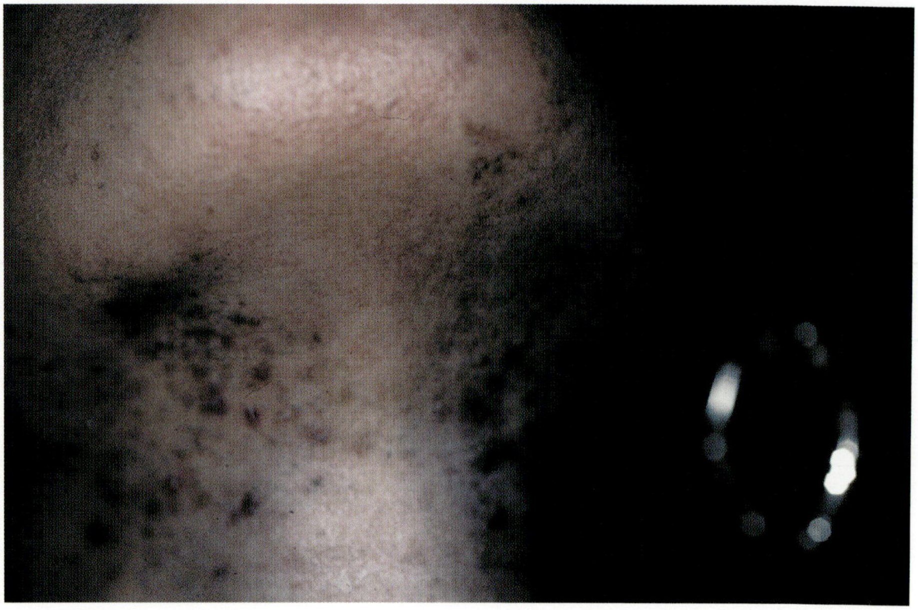

Figure 4.29. Hyperpigmentation associated with pseudofolliculitis barbae. This was not induced by laser hair removal

PAIN

Laser and light source optical heat-induced destruction of hair follicles is not pain-free. Pain thresholds vary throughout the body and from one individual to the next. Pain can be perceived differently at different times of the month. During menstruation, the skin appears to be more sensitive to pain.

Several laser-related factors have been found to be associated with pain during laser hair removal. The intensity of pain varies with the delivered fluence, utilized wavelength, pulse duration, spot size, repetition rate, laser interpulse spacing, and skin pigmentation. Regional body areas, such as the lip and groin, and chronically sun-exposed and tanned areas, also have been associated with differences in pain perception. Pain is the result of a polymodal activation of certain receptors, including nociceptive and non-nociceptive ones.[14–16]

At identical laser parameters, there is clearly greater pain with a large spot size than with a smaller spot size. Also, pain tends to increase the more prolonged is the hair removal session. Small treatment areas, taking very little time for treatment, are generally very well tolerated. Larger treated areas may lead to the requirement of topical anesthesia.

Likewise, a series of laser pulses delivered to adjacent skin areas with a high repetition rate will increase the perception of pain when compared to the perception of pain after only 1–2 laser pulses delivered to the same area. This phenomenon generally develops at repetition rates higher than approximately 0.5 Hz. The discomfort may become significant during treatment with laser systems having repetition rates higher than 1 Hz.

In one study,[17] two areas treated with the exact same parameters evoked different pain perceptions. The area treated earlier was always less painful than the later treated area.

Finally, with increasing wavelength and pulse durations, heat diffusion is likely to raise the temperature around the follicle and increase the level of pain.[1]

Several management procedures have been implemented to reduce pain and epidermal damage during laser hair removal treatments. These include appropriate sun protection and bleaching agents to decrease melanin content,[18] employing local and topical anesthesia,[17] lowering fluence levels,[19] decreasing the repetition rate,[20] and using an epidermal cooling device.[21,22] A variety of popular cooling devices include those that contact cool, air cool, or cool via a cryogen spray.

Laser hair removal associated with cryogen spurt durations of at least 20 milliseconds has been observed to provide pain reduction in all patients. In one study,[23] it was noted that, even with regard to Fitzpatrick skin type V patients, increasing cryogen spurt durations showed a marked lessening of pain. However, in skin types III and IV patients, cryogen delivery times greater than 20 milliseconds did not appreciably change pain perception.

Longer cryogen duration delivery times may also cause pain. Majaron and colleagues have found that after the applied cryogen dissipates from the skin, a layer of frost can develop which is dependent on condensation of associated ambient water vapor.[24] This frost formation may deposit latent heat to the target site, which not only significantly impairs cryogen cooling, but also may explain why some patients (skin types III and IV) experience more pain with increasing cryogen spurt duration.

The activation of cold thermoreceptors for pain, experienced with longer cryogen spurt durations, may be offset by the cooling and consequent lessening of heat thermoreceptors for pain. These observations suggest that the darkest skin types may benefit from longer cryogen spurt durations in order to alleviate pain. This benefit is less well defined in lighter skin. Finally, geographic spacing of laser pulses is essential to prevent thermal build-up, and the ability to reduce pain. Greater than 1.5 cm spacing between laser-delivered pulses allows the benefits of decreased pain to be seen with cryogen application. Pulsing rapidly with less than 1.5 cm anatomic areas between each pulse may negate the benefit of less pain that one would expect from cryogen cooling. This may be a consequence of the heated chromophore being re-heated through rapid diffusion by a subsequent laser pulse. It should be noted that the above research has been undertaken with cryogen cooling. Whether the same concepts apply to other forms of cooling has yet to be determined.

SCARRING AND TEXTURAL CHANGES

Despite the presence of severe macroscopic cutaneous damage, collagen and elastin networks in the dermis are found to be normal in the majority of patients after laser hair removal.[25]

Type 1 collagen constitutes the major type of collagen in the dermis. It has a tendency to change its fibrillar form at temperatures between 60°C and 70°C.[26] Collagen's normal appearance and distribution in the dermal layer after laser hair removal, support the clinical evidence that if laser-assisted hair removal is performed correctly scar formation rarely occurs.

The normal appearance and distribution of both collagen and elastin in laser-treated skin also suggest that textural changes in skin are unlikely after laser-assisted hair removal except in cases of over-aggressive treatment, inadequate cooling, or post-operative infection (Figures 4.30–4.56).

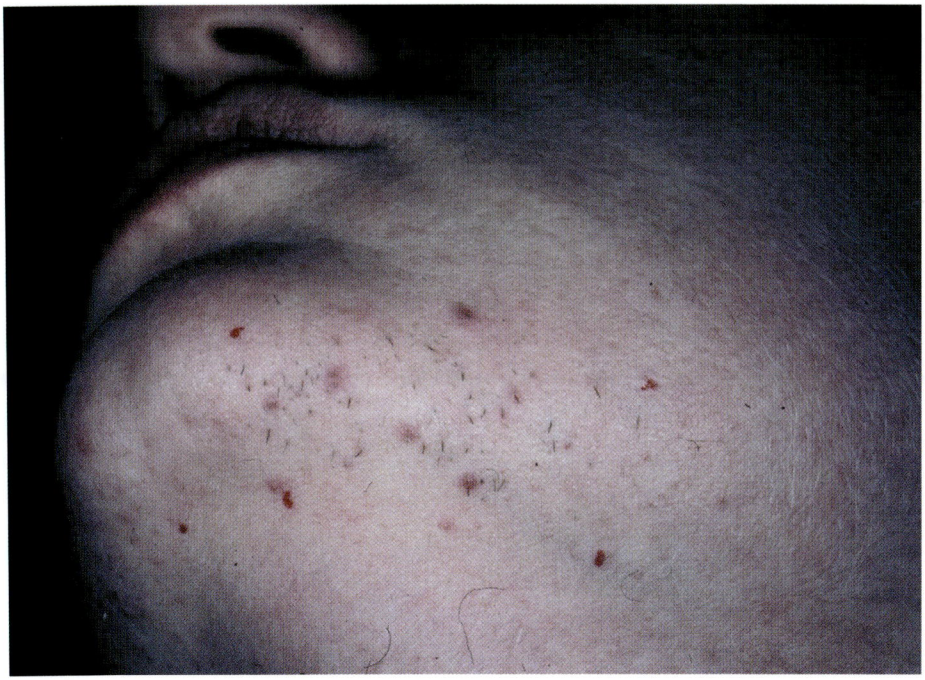

Figure 4.30. Chin hairs before treatment with an Nd:YAG laser

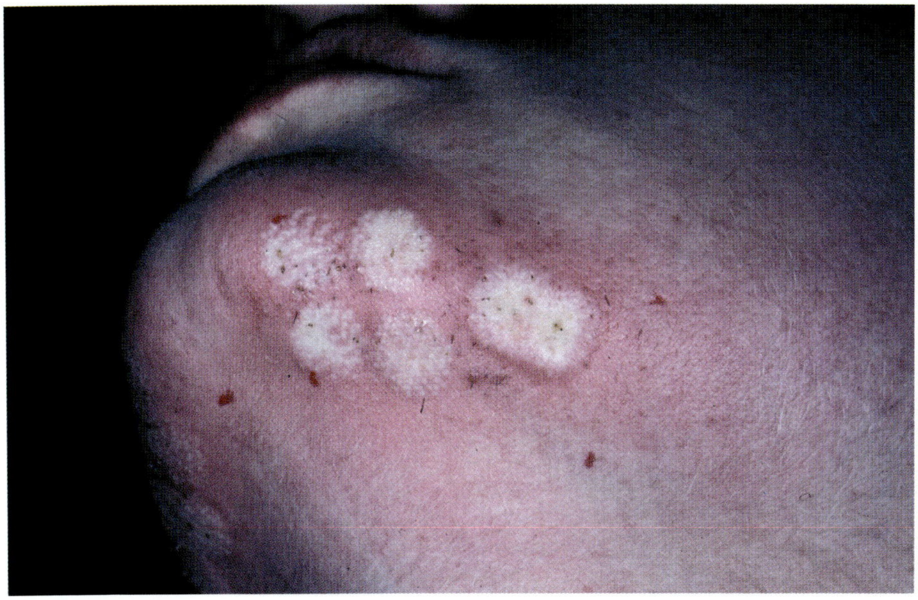

Figure 4.31. Epidermal whitening after Nd:YAG laser hair removal. Generally, this is seen with excessive fluences and inadequate epidermal cooling

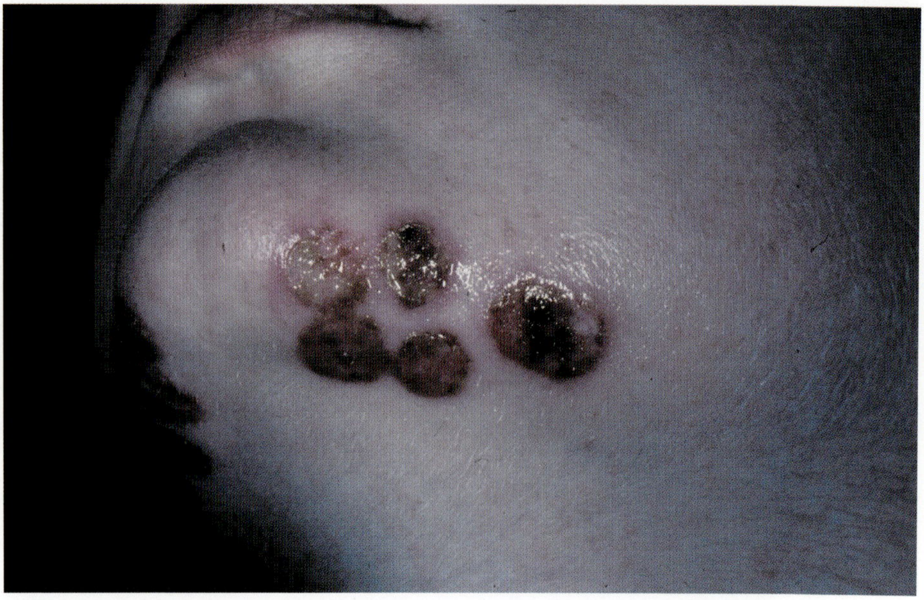

Figure 4.32. Ulcerations seen 1 week after treatment of patient seen in Figure 4.30

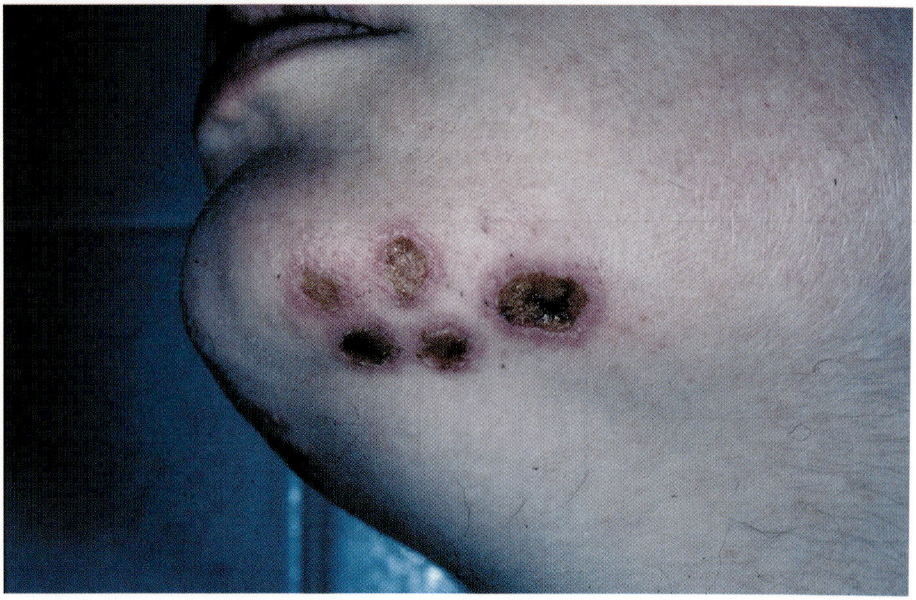

Figure 4.33. Ulcerations seen 2 weeks after treatment of patient seen in Figure 4.30

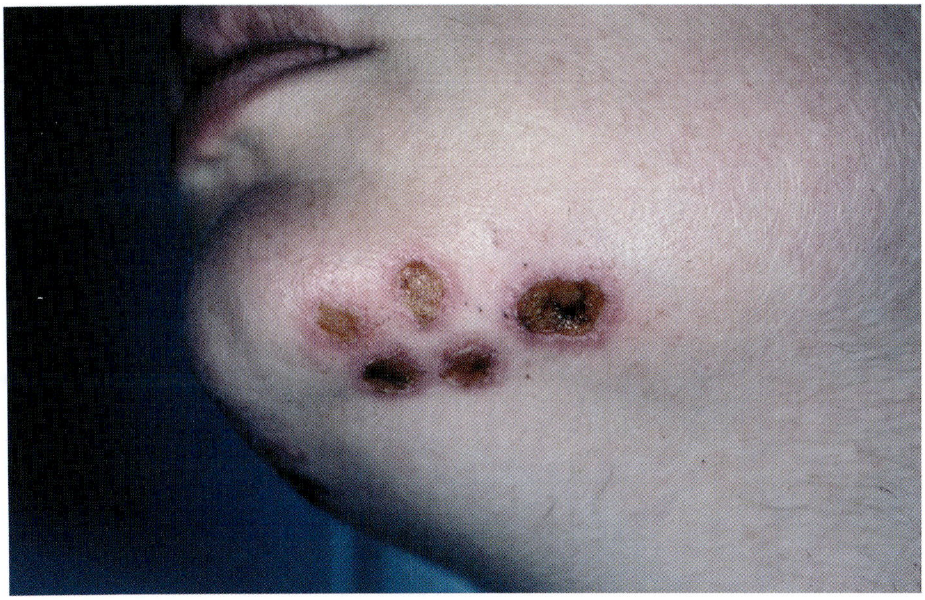

Figure 4.34. Ulcerations seen 3 weeks after treatment of patient seen in Figure 4.30

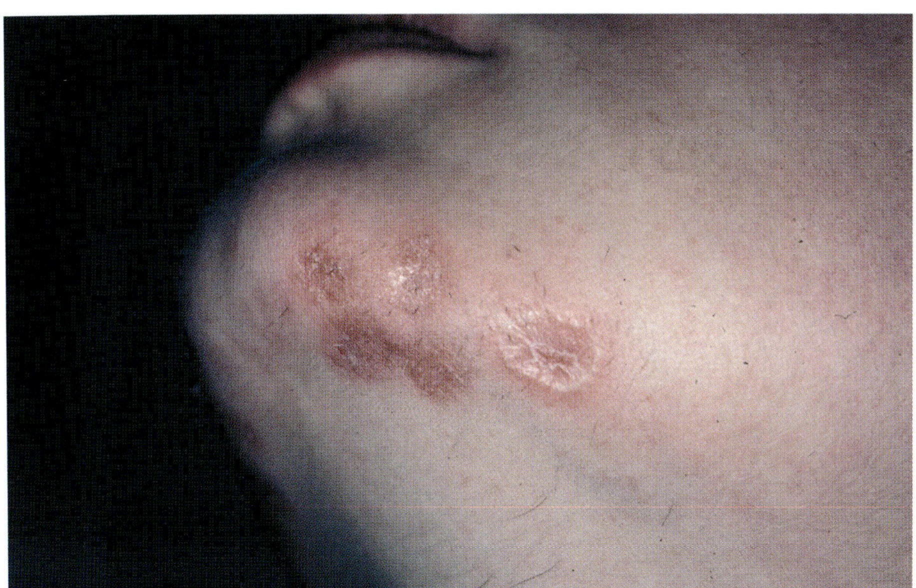

Figure 4.35. Scarring seen 3 months after treatment of patient seen in Figure 4.30

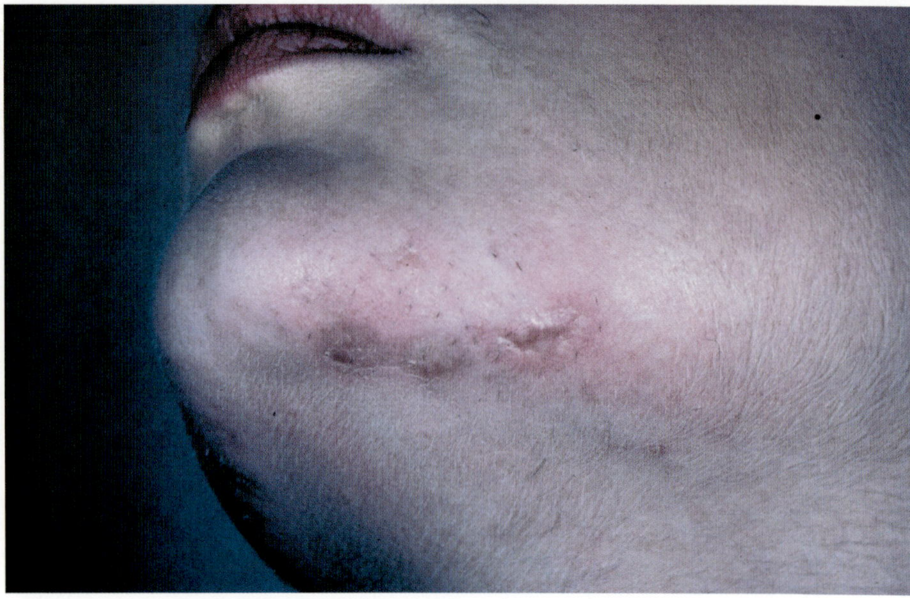

Figure 4.36. Scarring seen 6 months after treatment of patient seen in Figure 4.30

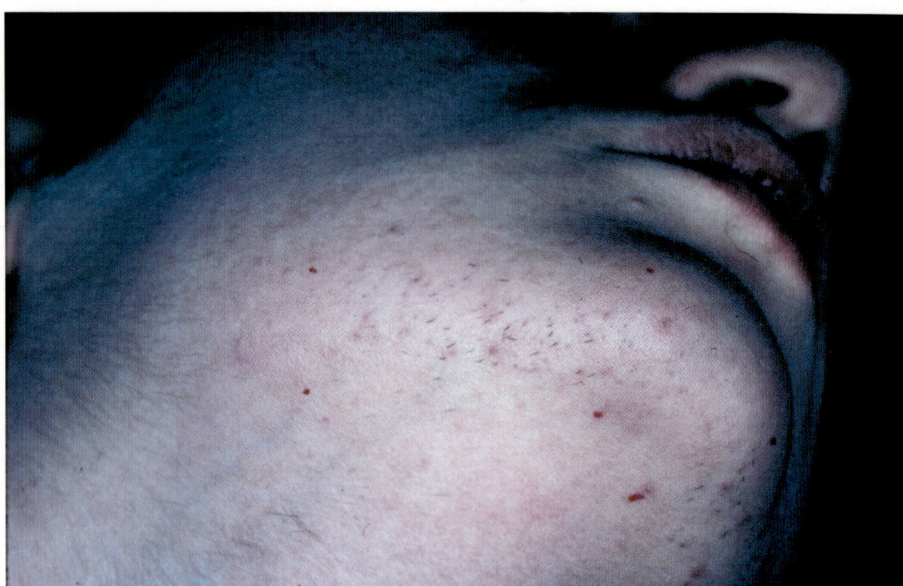

Figure 4.37. Chin hairs before treatment with an Nd:YAG laser

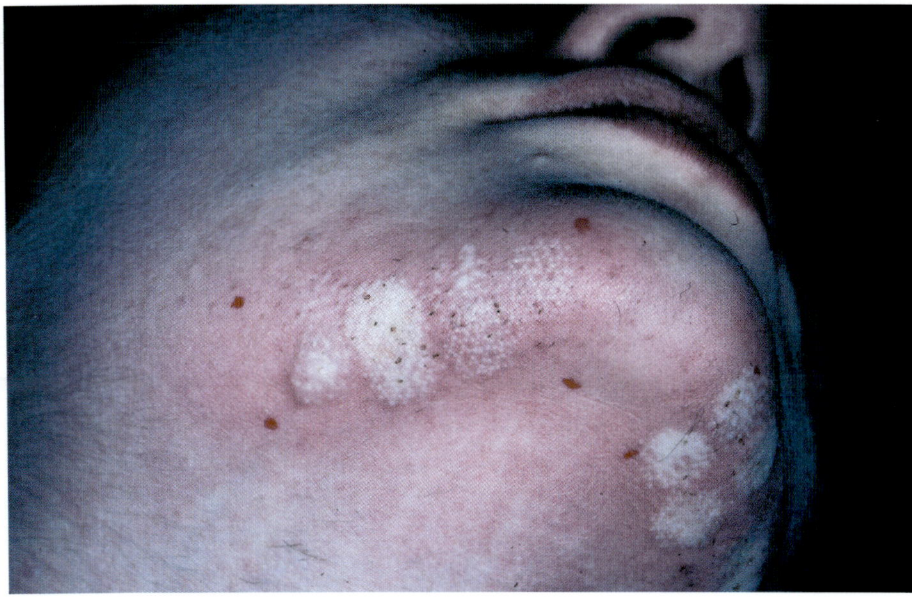

Figure 4.38. Epidermal whitening after Nd:YAG laser hair removal. Generally, this is seen with excessive fluences and inadequate epidermal cooling

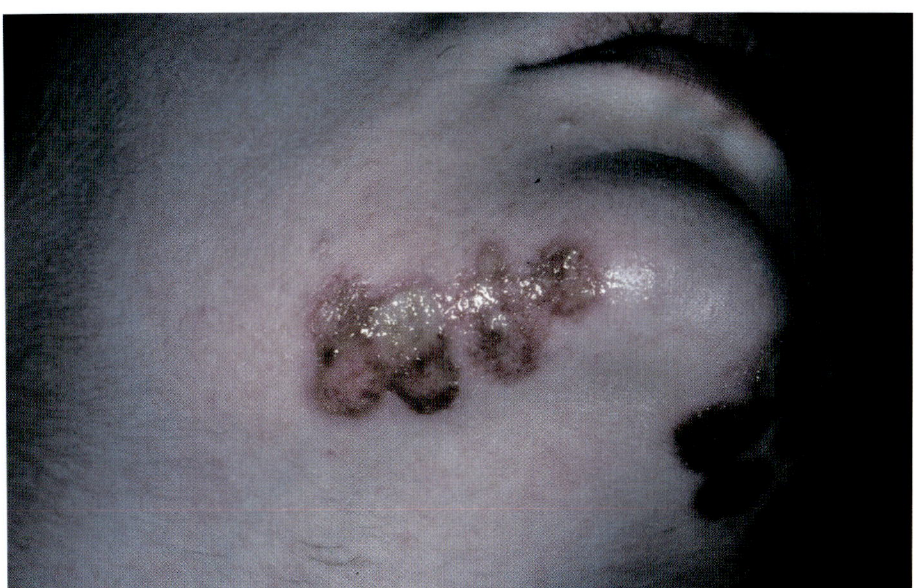

Figure 4.39. Ulcerations seen 3 days after treatment of patient seen in Figure 4.37

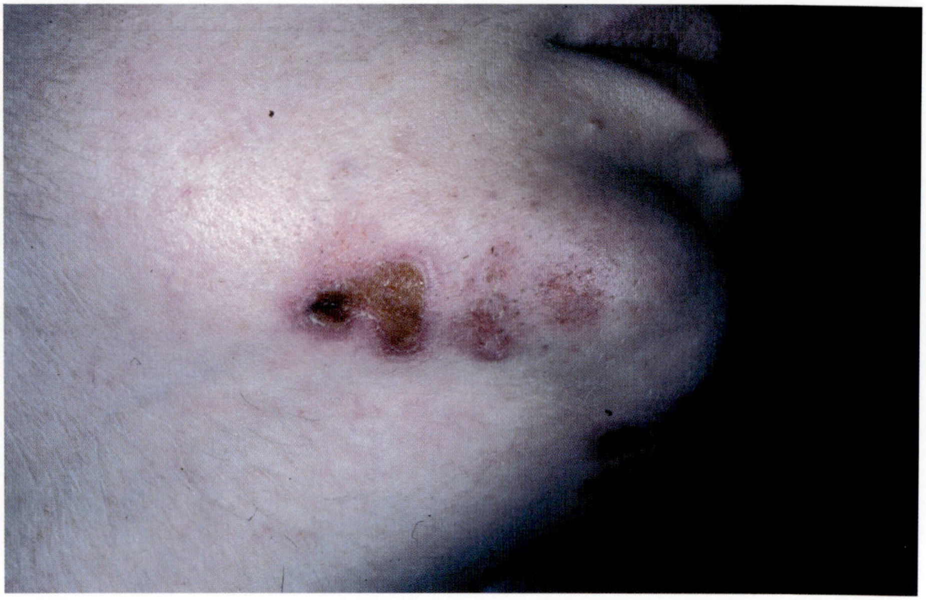

Figure 4.40. Three weeks after treatment of patient seen in Figure 4.37

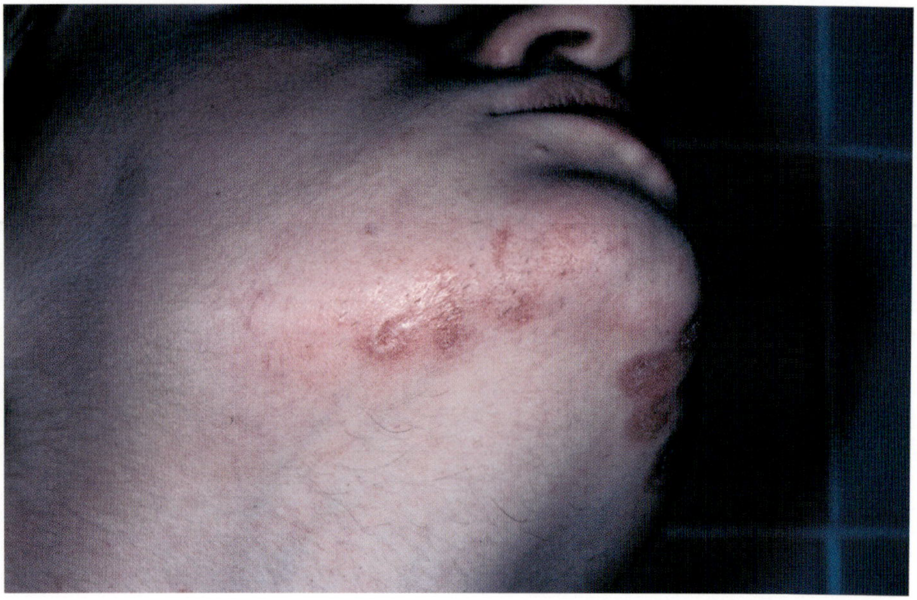

Figure 4.41. Scarring of chin 3 months after treatment of patient seen in Figure 4.37

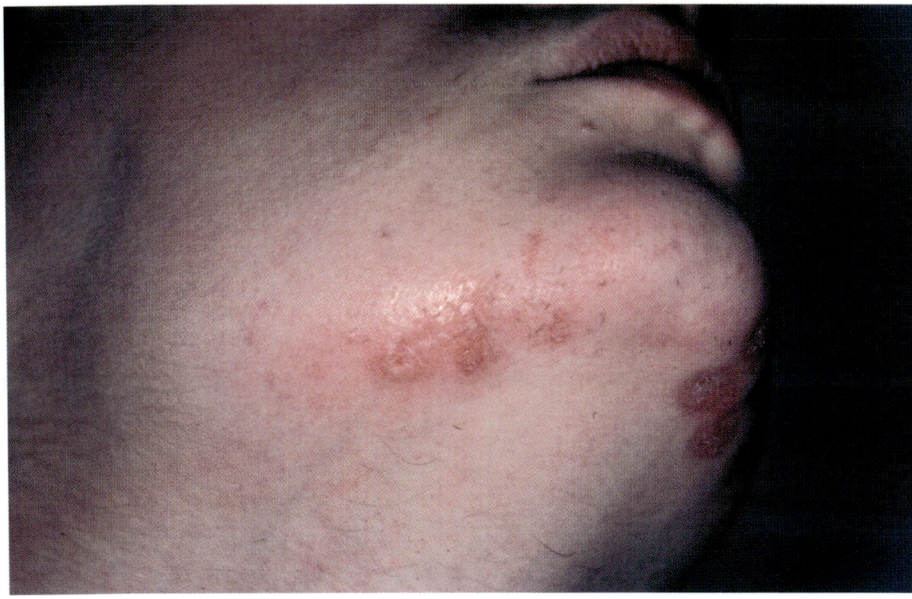

Figure 4.42. Scarring of chin 6 months after treatment of patient seen in Figure 4.37

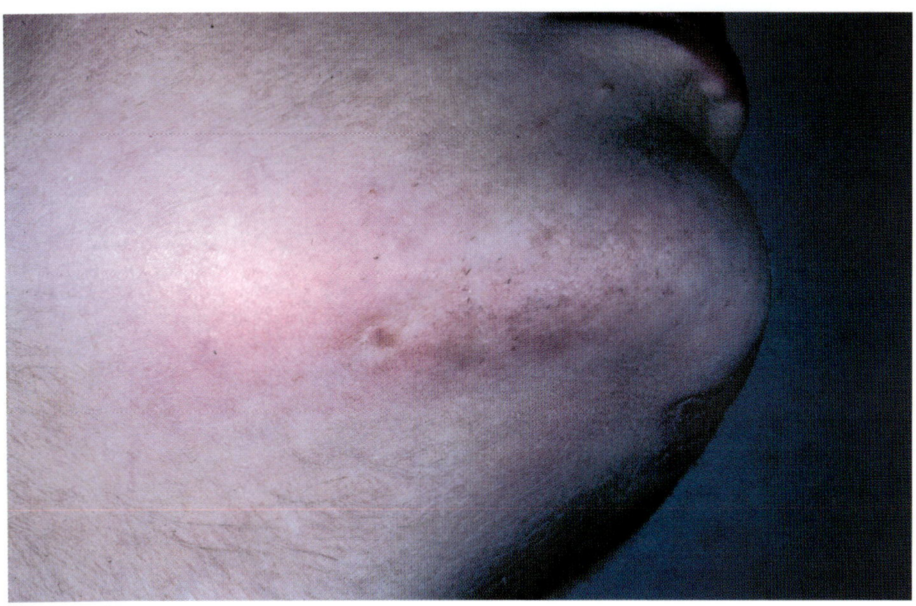

Figure 4.43. Scarring of chin 9 months after treatment of patient seen in Figure 4.37

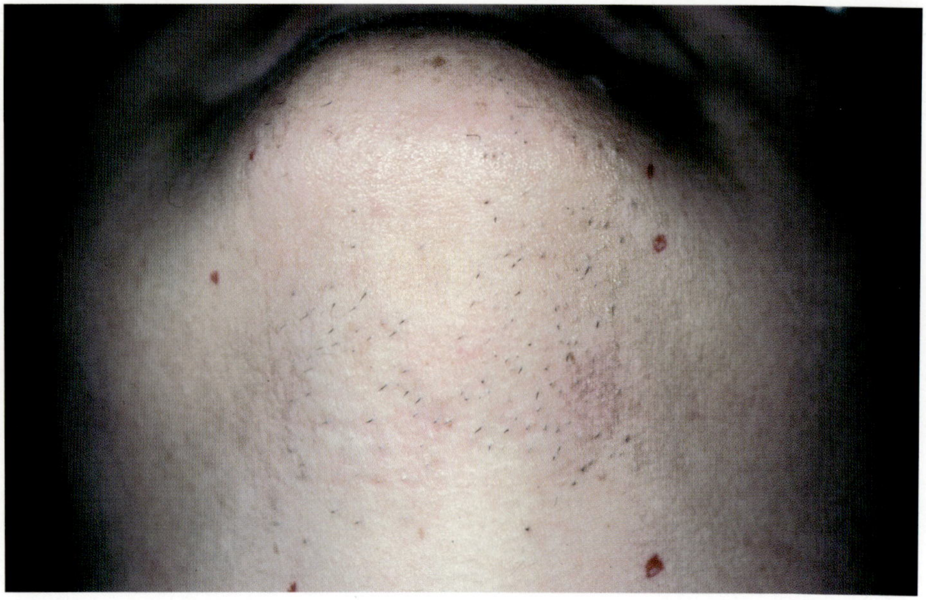

Figure 4.44. Chin hairs before treatment with an Nd:YAG laser

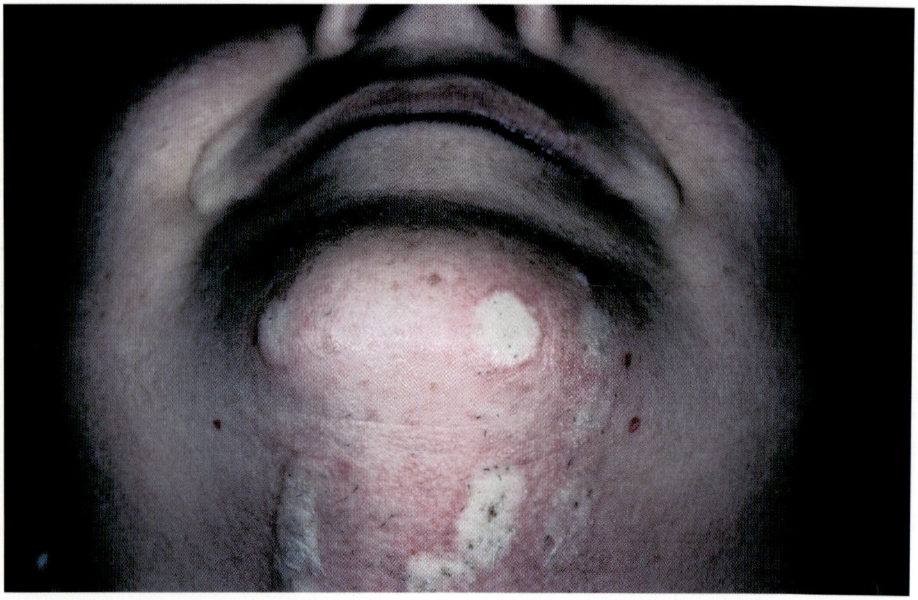

Figure 4.45. Epidermal whitening after Nd:YAG laser hair removal. Generally, this is seen with excessive fluences and inadequate epidermal cooling

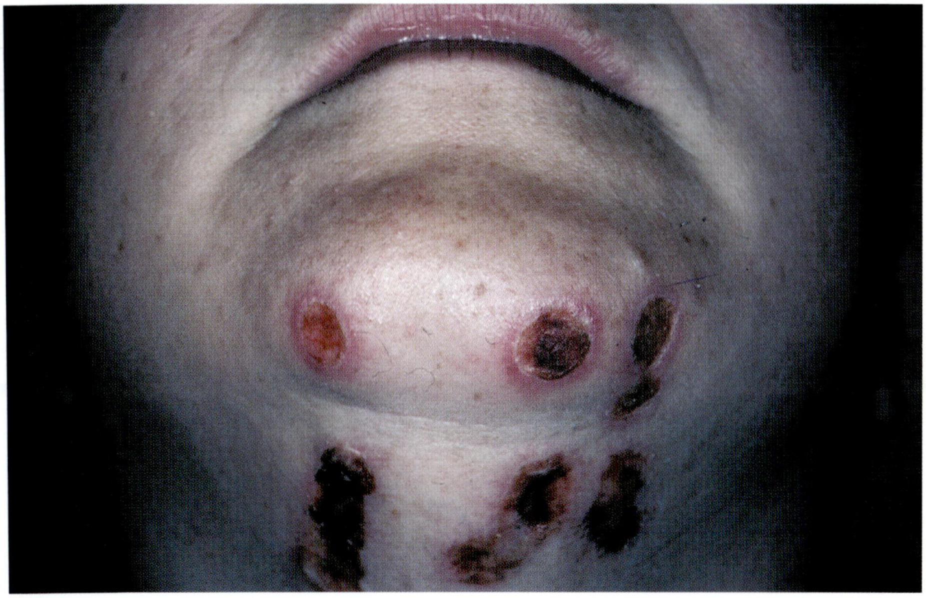

Figure 4.46. Ulcerations seen 1 week after treatment of patient seen in Figure 4.44

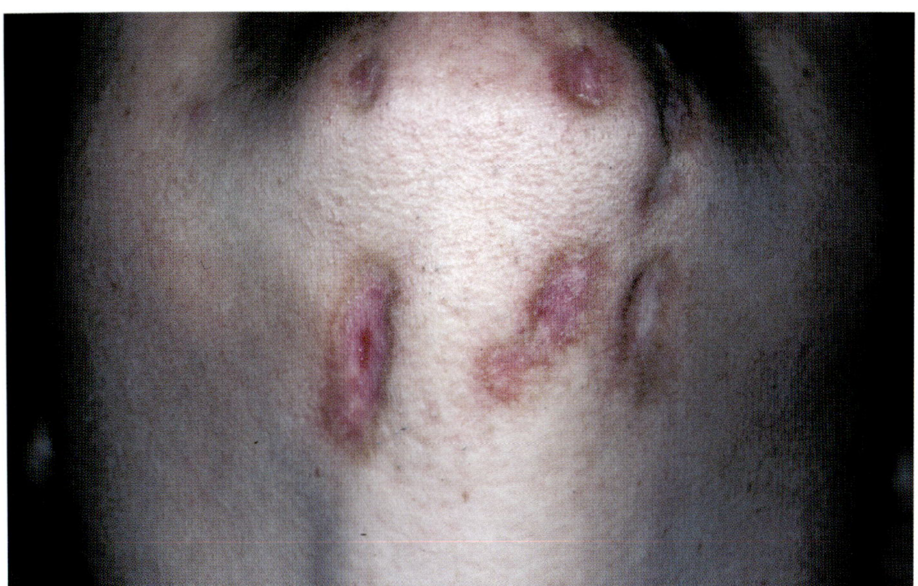

Figure 4.47. Three months after treatment of patient seen in Figure 4.44

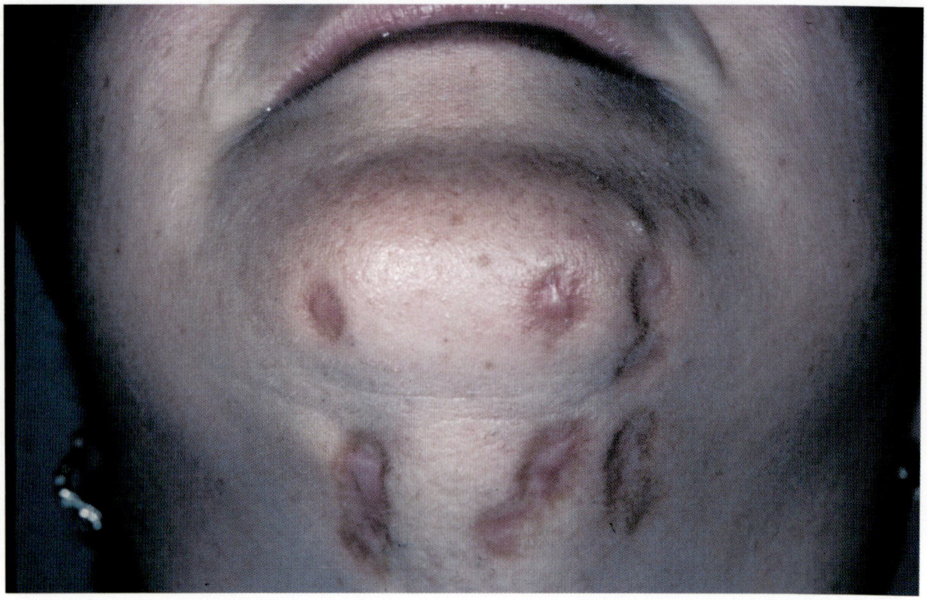

Figure 4.48. Scarring of chin 6 months after treatment of patient seen in Figure 4.44

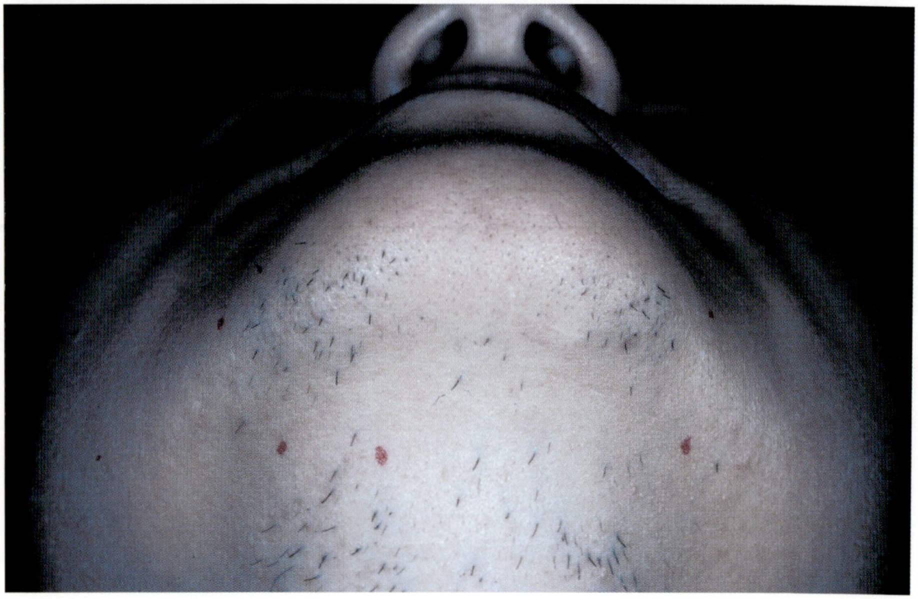

Figure 4.49. Chin hairs before treatment with an Nd:YAG laser

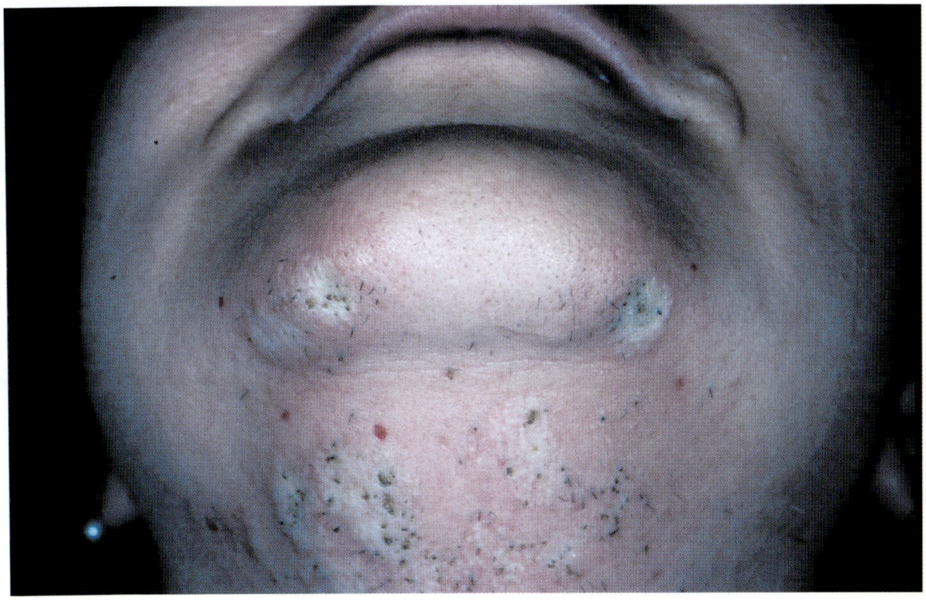

Figure 4.50. Epidermal whitening after Nd:YAG laser hair removal. Generally, this is seen with excessive fluences and inadequate epidermal cooling

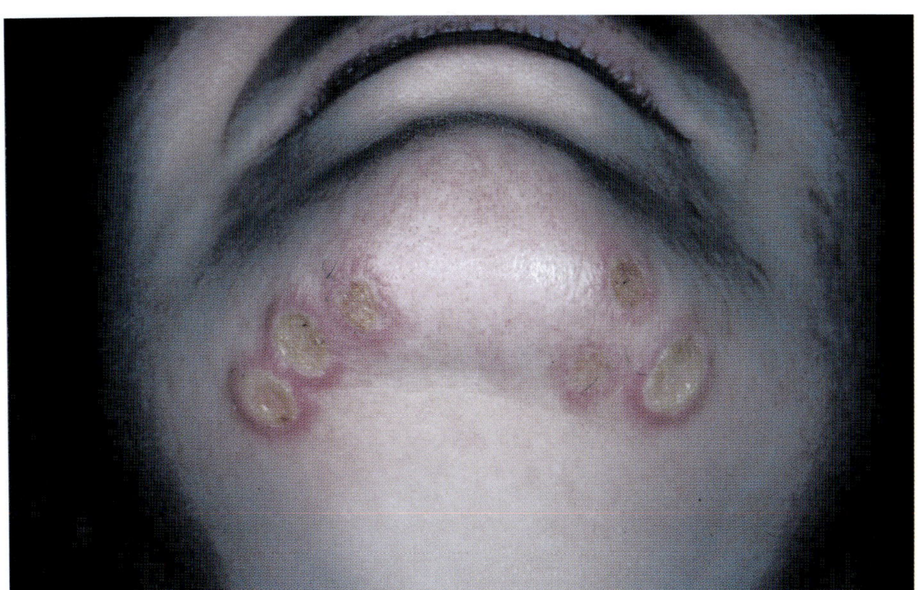

Figure 4.51. Ulcerations seen 1 week after treatment of patient seen in Figure 4.49

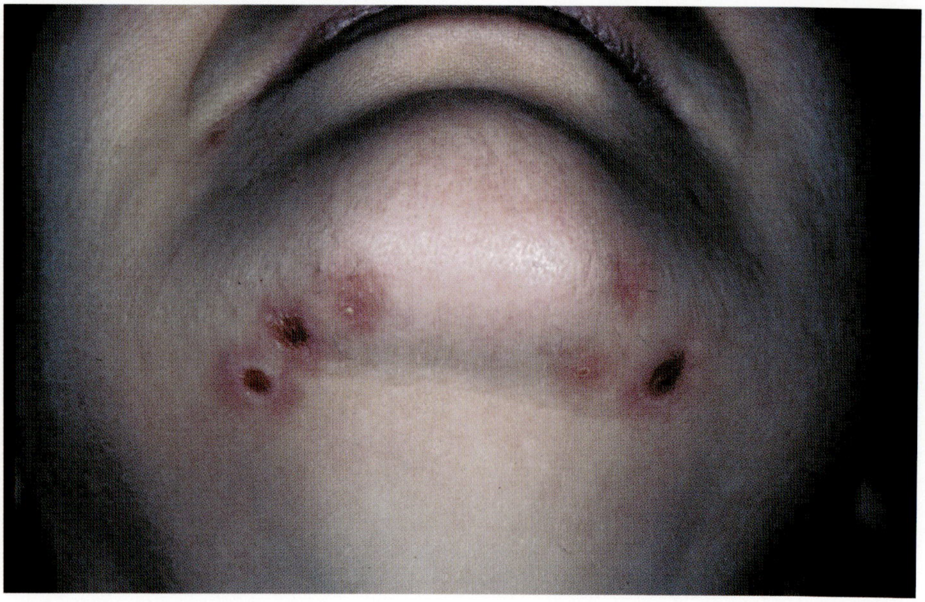

Figure 4.52. Three months after treatment of patient seen in Figure 4.49

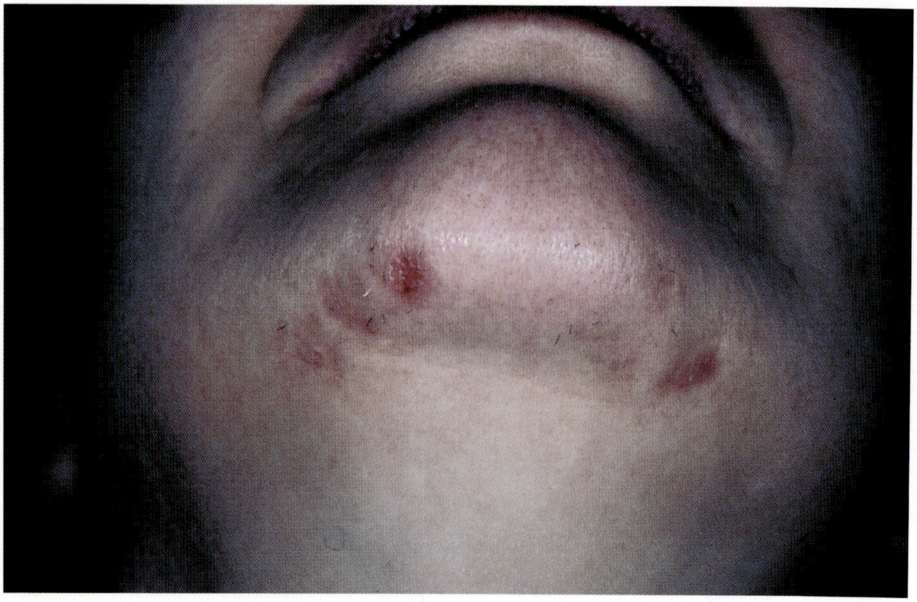

Figure 4.53. Scarring of chin 6 months after treatment of patient seen in Figure 4.49

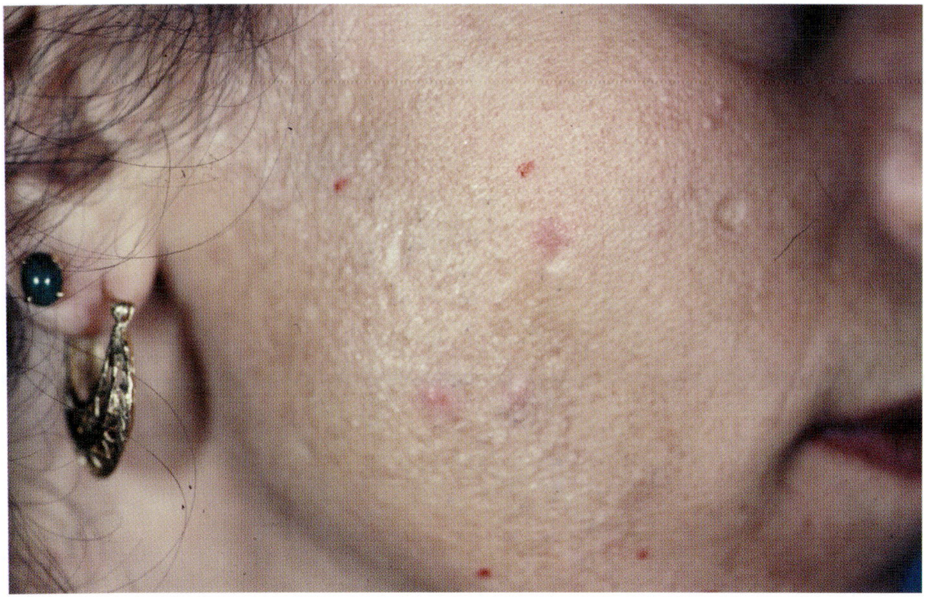

Figure 4.54. Facial hair before ruby laser hair removal

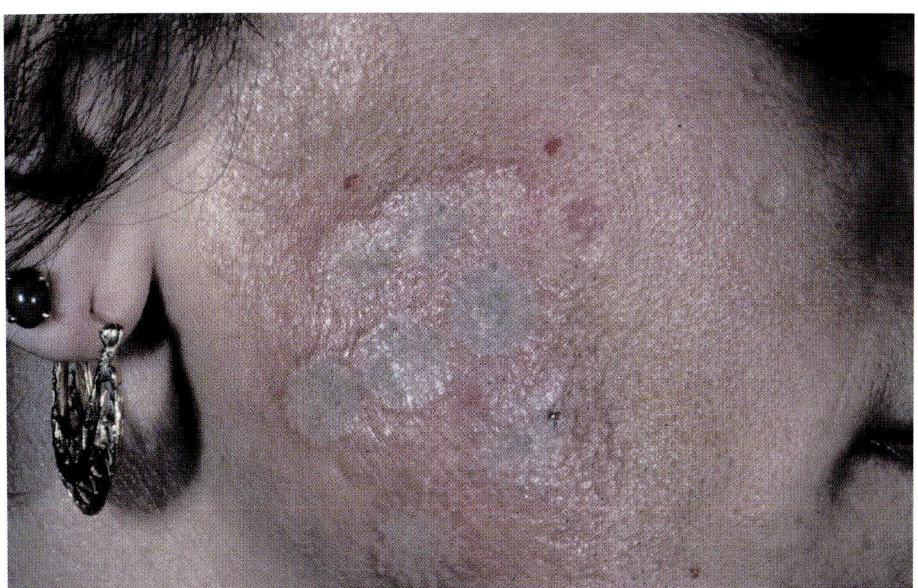

Figure 4.55. Facial hair immediately after treatment with a ruby laser. No cooling device was used

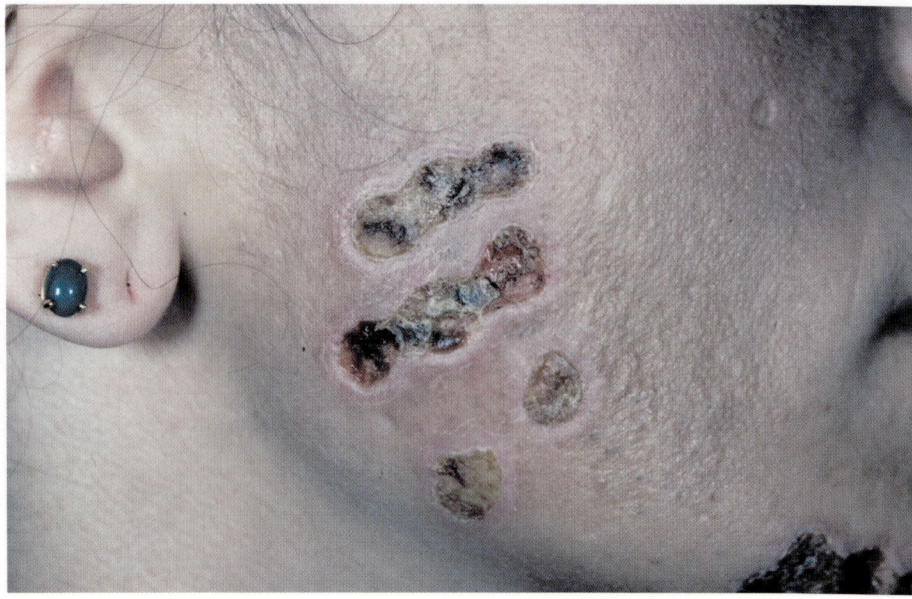

Figure 4.56. Ulceration leading to scarring 2 weeks after patient in Figure 4.54 was treated

EFFECTS ON TATTOOS AND FRECKLES

Lightening of tattoos and loss of freckles or pigmented lesions after laser-assisted hair removal is common. Freckles may eventually return, the removed tattoo pigment will not.

POTENTIAL LONG-TERM COMPLICATIONS

With current laser hair removal technology, it is essential that each patient is treated repeatedly to achieve optimal results. Hence, the potential long-term complications of this treatment need to be considered. Electromagnetic irradiation of melanin, particularly pheomelanin, has been reported to produce superoxides,[27] a free radical capable of deoxyribonucleic acid (DNA) damage and inducing carcinogenesis. However, melanin free radical production is more marked at shorter wavelengths of the electromagnetic spectrum and decreases markedly towards longer wavelengths, such as those typically used for laser hair removal.[28,29] In addition to free radical production, repeated induction of cellular hyperproliferation is also known to be important in tumor promotion. In the skin, the activation of keratinocytes by exogenous or endogenous stimuli is thought to provide a triggering event for skin inflammation and hyperproliferation, which can subsequently lead to tumor production.[30] Even in the absence of grossly evident damage to the epidermis, a single laser hair removal treatment can lead to an increase in basal layer keratinocytes.[25] However, this minimal damage has been shown to be insufficient to cause any detectable wound-healing response with associated increased epidermal proliferation, as judged by an expression of the hyperproliferation marker, keratin 16.[31] Work to establish a potential for mutagenesis has been performed and has proved that no such effect occurs.[32]

Suprabasal epidermal necrosis is seen in patients with blistering of skin after laser irradiation. This change is seen after blistering of any kind and is characteristic of superficial burns.[33,34] Although it is well established that 2% of squamous cell carcinoma and 0.5% of basal cell carcinoma arise in burn scars, with most squamous cell carcinoma occurring after a long latent period, it is highly unlikely that any burn associated with laser hair removal treatment will increase the risk of carcinogenesis.

LEUKOTRICHIA

According to some documented reports, as well as personal observations, some patients develop white hair following application of lasers or light source hair removal. It is not known whether leukotrichia development is determined by intrinsic or extrinsic factors.

Anderson and colleagues showed that the Q-switched ruby laser could produce leukotrichia.[35] Possibly, with this laser, heated melanin was selectively vaporized, leaving vacuoles in the hair shafts; however, the follicular units themselves survived. This would lead to leukotrichia. In another study,[36] some patients also developed white hairs following intense pulsed light hair removal.

Whitening of the hairs after laser hair removal treatment may be explained by destruction of the melanocytes within the hair follicles, without total destruction of the actual germinative cells. It is to be expected that absorption by melanocytes may lead to partial destruction of germinative cells and subsequent thinning of black hairs. White hairs that regrow after treatment may be perceived as being as thick as the remaining black hairs.

In some cases, mostly in younger patients, there is restoration of hair color over subsequent months. This may be explained by temporary arrest in melanin synthesis by damaged, but viable melanocytes. The melanocytes may ultimately become functional after time, leading to the restoration of hair color.

In those patients whose hair remains de-pigmented, there may be permanent destruction of the melanocytes. In older patients, a disproportionate increase in white hairs after laser hair removal treatments may be the result of a greater susceptibility of hair containing pigment-producing melanocytes to permanent thermal damage.[36]

Finally, it may be that the observed lighter-colored hairs seen after laser hair removal may simply be the result of a laser-induced preferential effect on darker hairs.

BLISTERING

Blistering or crusting may occur in 10–15% of patients.[37] Histologic suprabasal epidermal necrosis is seen in all patients with clinical blistering of the skin after laser hair irradiation. These changes, as described above, are typical for those seen after a superficial burn.[33,34] The noted effects are thought to be due to a direct thermal injury. In general, the maximum tolerated fluence leading to the end-point of a burn is greater for a smaller spot size than is seen with a larger spot size. That is, a lower fluence may lead to a burn when a larger spot size is used; yet the same parameters with a smaller spot size would not create the same effect (Figures 4.1, 4.5–4.7, 4.57).[17]

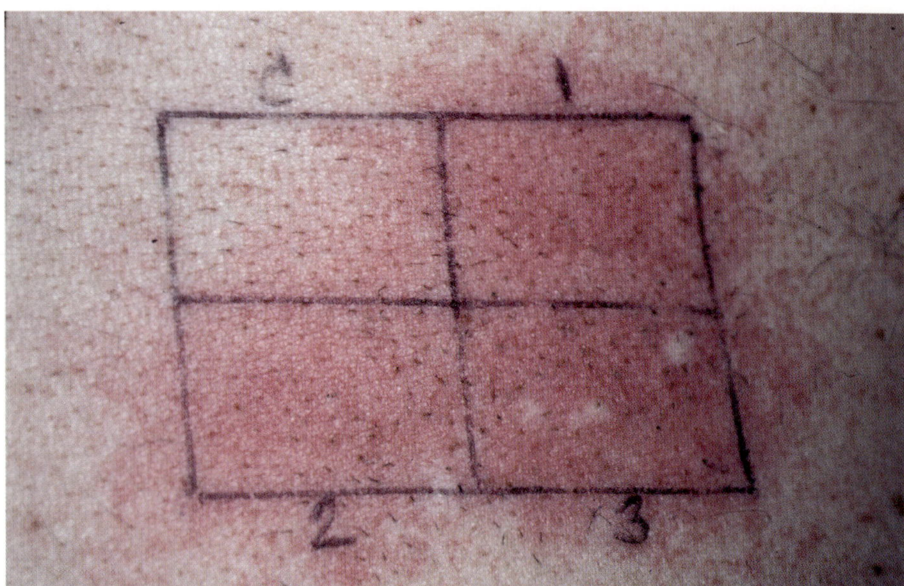

Figure 4.57. Test spots using various Nd:YAG laser fluences. Note early blistering at site 3. This site might lead to a scar

EFFECTS ON SEBUM EXCRETION

Preliminary studies suggest that sebum secretion may be affected by laser hair removal.[38]

Histologically, a decrease in glandular size is observed at all three anatomic levels of sebaceous glands (most significantly at the portion of the isthmus). Sporadic damage to sebaceous glands can be seen immediately after laser irradiation.

Human sebaceous glands contain no pigmented melanocytes.[39] Thus, laser hair removal wavelengths are poorly absorbed by the sebaceous gland. A primary thermal effect is unlikely. A possible explanation for the decreased sebum noted after laser hair removal is the smaller observed sebaceous glands associated with the miniaturization of hair shafts after laser treatment.

Increased sebocyte proliferation has been reported after non-specific injury to the superficial portion of pilosebaceous apparatus.[40,41] With laser hair removal, a focal documented histologic injury to the sebaceous glands can be seen. However, one does not see a laser hair removal-induced stimulation of sebaceous glands. Thus, a sebaceous gland proliferative response to injury is not consistent with the noted post-laser hair removal reduction of sebaceous gland size.

PURPURA

Purpura, occasionally seen after laser hair removal, and mostly observed on the lower extremities, probably reflects the influence of gravity and higher hydrostatic pressure in these anatomic regions (Figure 4.58).

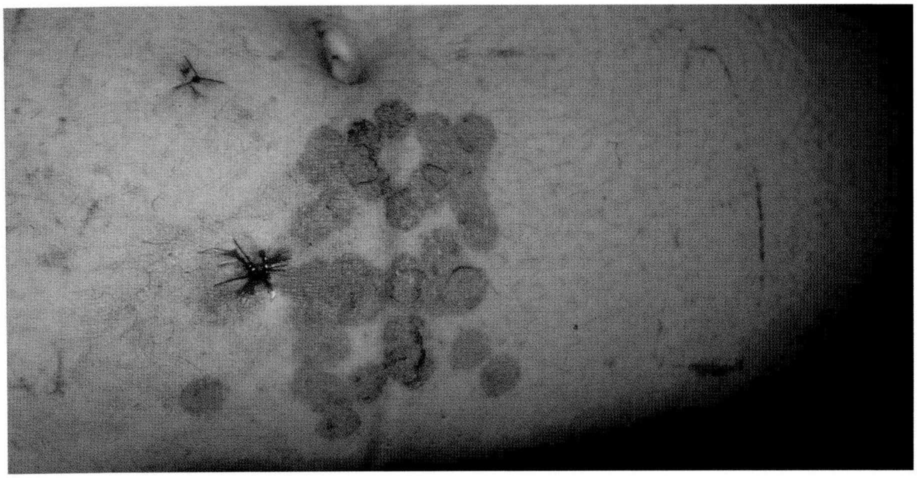

Figure 4.58. Purpura after treatment with a ruby laser

INFECTIONS

Herpex Simplex Virus

Herpes simplex virus (HSV) outbreaks are uncommon after laser and light sources treatment of hair removal, but may occur especially in patients with a strong history of outbreaks. Such infections are most commonly seen on, or around, the lips.

Bacterial Infection

Although the risk of bacterial infection is extremely low, it may occur following epidermal damage induced by any form of trauma, including aggressive laser hair removal.

PLUME

The plume generated by the vaporized hair shafts has a typical sulfur smell and in large quantities can be irritating to the respiratory tract. Smoke evacuators can be helpful.

CONCLUSION

Complications following laser hair removal are rare.[42] However, they do occur. Most commonly, one sees transient hyper- or hypopigmentation that improves with time.

REFERENCES

1 Ross EV, Ladin Z, Kreindel M, Dierickx C. Theoretical considerations in laser hair removal. Dermatol Clin 1999;17:333–355.

2 Liew SH. Laser hair removal: Guidelines for management. Am J Clin Dermatol 2002;3:107–115.

3 Welch A, Wissler E, Priebw L. Significance of blood flow in calculations of temperature in laser irradiated tissue. IEEE Trans Biomed Eng 1980;27:164–166.

4 Liew SH. Ruby laser-assisted hair removal: clinical efficacy and evaluation of cutaneous changes [doctoral thesis]. London: University College London; 2000.

5 Haedersdal M, Egekvist H, Efsen J, Bjerring P. Skin pigmentation and texture changes after hair removal with the normal-mode ruby laser. Acta Derm Venereol 1999;79:465–468.

6 Anderson RR. Laser-tissue interactions. In: Baxter SH, ed. Cutaneous Laser Surgery. The Art and Science of Selective Photothermolysis. St. Louis, MO: Mosby; 1994:1–19.

7 Grossman MC, Dierickx C, Farinelli W, Flotte T, Anderson RR. Damage to hair follicles by normal-mode ruby laser pulses. J Am Acad Dermatol 1996;35:889–894.

8 Bjerring P, Zachariae H, Lybecker H, Clement M. Evaluation of the free-running ruby laser for hair removal. Acta Dermatol Venereol 1998;78:48–51.

9 Williams R, Havoonjian H, Isagholian K, et al. A clinical study of hair removal using the long-pulsed ruby laser. Dermatol Surg 1998;24:837–842.

10 Liew SH, Grobbelaar AO, Gault DT, et al. Ruby laser hair removal: Clinical efficacy in Fitzpatrick skin type I–V and histological changes in epidermal melanocytes. Br J Dermatol 1999;140:1105–1109.

11 Liew SH, Grobbelaar AO, Gault DT, et al. Ruby laser-assisted hair removal: Repeated treatments and clinical efficacy. Eur J Plast Surg 2000;23:121–126.

12 McDaniel DH. Clinical usefulness of the hexascan. J Dermatol Surg Oncol 1993; 19:312–317.

13 Weeland RG. Clinical uses of lasers in dermatology. Lasers Surg Med 1995;16:2 [abstract].

14 Defrin R, Ohry A, Blumen N, Urca G. Sensory determinants of thermal pain. Brain 2002;125:501–510.

15 Drummond PD. The effect of sympathetic activity on thermal hyperalgesia in capsaicin-treated skin during body cooling and warming. Eur J Pain 2001;5:59–67.

16 Pieran FK, Torrey P, Carpenter DO. Afferent nerve fiber activity responding to temperature changes of scrotal skin of the rat. J Neurophysiol 1975;38:601–612.

17 Eremia S, Newman N. Topical anesthesia for laser hair removal: Comparison of spot sizes and 755 nm vs 800 nm wavelengths. Dermatol Surg 2000;26:667–669.

18 Garcia C, Alamoudi H, Nakib M, Zimmo S. Alexandrite laser hair removal is safe for Fitzpatrick skin types IV–VI. Dermatol Surg 2000;26:130–134.

19 Waldorf HA, Alster TS, McMillan K, et al. Effects of dynamic cooling on 585 nm pulsed dye laser treatment of port-wine-stain birthmarks. Dermatol Surg 1997;23:657–662.

20 Nanni CA, Alster TS. Laser-assisted hair removal: Side effects of Q-switched Nd:YAG, long-pulsed ruby, and alexandrite lasers. J Am Acad Dermatol 1999;41:165–171.

21 Anvari B, Tanenbaum BS, Milner TE, et al. A theoretical study of the thermal response of skin to cryogen spray cooling and pulsed laser irradiation: Implications for treatment of port-wine-stain birthmarks. Phys Med Biol 1995;40:1451–1465.

22 Eremia S, Li SY, Umar SH, Newman N. Laser hair removal: long term results with a 755 nm alexandrite laser. Dermatol Surg 2001;27:920–924.

23 Nahm WK, Tsoukas MM, Falanga V, et al. Preliminary study of fine changes in the duration of dynamic cooling during 755 nm laser hair removal on pain and epidermal damage in patients with skin types III–V. Lasers Surg Med 2002: 31:247–251.

24 Majoran B, Kimel S, Verkruysse W, et al. Cryogen spray cooling in laser dermatology: Effects of ambient humidity and frost formation. Lasers Surg Med 2001;28:469–476.

25 Liew SH, Cerio R, Sarathchandra P, et al. Ruby laser-assisted hair removal: An ultrastructural evaluation of cutaneous damage. Br J Plast Surg 1999;52:636–643.

26 Anderson RR. Laser–tissue interactions. In: Goldman MP, Fitzpatrick RE, eds. Cutaneous Laser Surgery: The Art and Science of Selective Photothermolysis. St. Louis, MO: Mosby; 1984:1–18.

27 Menon IR, Persad S, Ranadive NS, et al. Role of superoxide and hydrogen peroxide in cell lysis during irridiation of in-vitro Ehrlich ascitic carcinoma cells in the presence of melanin. Can J Biochem Cell Biol 1985;63:278–283.

28 Sarna T, Sealy RC. Free radicals from eumelanin: Quantum yields and wavelength dependence. Arch Biochem Biophys 1984;232:574–583.

29 Chekdekel MR, Agin PP, Sayre RM. Photochemistry of pheomelanin: Action spectrum for superoxide production. Photochem Photobiol 1980;34:553–555.

30 Marks F, Furstenberger G, Heinzelmann T, et al. Mechanisms in tumour promotion: Guidance for risk assessment and cancer chemoprevention. Toxicol Lett 1995;82/83:907–917.

31 Liew SH, Grobbelaar AO, Gault DT, et al. The effect of ruby laser light on cellular proliferation of epidermal cells. Ann Plast Surg 1999;43:519–522.

32 Logan ID, McKenna PG, Barnett YA. An investigation of the cytotoxic and mutagenic potential of low intensity laser irridiation in Friend erythroleukaemia cells. Mutat Res 1995;347:67–71.
33 Foly FD. Pathology of cutaneous burns. Surg Clin North Am 1970;50:1210–1220.
34 Kennedy CTC. Reactions to mechanical and thermal injury. In: Campion RH, Burton JL, Ebling FJG, eds. Textbook on Dermatology. Oxford: Blackwell; 1992:808–818.
35 Anderson RR, Margolis RJ, Watenabe S, et al. Selective photothermolysis of cutaneous pigmentation by Q-switched Nd:YAG laser at 1064, 532, and 355 nm. J Invest Dermatol 1989;93:28–32.
36 Radmanesh M, Mostaghimi M, Yousefi I, et al. Leukotrichia developed following application of intense pulsed light for hair removal. Dermatol Surg 2002;28:572–574.
37 Nanni CA, Alster TS. A practical review of laser-assisted hair removal using the Q-switched Nd:YAG, long-pulsed ruby, and long-pulsed alexandrite lasers. Dermatol Surg 1998;24:1399–1405.
38 Manuskiatti W, Dierickx CC, Gonzalez S, et al. Laser hair removal affects sebaceous glands and sebum excretion: A pilot study. J Am Acad Dermatol 1999;41:176–180.
39 Montagna W. The sebaceous glands in man. In: Montagna W, Ellis RA, Silver AF, eds. The Sebaceous Glands: IV. Oxford: Pergamon; 1963:19–31.
40 Eisen AZ, Holyoke JB, Lobitz WC. Responses of the superficial portion of the human pilosebaceous apparatus to controlled injury. J Invest Dermatol 1955;25:145–156.
41 Moore GP, Panaretto BA, Carter NB. Epidermal hyperplasia and wool follicle regression in sheep infused with epidermal growth factor. J Invest Dermatol 1985;84:172–175.
42 Goldberg DJ. Laser Hair Removal. London: Martin Dunitz; 2000.

5 COMPLICATIONS IN LASER TREATMENT OF VASCULAR LESIONS

KEY POINTS

(1) The flashlamp pulsed dye laser (FLPDL) is the most commonly used vascular lesion laser
(2) Atrophic and hypertrophic scarring can occur after vascular lesion laser treatment. These complications are rare after FLPDL treatment
(3) Pigmentary changes after FLPDL treatment are more common in darker skin types and in those patients treated with higher fluences
(4) Although complications after treatment with the newer near infrared vascular lesion lasers have yet to be reported, they must be considered when these lasers are used

INTRODUCTION

Benign cutaneous vascular lesions, such as hemangiomas and vascular malformations, are almost never life-threatening. Treatment is generally sought for cosmetic reasons. Various treatments have been used to remove such lesions including surgery, ionizing radiation, cryotherapy, sclerotherapy, tattooing with flesh-colored pigments, dermabrasion, electrocautery, intralesional or systemic steroids, and cosmetic camouflage.[1–4]

Lasers have been used in the treatment of benign cutaneous vascular lesions since the mid 1960s. As discussed earlier in this book, the long-pulsed ruby laser, with its 694 nm wavelength, was among the first lasers used to treat skin lesions.[5] Because of the poor hemoglobin absorption at this wavelength, the ruby laser lacked vascular specificity. Non-specific thermal injury of the irradiated site was to be expected. The ruby laser was ultimately replaced by the argon laser with its wavelengths in the blue and green spectrum: 80% of the argon laser's emitted light is from 458 nm to

514 nm providing a fair degree of selectivity for the vascular target.[6–9] This laser, although no longer in popular use, was traditionally employed with shuttered pulse durations of 50 milliseconds to 300 milliseconds at an energy of 0.8–2.9 watts of power. Utilized spot sizes were generally 0.1–1.0 mm, with or without a scanning device, to produce the end-point of tissue blanching. Although the results with the argon laser were good to excellent in 60% of patients, adverse effects, such as the risk of pigmentary changes and hypertrophic scarring (most commonly seen in children),[7,10–14] remained a problem. Persistence of treated vascular lesions was related to the destruction of blood vessels in the superficial papillary dermis, leaving ectatic middle and deep reticular dermal vessels intact.[15] In an effort to lessen the incidence of complications different argon laser treatment methods were used, such as treatment of only small areas,[16] treatment in alternating stripes,[17,18] chilling of the lesion before therapy,[19] careful selection of both patients and lesions,[7,20,21] low energy treatment,[14,22] mechanical scanning devices,[23] and meticulous tracing of vessels with a very small diameter beam.[24] Even with the use of a combination of these techniques, the incidence of hypertrophic scarring was still unacceptably high.[25]

Because of the limitations inherent with the argon laser, attention was focused on developing lasers with more specific absorption characteristics for intravascular oxyhemoglobin (HbO_2), the treatment chromophore. Early experimental, in vitro studies demonstrated that 50 µm vessels containing HbO_2, 1 mm below the epidermal granular layer, highly absorb 577 nm laser irradiation.[26] Endothelial cells are also damaged at this wavelength independent of their HbO_2 absorption. However, this effect is minimal. It was this set of findings that led to the development of lasers having a wavelength of 577 nm. This ultimately led to the genesis of today's flashlamp pulsed dye lasers (FLPDLs). While initial FLPDLs emitted only 577 nm laser irradiation, newer models emit wavelengths up to 595–600 nm.

It should be noted that non-specific CO_2 laser vaporization had, at one time, been advocated for the treatment of vascular lesions, such as port wine stains (PWSs). However, because the chromophore for this 10 600 nm laser is water, and not hemoglobin, damage caused by this laser is non-specific. Results were poor and scarring was common.

KTP lasers, having a hemoglobin absorbing wavelength of 532 nm, are also popular for the treatment of some vascular lesions. The minimal side effect profile observed following use of this technology makes the KTP laser particularly attractive for the treatment of facial telangiectasias. In one study, facial telangiectasia patients expressed a preference for repeated treatments with the KTP laser as opposed to a single FLPDL treatment. This was due to the FLPDL-associated purpura and possible subsequent laser-induced hyperpigmentation.[27]

The factors that determine how cutaneous blood vessels are altered by lasers appear to be both laser- and patient-related. The inappropriate combination of these factors could be responsible for many potential adverse effects. These adverse effects have encouraged several investigators to examine and manipulate laser exposure and tissue reactions, such as energy density,[10] spot size,[28] exposure duration,[29] treatment technique,[8,30] tissue temperature,[12] age of treated patients,[8] and skin types – all in an attempt to reduce the risk of complications.

The risk of significant complications from the FLPDL is minimal. At suprathreshold exposures to FLPDL treatment, the shorter the emitted pulse duration, the greater is the degree of subsequent vessel obliteration. This results from the observed moderate to massive hemorrhage seen in many papillary and upper reticular dermal vessels. The affected vessels appear shattered with fragmented red cells scattered in the perivascular region. Irradiation with the same delivered fluence but using a longer pulsewidth, rarely results in hemorrhage. Vascular architecture appears preserved. Yet, with both short and long pulses a highly selective vascular injury, with subsequent vasculitis, can be seen.

Not only is there greater vascular damage at shorter FLPDL-delivered pulsewidths, there is also a potential for greater epidermal damage at these short pulsewidths. Thus, epidermal separation is more prominent as the laser pulse duration is decreased.

Laser-induced vascular and epidermal changes vary with skin pigmentation. Melanin absorption occurs over a broad spectrum of wavelengths. Its absorption increases steadily towards shorter wavelengths.[31] Beyond 1100 nm absorption however, absorption by melanin is essentially negligible.

The predominance of vascular over epidermal damage in lighter skin types is often reversed in those subjects with heavily pigmented skin. The majority of blood vessels in the dermis lie immediately below the epidermal pigment cell layer in the form of an extensive network of capillaries, venules, and arterioles. In Fitzpatrick skin types I and II, selective absorption of laser irradiation by papillary loop capillaries and horizontal plexus vessels appear to result in highly selective vascular thermal damage. However, in darker skin types, epidermal melanocytic competition for visible light laser irradiation results in both vascular damage and selective damage to the pigmented epidermal basal cell layer. As melanin pigment concentration increases in the skin, there is a corresponding reduction in dermal vascular damage with an increase in epidermal damage. In Fitzpatrick skin types V and VI, the increased pigment concentration, and subsequent laser absorption, is such that very few clinical and histological changes are detected in the underlying blood vessels. Major histologic damage occurs in the heavily pigmented epidermal basal cell layer.

There also appears to be a patient-specific energy dose therapeutic window. Any energy above a certain level, in a particular treated patient, is likely to result in undesired cutaneous damage. Any energy below a certain dose will lead to insufficient lesional lightening. Logic would suggest that laser test spot evaluation might determine a specific patient's response. Unfortunately, scarring may occur even in patients who have had successful initial tests.

The reasons why these side effects manifest themselves inconsistently remain unknown. Factors that may be considered include blood vessel heterogeneity in treated port wine stains. Since port wine stains can be composed of a wide range of vessel sizes, one might expect a differential vessel response to laser treatment. In addition, subclinical infection or mild local trauma may interfere with the normal healing process. Uneven laser irradiation and transmission parameters, as well as varying skin types may also contribute.[32,33]

SCARRING

Scarring as manifest by a permanent raised hypertrophic, atrophic, or depressed laser-treated site, is the most undesirable observed complication seen after laser and non-laser intense pulsed light treatment of vascular lesions.

Various studies have shown the clinical and histologic effects of ruby, argon, carbon dioxide (CO_2), KTP, and pulsed dye lasers after the treatment of vascular lesions differ significantly. This difference reflects differences in post-laser heat deposition. Because the basic mechanism of current laser therapy is photothermal, scarring appears to be largely related to the degree of primary thermal damage.[34] Injuries caused by CO_2 and argon lasers have been shown to be non-specific. Full-thickness tissue can be thermally destroyed. 'Repair' of such injuries results in fibrosis and scar tissue formation.

Despite good CO_2 and argon laser optical absorption, non-vascular as well as vascular structures in the skin are damaged by these lasers; scarring results. The incidence of scarring will vary with the treated patient population and the chosen laser and technique.

Upper lip, nasolabial areas, and chest are reported as high-risk sites, but sites, such as the periungual area and the feet, can also develop hypertrophic scars. Forehead, eyelid, temple, neck, and earlobe are found to be less prone to scarring. Because significantly greater amounts of heat can be generated by non-laser intense pulsed light sources and newer deeper penetrating near infrared lasers, (1064 nm Nd:YAG), one would expect the incidence of scarring to be higher with such technologies (Figures 5.1–5.7).

Hypertrophic Scarring

Hypertrophic scarring has been reported following treatment with a variety of vascular lasers. It is quite common after argon laser treatment, with 69% of physicians using this laser reporting at least one case of hypertrophic scarring.

Treatment of children with the argon laser, particularly infants, leads to the highest incidence of hypertrophic scarring. This complication has been reported in as many as 38% of patients under the age of 12 years.[8] Because of this high rate of hypertrophic scarring, argon laser treatment of patients younger than 17 years was not recommended.[6,21]

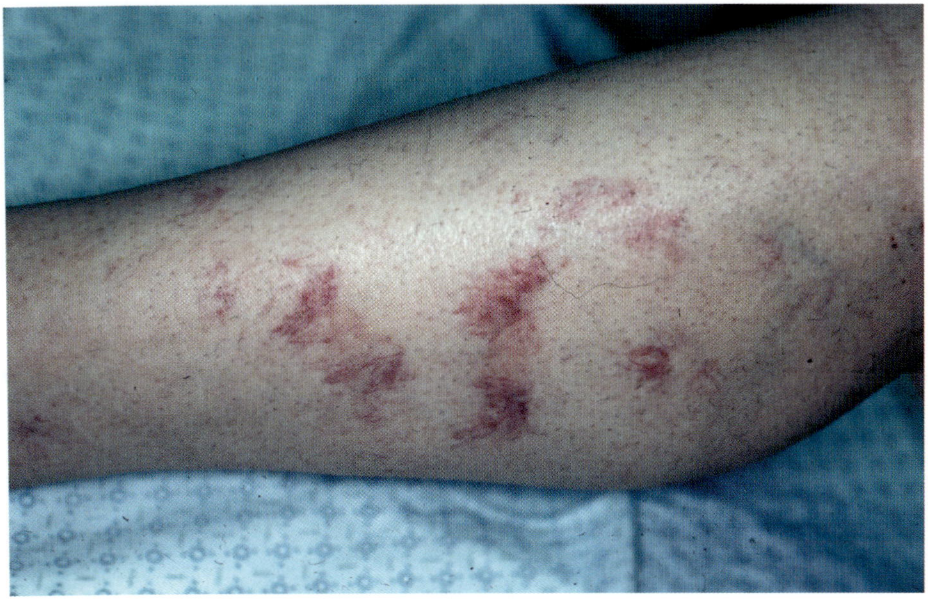

Figure 5.1. Small spider vessels on the leg before treatment

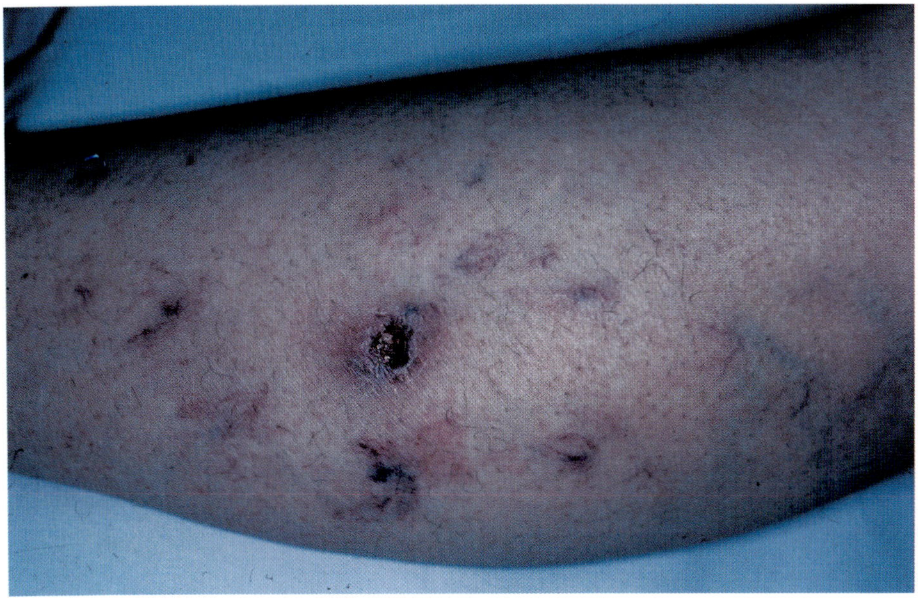

Figure 5.2. Ulceration after treatment of patient in Figure 5.1 with an Nd:YAG laser

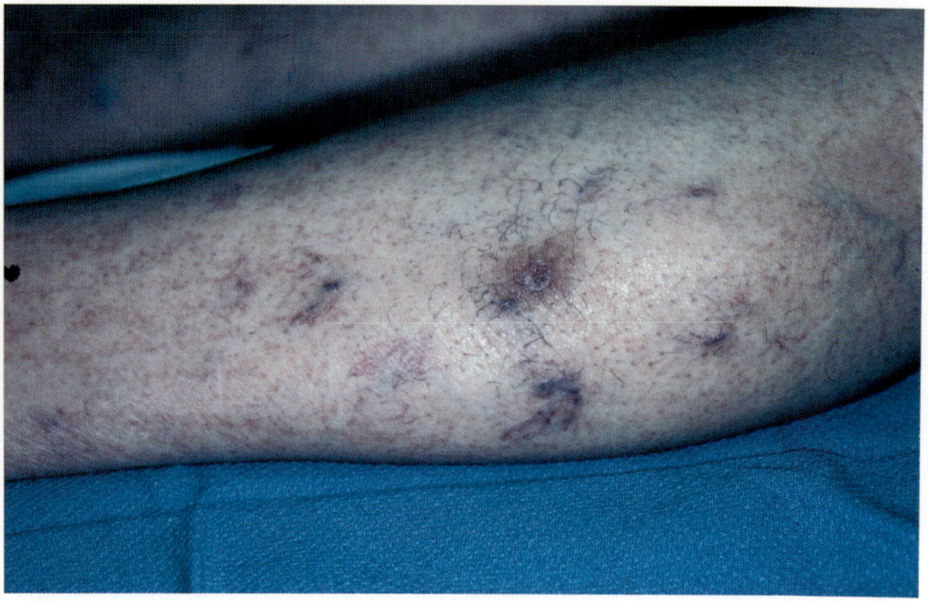

Figure 5.3. Patient in Figure 5.1, 6 months after treatment. Note mild atrophy at ulceration site

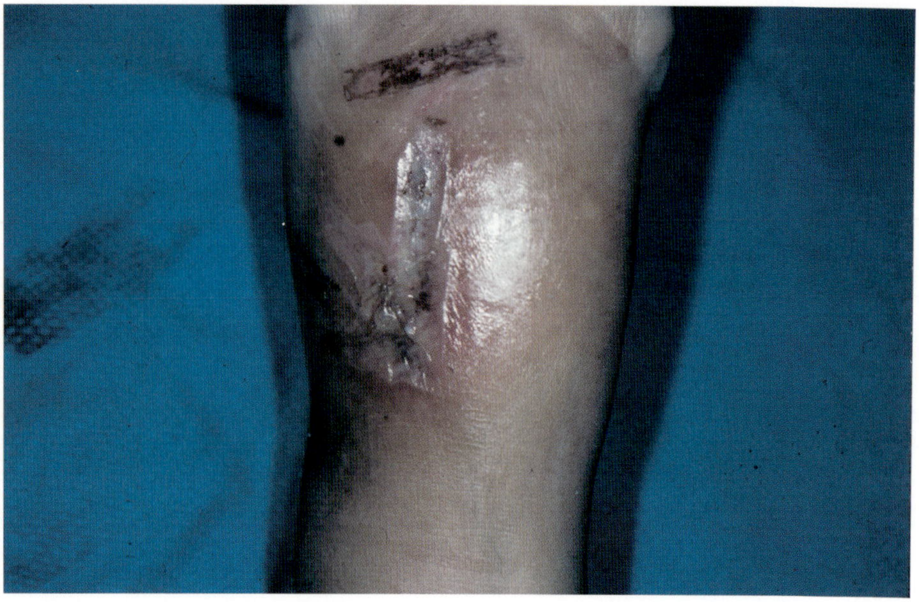

Figure 5.4. Intense pulse light-induced ulceration 5 days after treatment on the leg

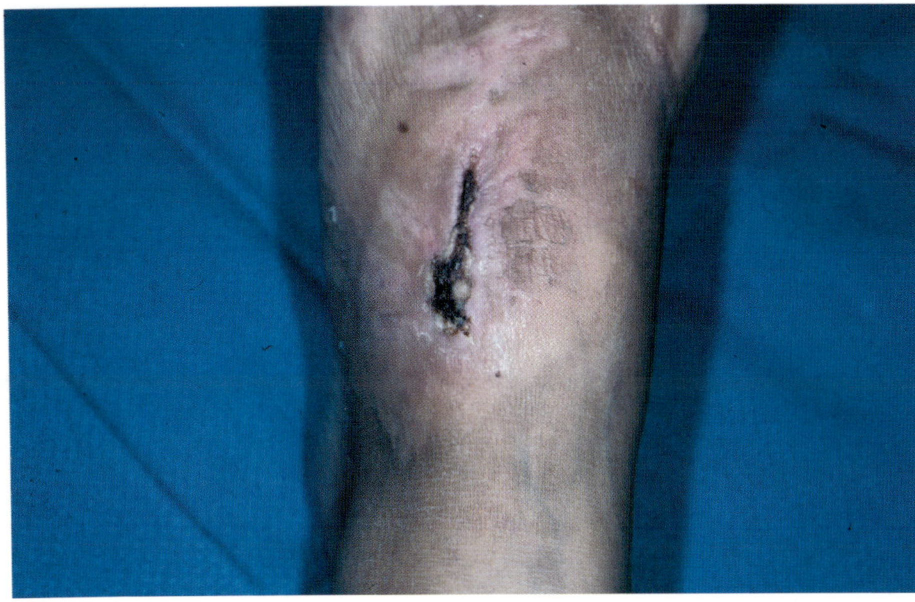

Figure 5.5. Scarring and persistent crusting 6 weeks after treatment of patient in Figure 5.4

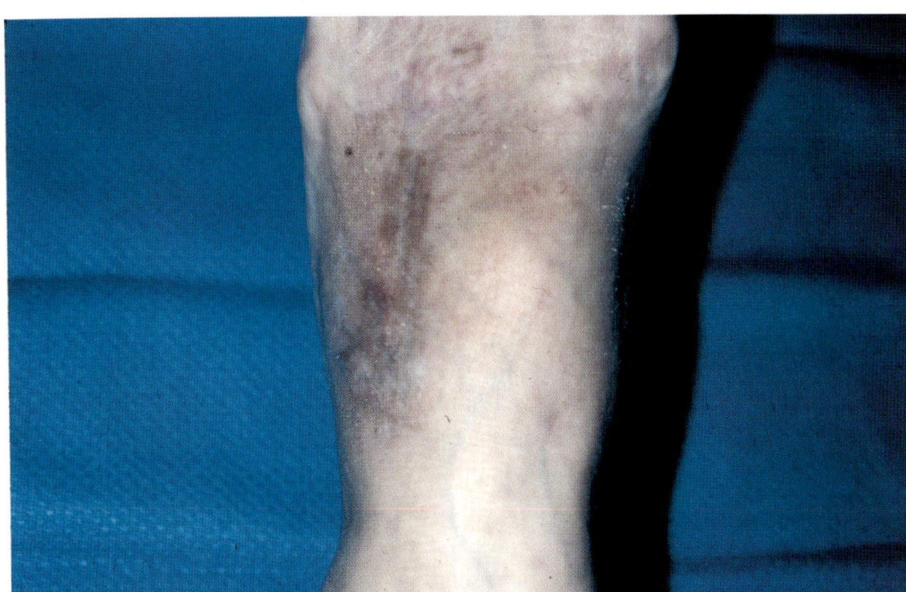

Figure 5.6. Scarring 6 months after treatment of patient in Figure 5.4

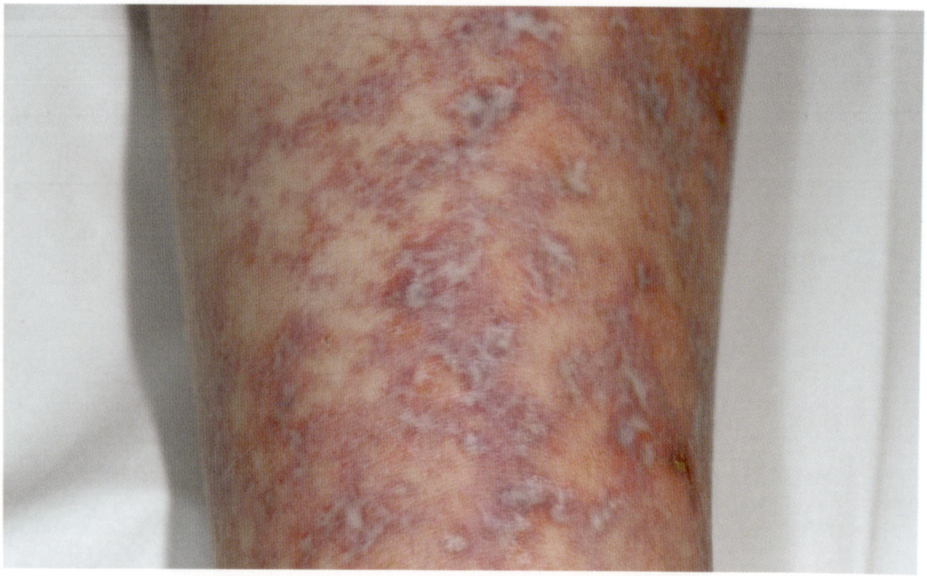

Figure 5.7. Extensive atrophic scarring after FLPDL treatment of a port wine stain (PSW). Such findings are distinctly unusual

The CO_2 laser has been used to treat port wine stains (PWS). However, because of the non-specific nature of this laser, a poor response in most patients, and a 9% reported post-laser treatment incidence of hypertrophic scars, this laser is rarely used for the treatment of vascular lesions.[35]

Today, the gold standard for the treatment of PWS is the 577–595 nm FLPDL. Unlike the CO_2 and argon lasers, the FLPDL leads to a highly selective vascular injury in normal human skin,[36–42] without much damage to the epidermis or to the non-vascular dermal structures. Thermal vascular damage caused by this pulsed laser results from heat generated within the treated dermal blood vessels. Unlike the damage seen after CO_2, and occasional argon laser treatment, FLPDL treatment does not generally lead to full-thickness epidermal and dermal coagulative necrosis.

Despite the lack of obvious clinical and histologic evidence of epidermal damage after FLPDL, such damage may have been after NBTC staining. The degree of damage, ranging from elongation and ballooning of single keratinocytes to diffuse epidermal coagulation with blistering, is directly dependent on the intensity of epidermal penetration. Increased epidermal pigmentation leads to greater post-FLPDL treatment NBTC staining, an increased risk of scarring, and a corresponding decrease in observed clinical results.[43,44]

Hypertrophic scarring seen after FLPDL treatment is extraordinarily rare. When it occurs, it is most commonly caused by localized infection, excessive overlapping of delivered laser pulses, or the repetitive pinpoint thermal damage to the superficial dermis and epidermis of multiply treated PWS.[43]

Atrophic Scars

Some slight treatment site vascular laser-induced atrophy has been reported in patients treated with a variety of different vascular lasers and intense pulsed light sources. It can occur in up to 11% of patients with an equal male and female incidence. However, female patients with an olive complexion have been found to have a 2.5 times greater incidence of such scars. Atrophic, depressed scars can occur in all age groups. They are most commonly seen after the treatment of mature PWS.[18]

It has been suggested that post laser-induced cutaneous atrophy is generally caused by excessive delivery of energy, overlapping of laser treatment sites,[45–47] trauma,[48] and/or foci of sub-clinical infection.[49] Atrophy can also occasionally occur without apparent reason.

PURPURA

Purpura is generally the most immediate visible response of the FLPDL treatment. It appears within a few seconds to a minute at the site of FLPDL impact. There is usually no epidermal damage. Purpura generally disappears within 1–2 weeks after laser treatment. Although the bruise-like purpura is a transient side effect, it is often a major cause of morbidity and individual distress. FLPDL-induced purpura leads to 43% of patients severely restricting their lifestyle after laser treatment (Figures 5.8–5.34).[50]

It is generally accepted that purpura is caused by damage imparted to small capillaries throughout the normal dermis.[40] These vessels are of diameters in the range 20 µm to 60 µm.[40]

There are conflicting opinions as to the clinical necessity of post-treatment purpura. It is occasionally stated that good vascular lesion clearance can be seen without purpura. However, it is also generally accepted that at least a deep transient red or violet discoloration is a threshold response indicating vascular damage.

The energy required to produce clinical purpura varies with skin types, vessel size, pulse durations, and emitted laser wavelengths.

As epidermal melanin increases, more laser energy is required to produce purpura. Unfortunately, epidermal cell damage also becomes more marked as melanin concentration increases (Fitzpatrick skin types IV–VI). There is a progressive increase in the degree of vascular damage with increasing delivered fluences. Correspondingly, the intensity of the purpura is directly proportional to the delivered fluence. As the fluence is increased, a more intense purpura is observed.

The threshold for inducing purpura also increases with increasing laser-delivered pulsewidth. This can be best explained by the heat transfer occurring from microvessels during laser exposure.

Significant heat loss occurs from selectively heated vessels when treated with pulsewidths equal to or greater than the vessel's thermal relaxation time. The selective

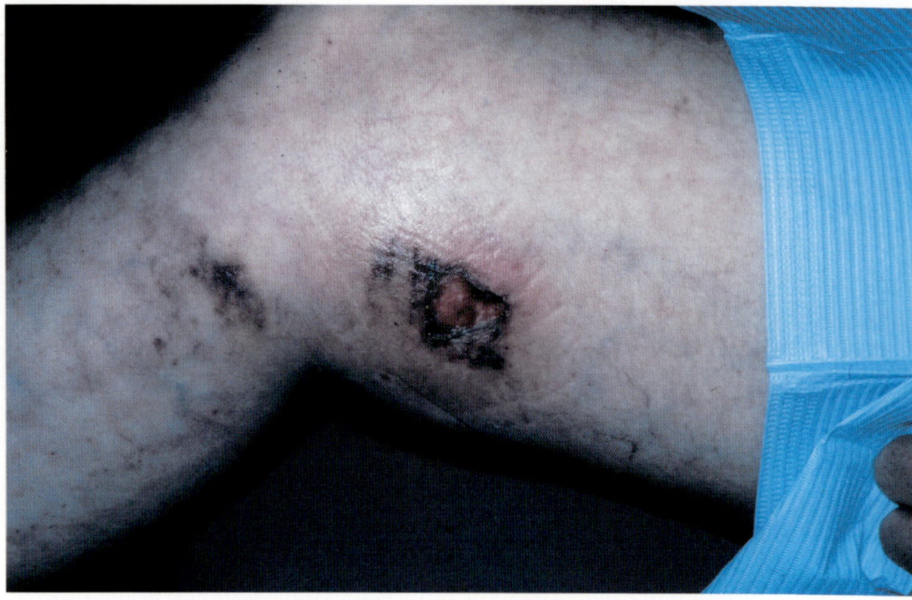

Figure 5.8. Purpura and ulcerations seen 5 days after treatment with the FLPDL

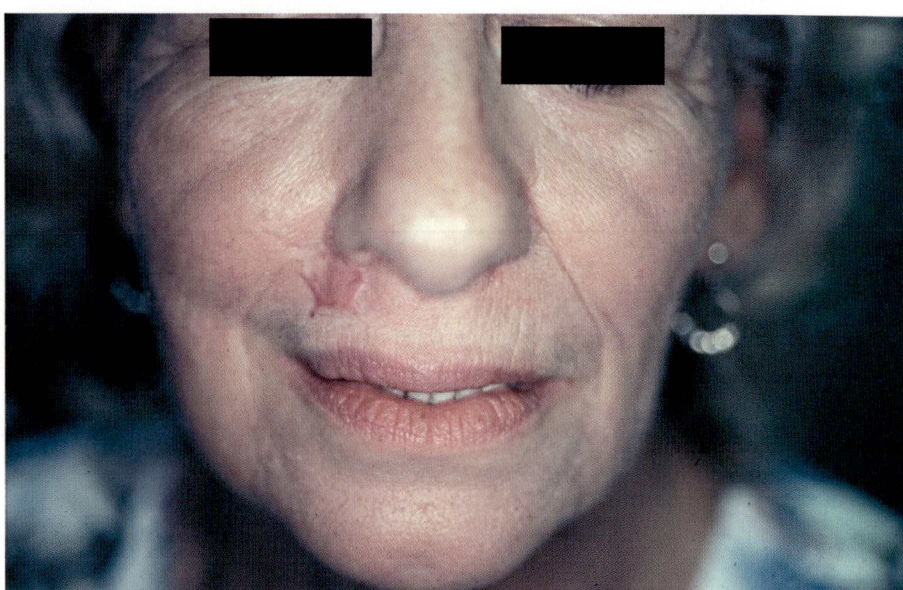

Figure 5.9. Scar on upper lip before treatment with the FLPDL

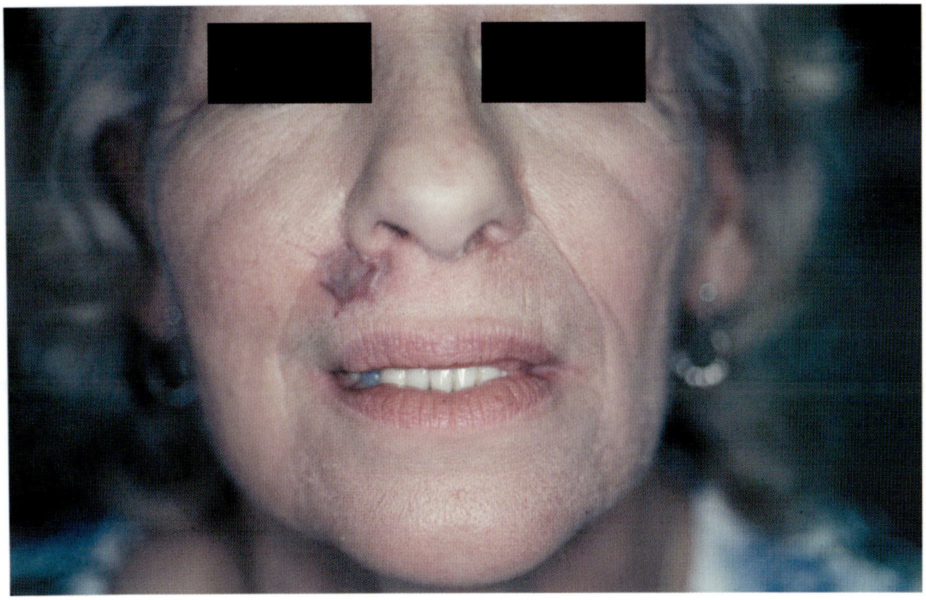

Figure 5.10. Purpura seen immediately after treatment with the FLPDL

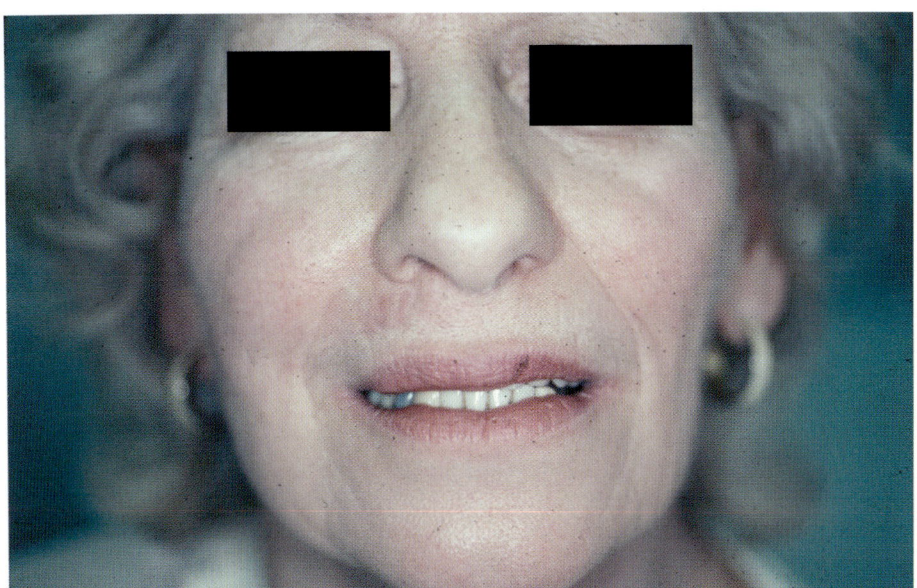

Figure 5.11. Improvement in scar after treatment with the FLPDL

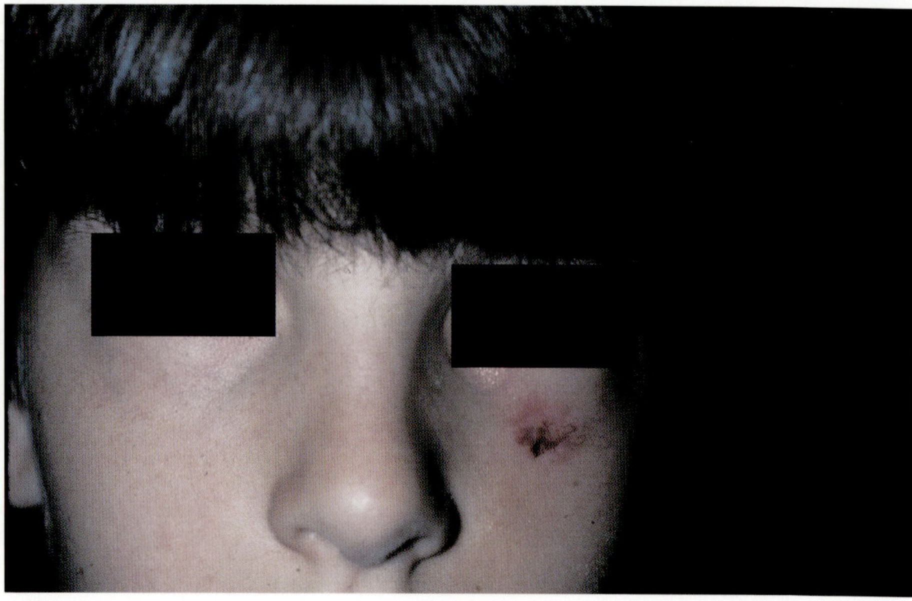

Figure 5.12. Purpura and blisters after telangiectasia was treated with the FLPDL

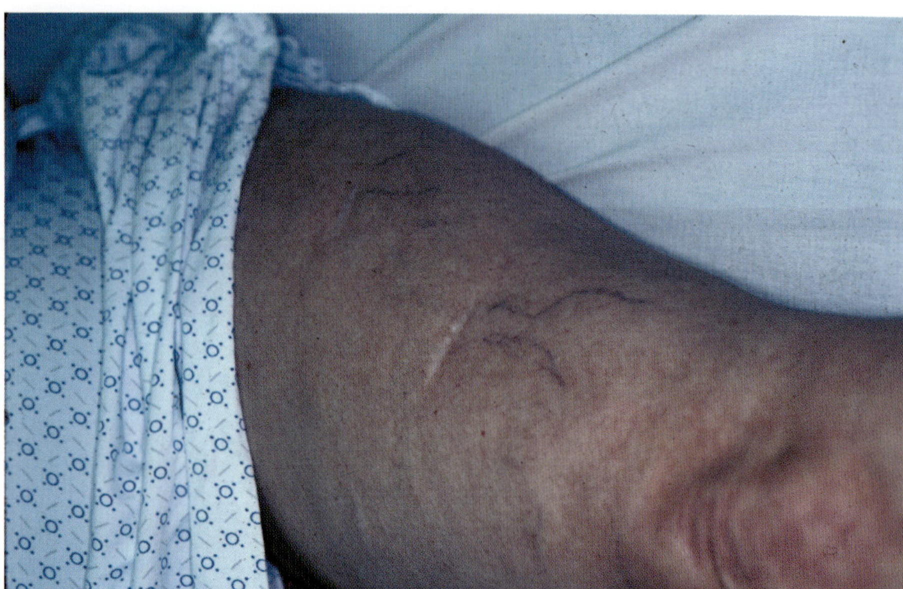

Figure 5.13. Spider veins before treatment with the FLPDL

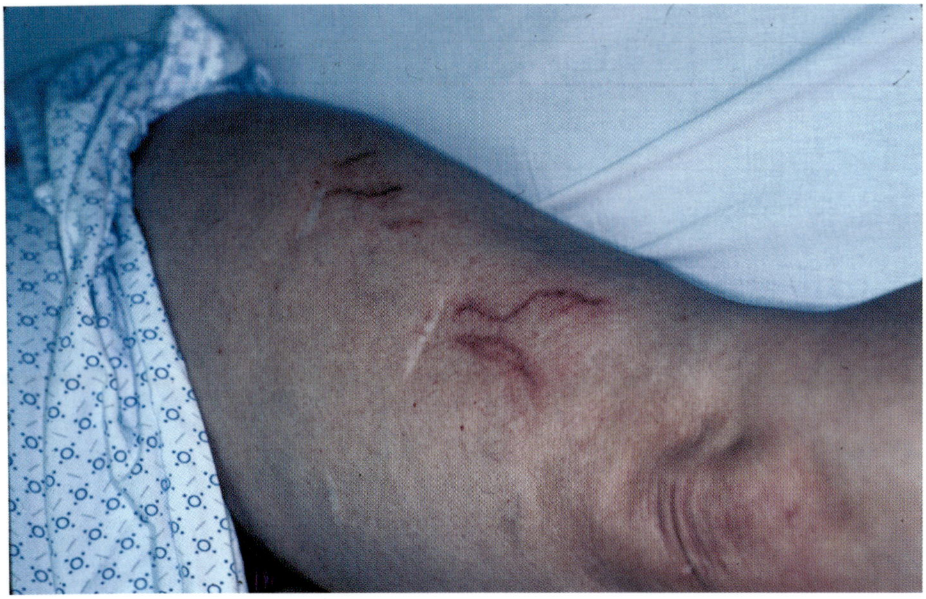

Figure 5.14. Pulsed dye laser-induced purpura immediately after treatment of spider veins

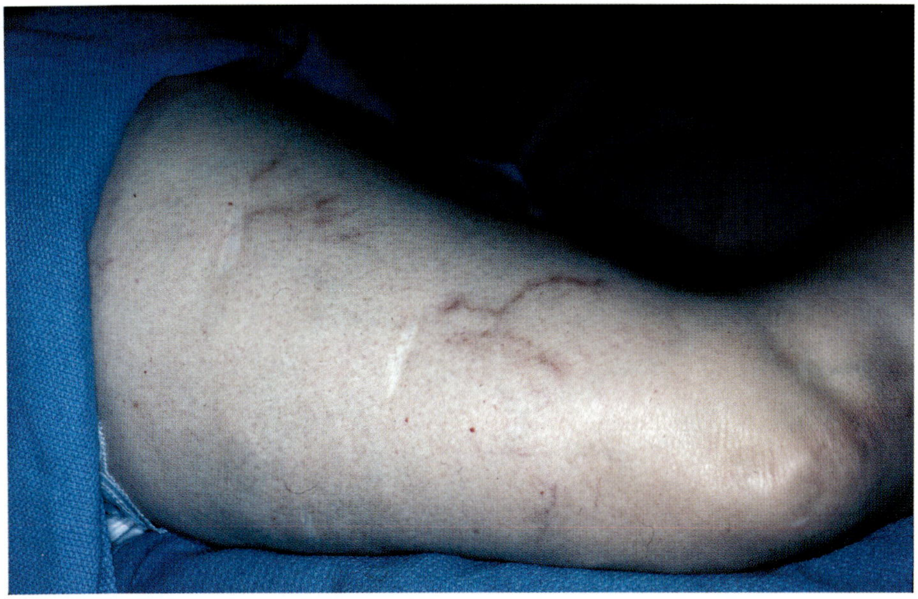

Figure 5.15. Purpura after FLPDL treatment of spider veins. Note nearby scarring and hypopigmentation from previous intense pulsed light treatment

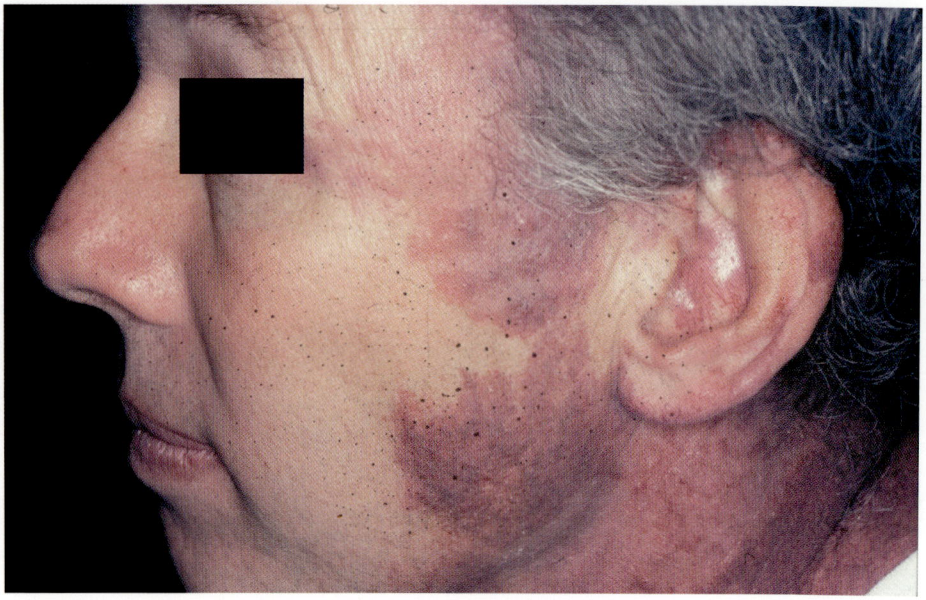

Figure 5.16. Port wine stain before treatment with FLPDL

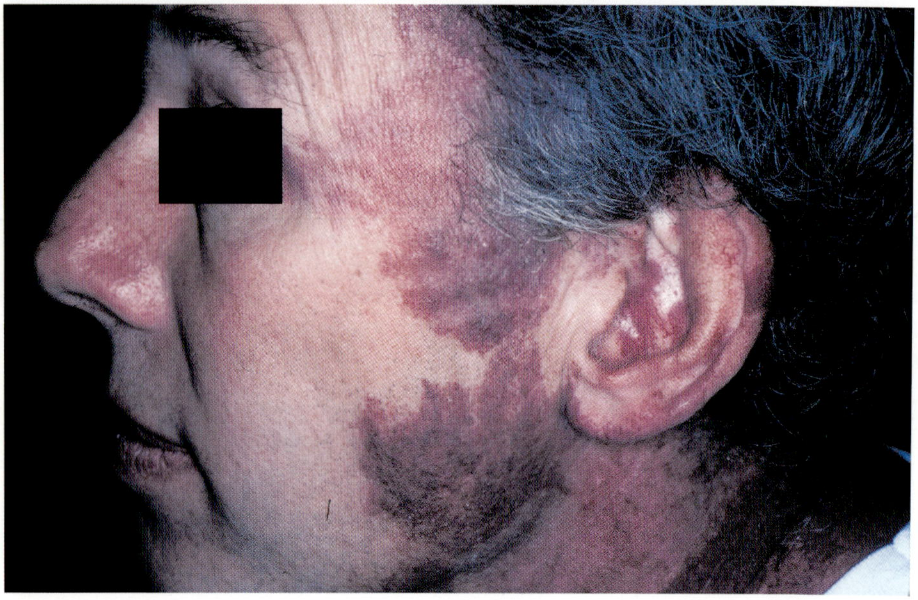

Figure 5.17. FLPDL-induced purpura

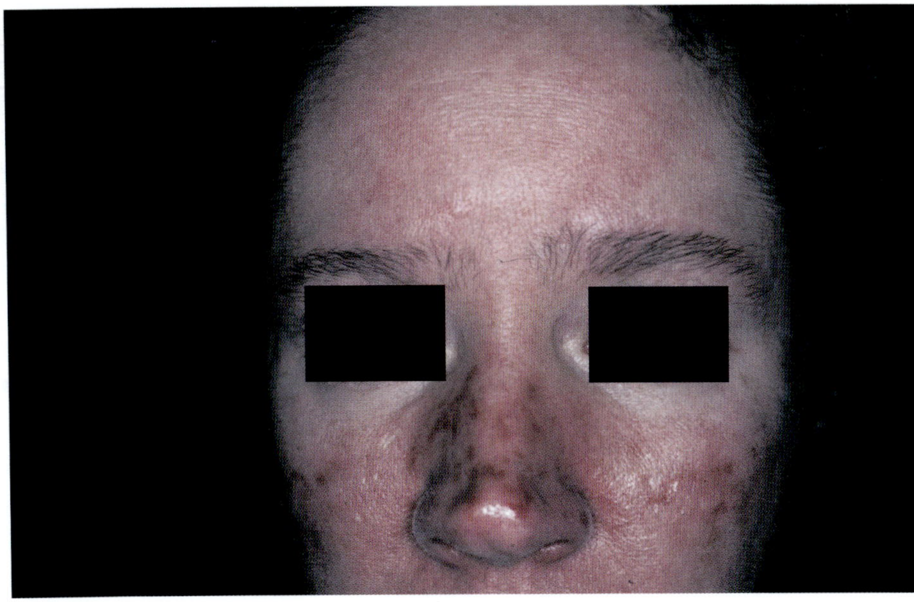

Figure 5.18. Persistent purpura 1 week after FLPDL treatment

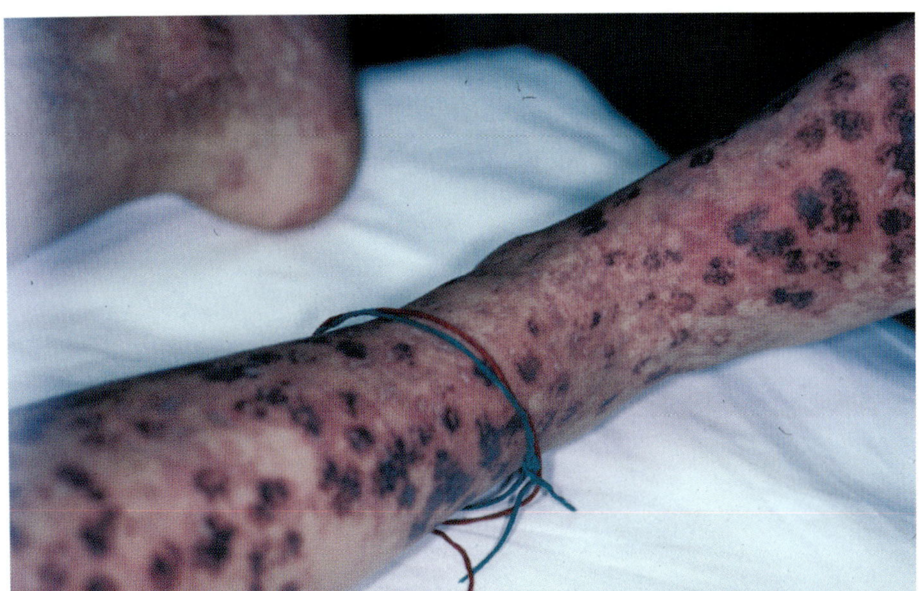

Figure 5.19. Extensive purpura of leg immediately after FLPDL treatment

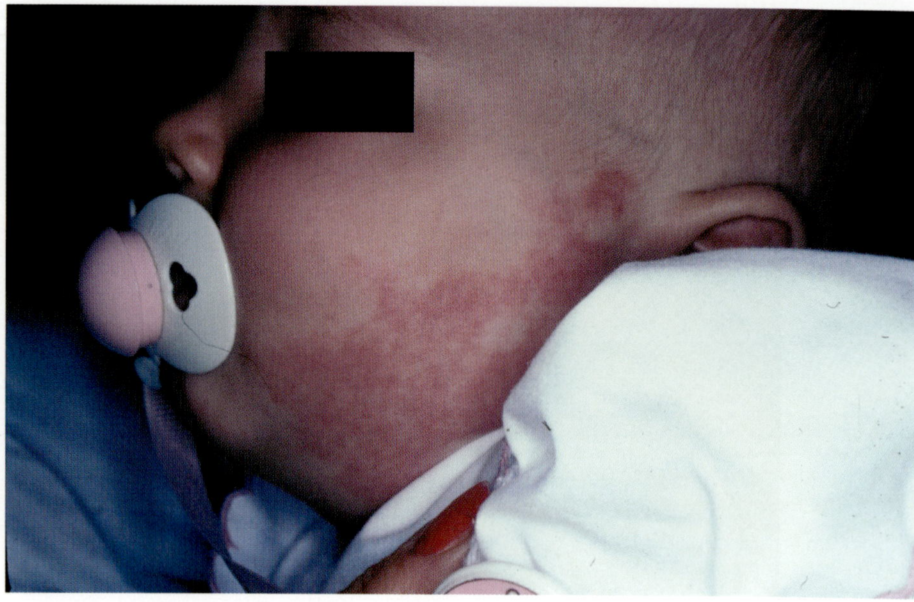

Figure 5.20. Port wine stain before treatment with the FLPDL

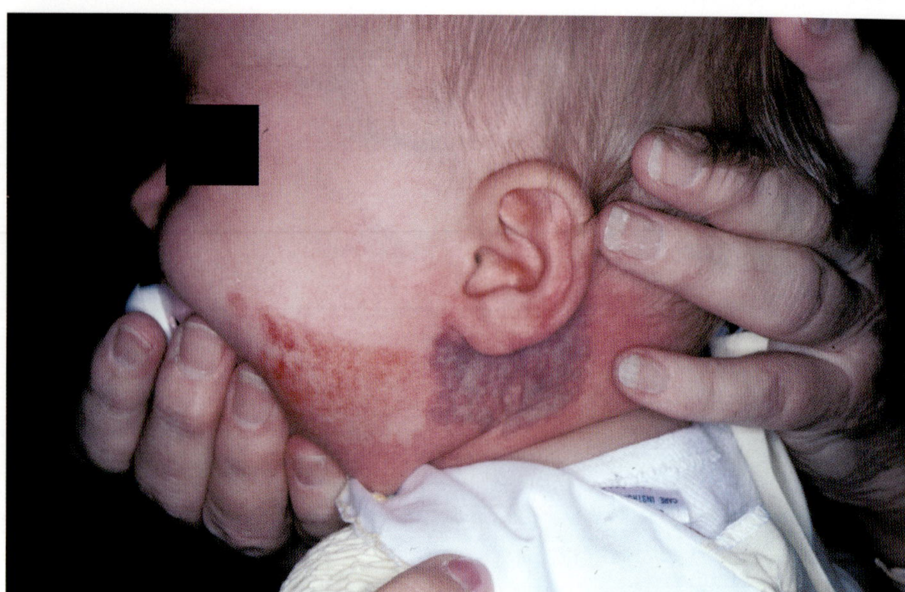

Figure 5.21. Purpura immediately after treatment with the FLPDL

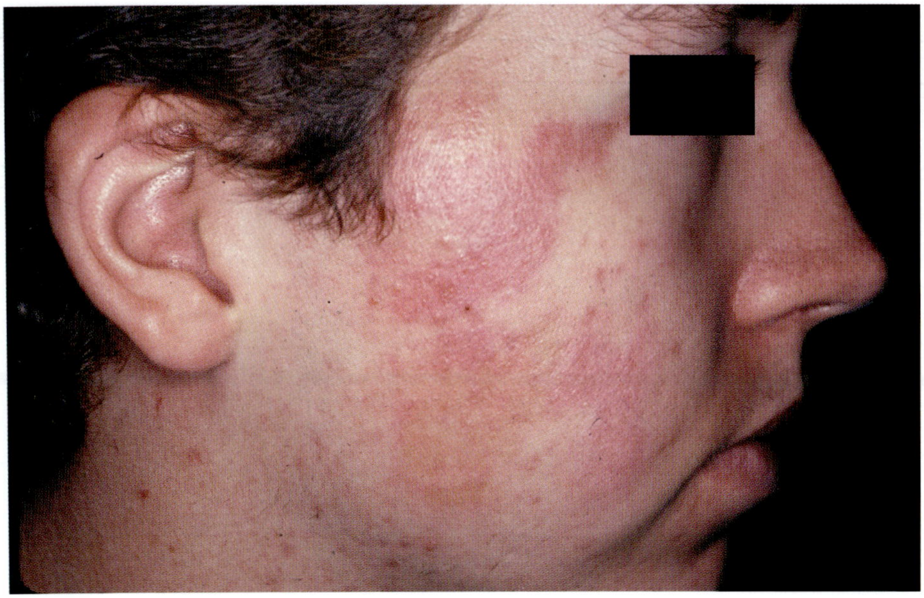

Figure 5.22. Port wine stain before FLPDL treatment

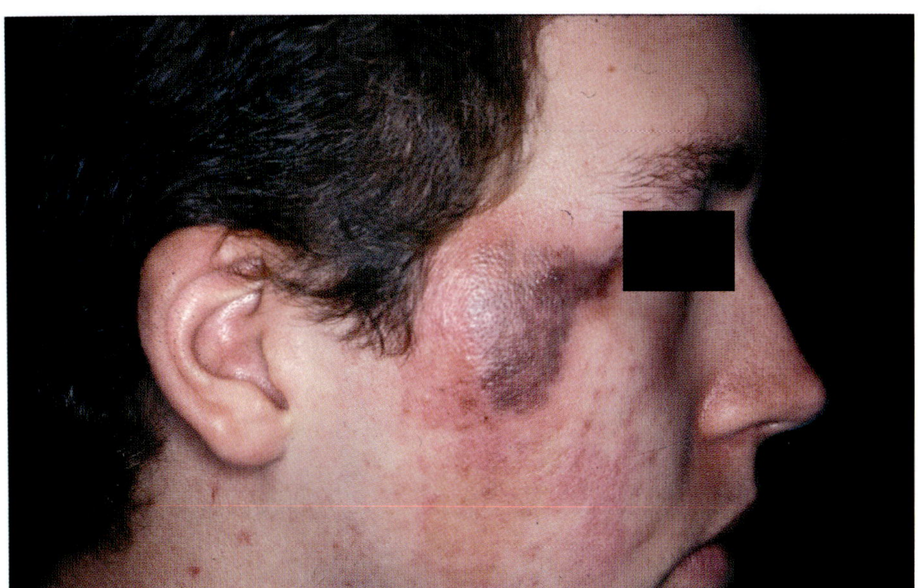

Figure 5.23. Purpura immediately after treatment with the FLPDL

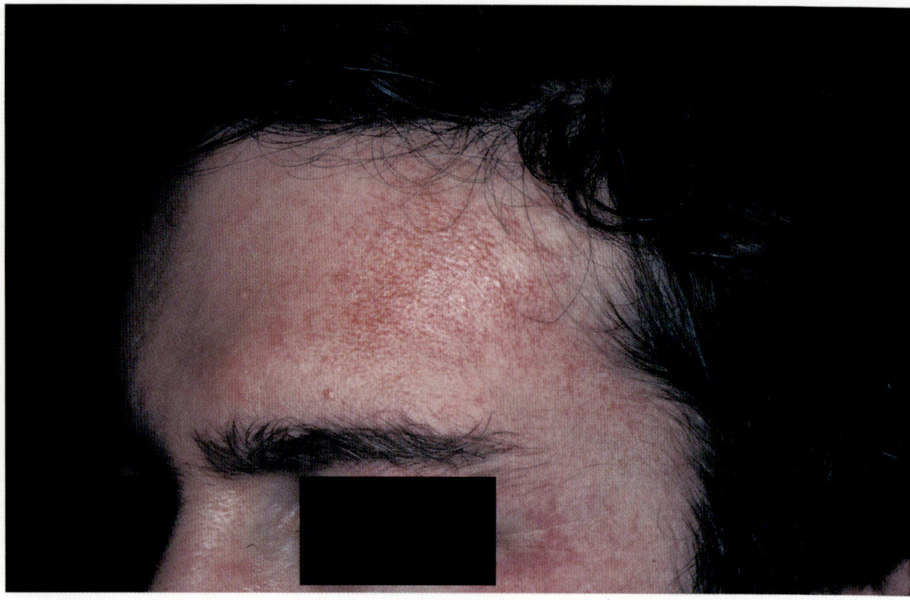

Figure 5.24. Port wine stain before FLPDL treatment

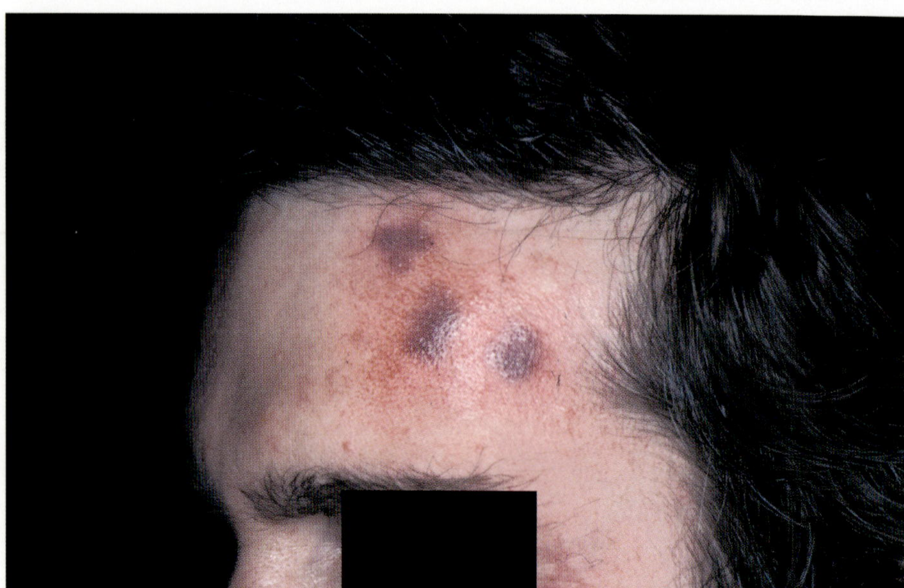

Figure 5.25. Purpura immediately after treatment with the FLPDL

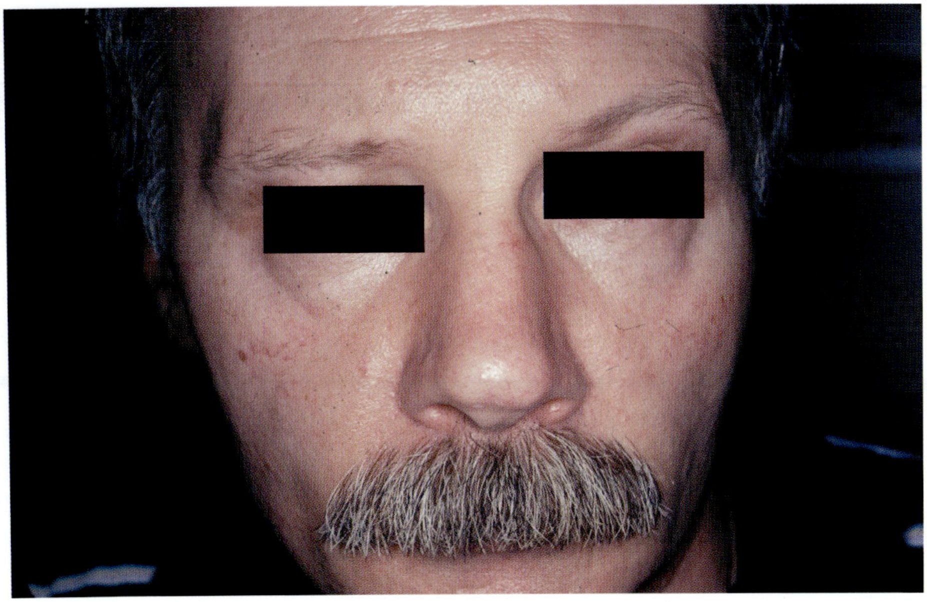

Figure 5.26. Telangiectasias before FLPDL treatment

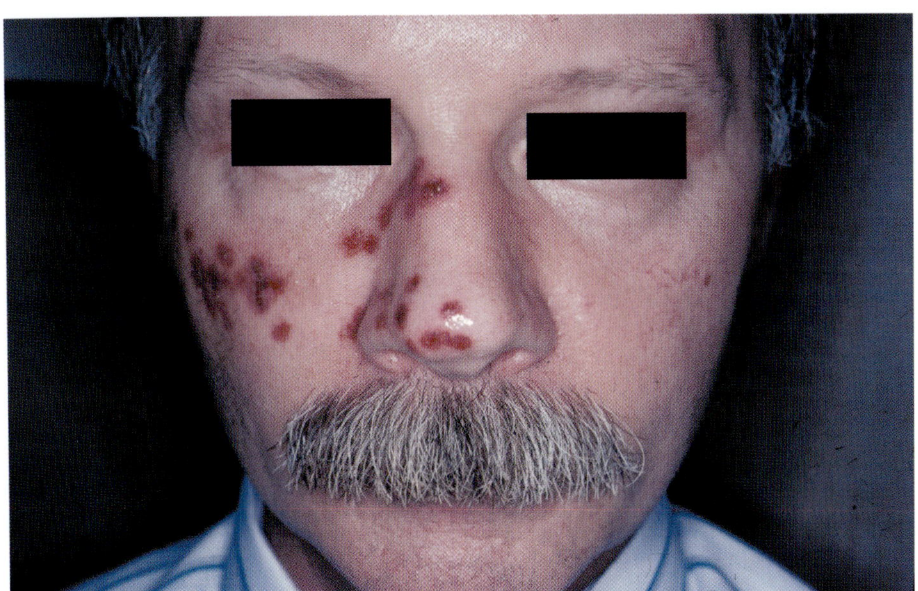

Figure 5.27. Purpura immediately after treatment with the FLPDL

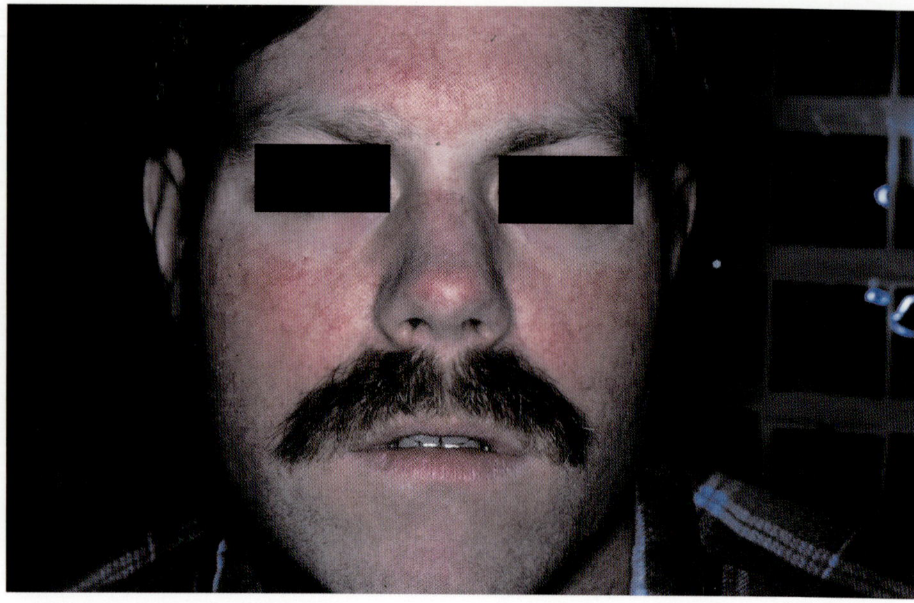

Figure 5.28. Rosacea before FLPDL treatment

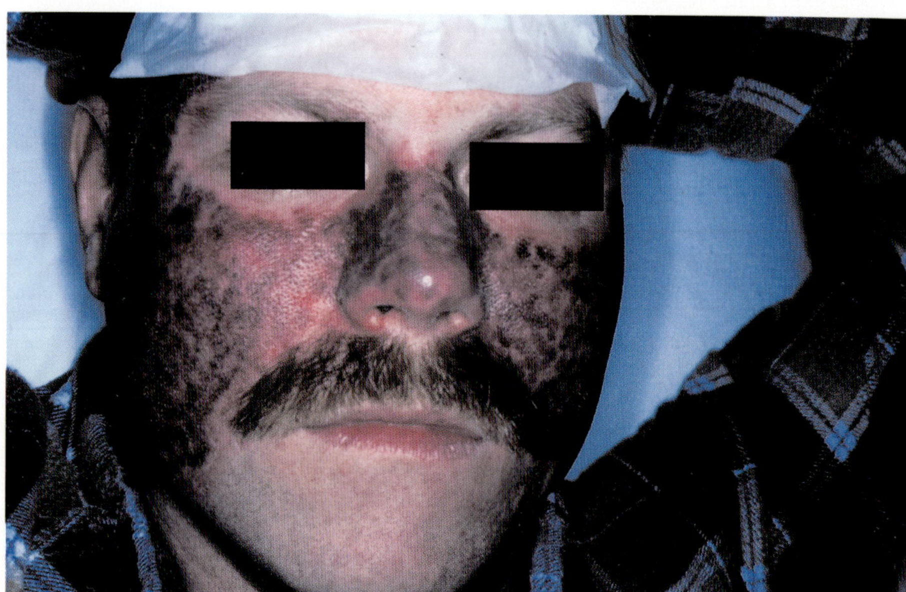

Figure 5.29. Purpura immediately after treatment with the FLPDL

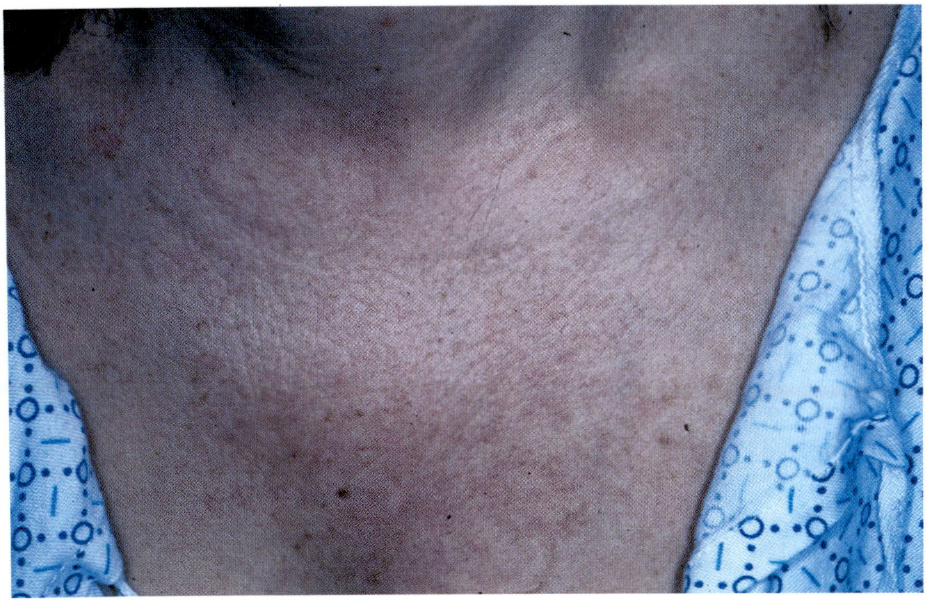

Figure 5.30. Poikiloderma of the neck before FLPDL treatment

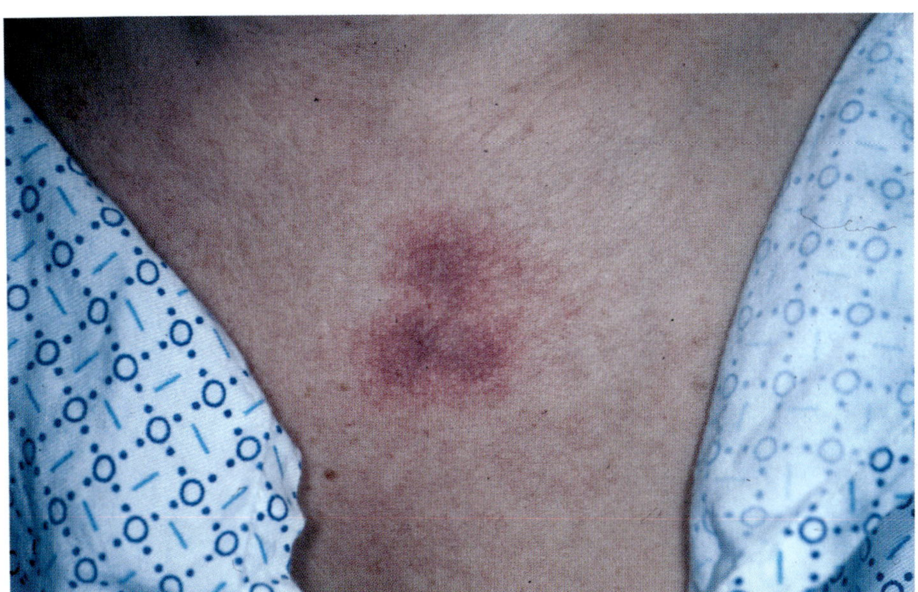

Figure 5.31. Purpura after FLPDL treatment of poikiloderma of the neck

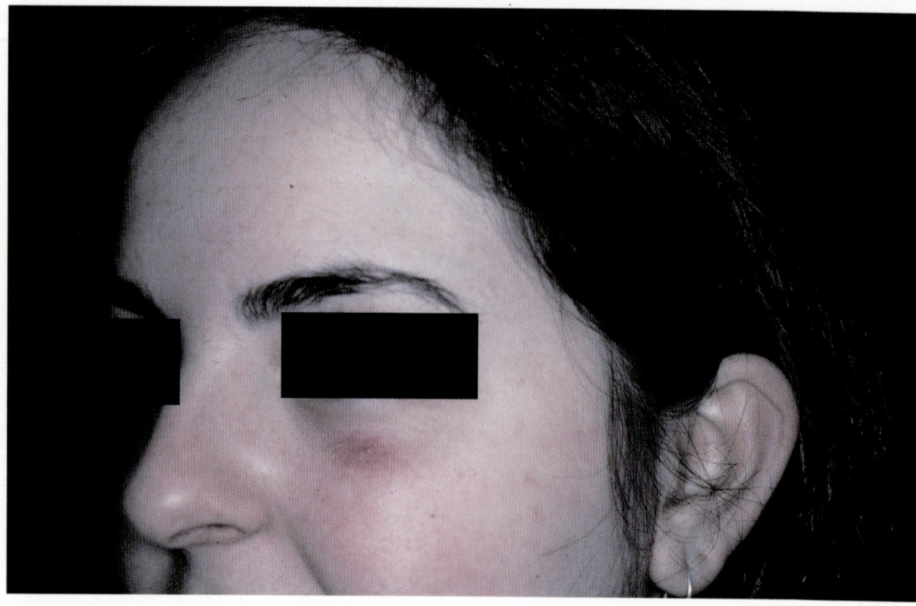

Figure 5.32. Facial telangiectasia before treatment with the FLPDL

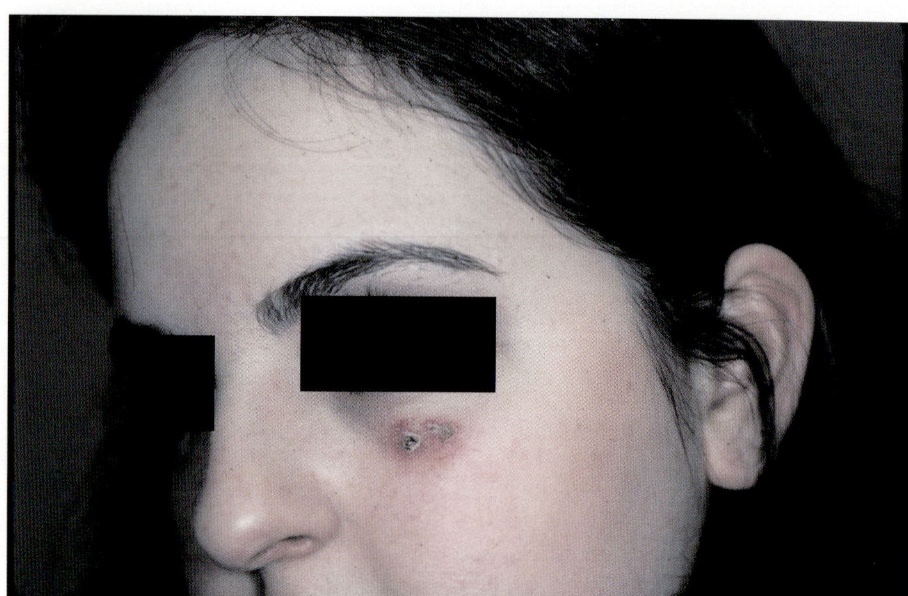

Figure 5.33. Purpura and crusting after treatment with the FLPDL

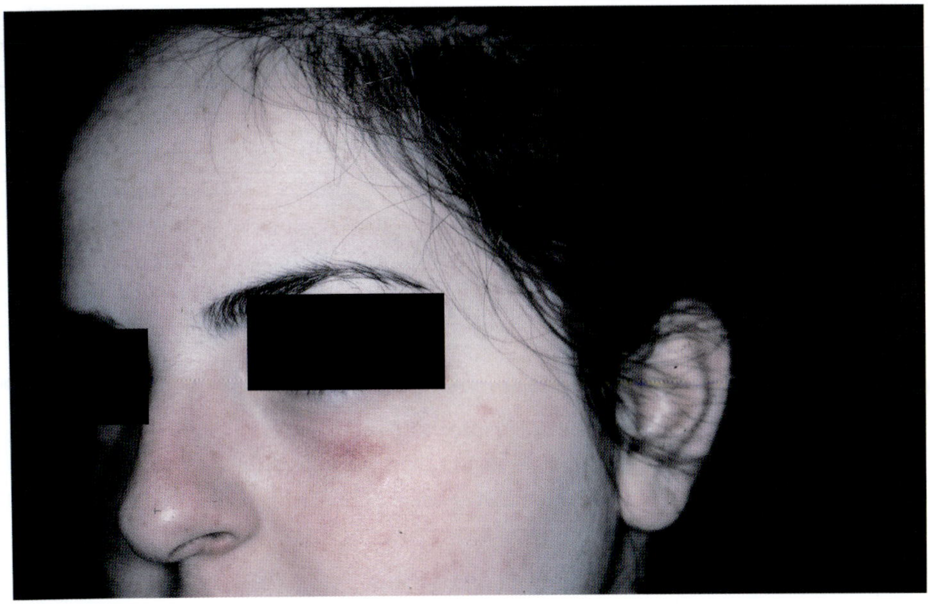

Figure 5.34. Resolution of purpura and crusting after treatment with the FLPDL

heating process, therefore, becomes less significant as pulsewidth is increased beyond the thermal relaxation time. In this situation, a greater exposure dose becomes necessary to reach therapeutic damaging temperatures.

Newer FLPDLs provide several shorter sub-pulses that extend over a time interval of up to 40 milliseconds. With these longer pulse durations, the character of the laser-induced purpura is somewhat different. It now appears more red in appearance and less purple, maroon, or violet-colored than is seen with older shorter pulsed systems.

KELOID FORMATION AND ORAL ISOTRETINOIN INTAKE

Case reports have described rare keloid formation occurring in the areas treated with either argon or pulse dye lasers during and even up to 9 months following cessation of oral isotretinoin therapy.[51–53] Controversy remains as to whether there is a true causal effect.

The most common areas of involvement are the chest, shoulders, and back, followed by the head and neck. Dark-skinned individuals are more likely to develop keloids, notably on the head and neck. Areas of skin under tension are thought to be more prone to scar formation.

Retinoids have been shown to inhibit collagenase synthesis in fibroblast cultures.[54] In addition, the retinoid induced alteration in the pilosebaceous unit, an important structure in the normal process of wound-healing, may contribute to the formation of keloids. The mechanism of action of the proposed laser/oral isotretinoin keloid formation is unclear. Although vascular lasers are theoretically selectively absorbed by hemoglobin within vascular spaces, an indirect effect on collagen may also occur due to fibroblast absorption at wavelengths of 585–595 nm.

In line with this controversy is the fact that the amount of time needed between the cessation of isotretinoin therapy and the beginning of laser therapy, to eliminate the risk of keloid formation, is not known. Although the drug is eliminated from the body (half-life <20 hours) within weeks of cessation, the effect of isotretinoin in the pilosebaceous unit generally persists for many months, as has been seen in the treatment of acne.

PIGMENTARY CHANGES

Laser-induced pigmentary changes, or dyspigmentation, is defined as a transient (resolving with in 1 year post-treatment) or permanent change in skin color on laser-treated sites as compared to adjacent normal skin. In one survey,[55] 43% of physicians reported unexpected pigmentary changes after vascular laser therapy. Usually, these changes resolve within 6 months. However, in some cases, these may persist for a longer period of time.

There is a clear association between epidermal damage and blistering and/or crust formation after FLPDL treatment.[43,56] The frequency of post laser-induced transient hyper- and hypopigmentation, is in the range of 57% and 10%, respectively.[48,49,57–59] Localization of hyperpigmentation/hypopigmentation does not show a predilection for any specific body site. Avoidance of sun exposure before and during FLPDL therapy for port wine stains (PWS) will minimize post-treatment blistering and lower the incidence of hyper- and hypopigmentation.

Hyperpigmentation

The exact pathogenesis of post laser-induced hyperpigmentation is still obscure. Hyperactive melanocytes may result from melanocyte injury. Arachidonic acid metabolites and histamine, which are found in increased concentration in inflamed skin, are also thought to play a key role in the induction of post-inflammatory hyperpigmentation.[60]

Post-laser treatment hyperpigmentation, when seen without associated epidermal injury, is likely due to laser or intense pulsed light source induced extravasation of erythrocytes through the injured vessels with resultant hemosiderin deposition and perivascular inflammation (Figures 5.35–5.42).[61]

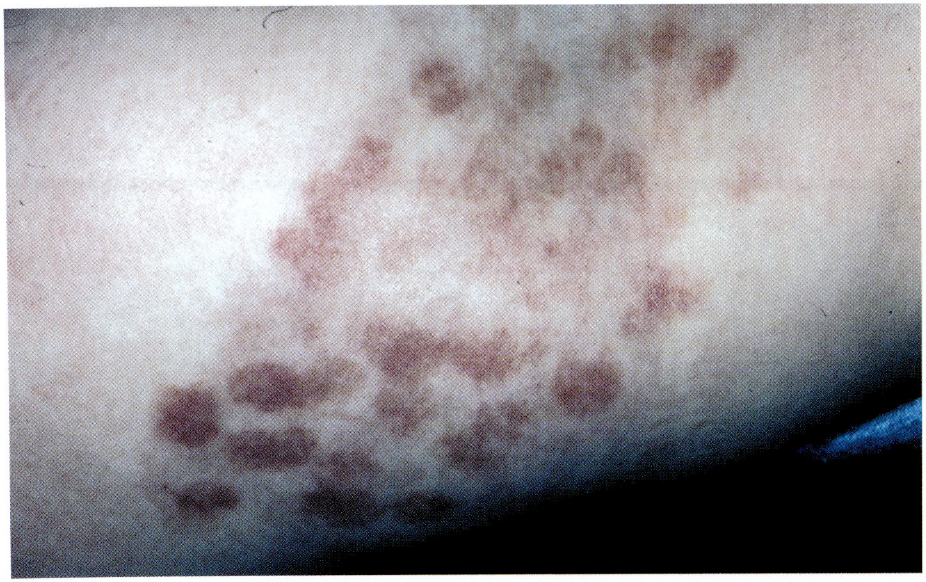

Figure 5.35. Post-inflammatory hyperpigmentation 6 months after treatment with the FLPDL

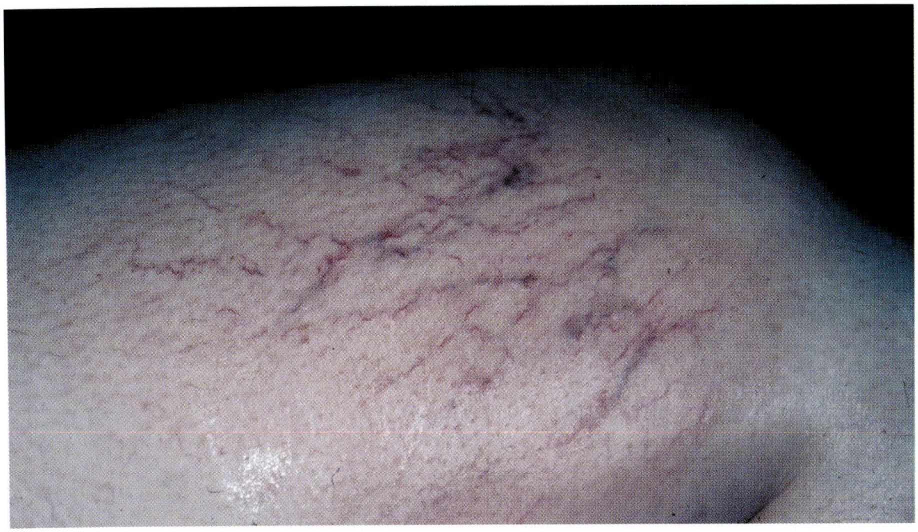

Figure 5.36. Spider veins before treatment with the Nd:YAG laser

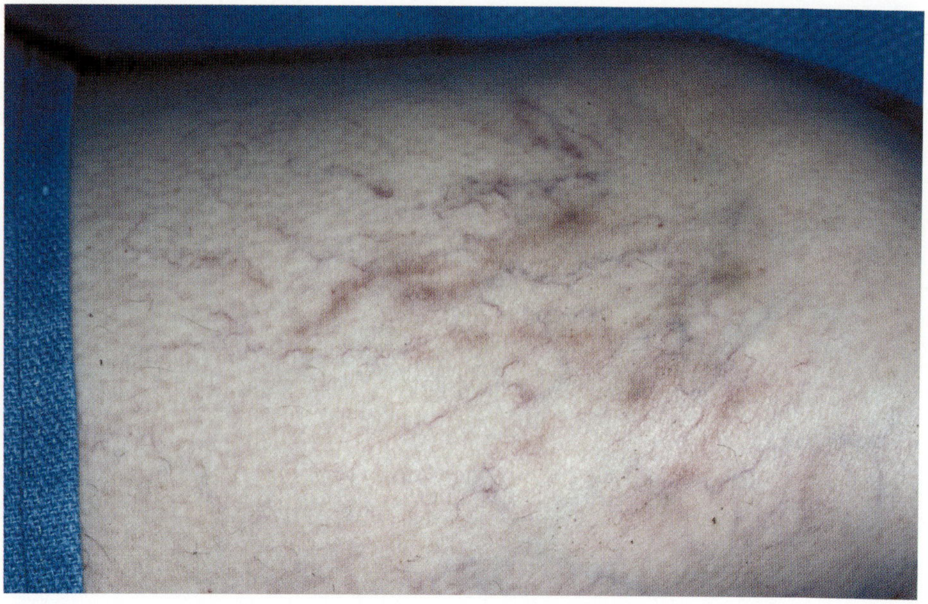

Figure 5.37. Post-inflammatory hyperpigmentation 2 months after treatment with the Nd:YAG laser

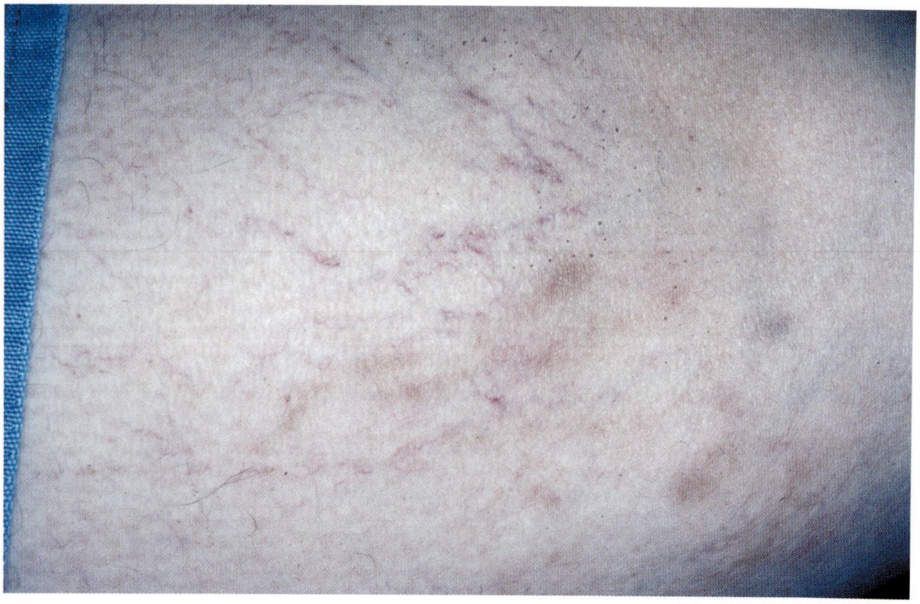

Figure 5.38. Post-inflammatory hyperpigmentation 3 months after treatment with the Nd:YAG laser

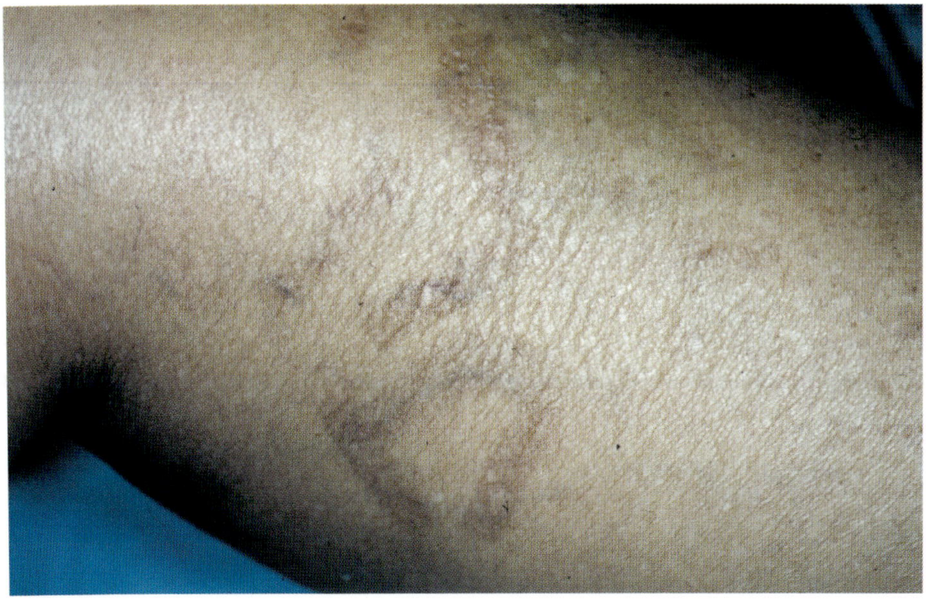

Figure 5.39. Post-inflammatory hyperpigmentation after treatment of spider veins with an intense pulsed light source

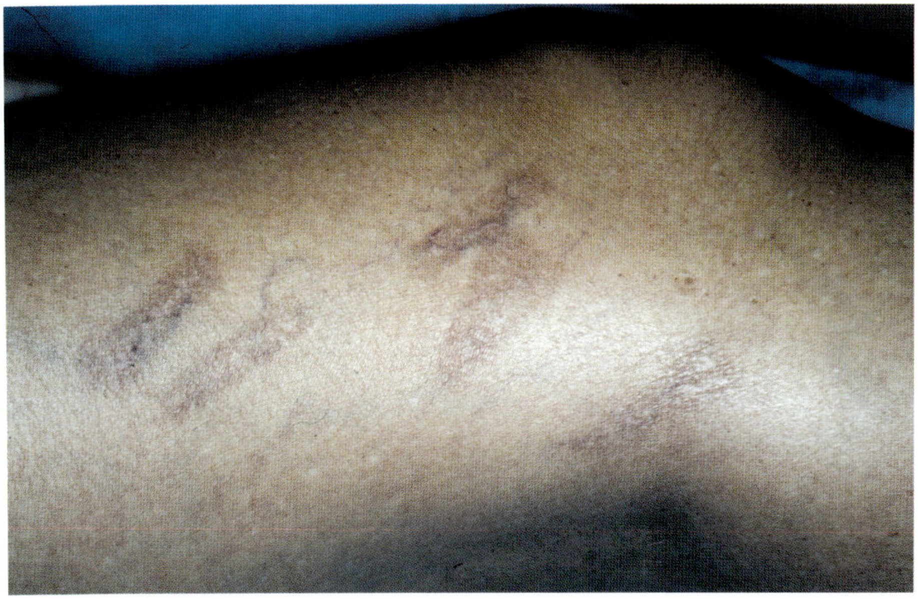

Figure 5.40. Post-inflammatory hyperpigmentation after treatment of spider veins with an intense pulsed light source

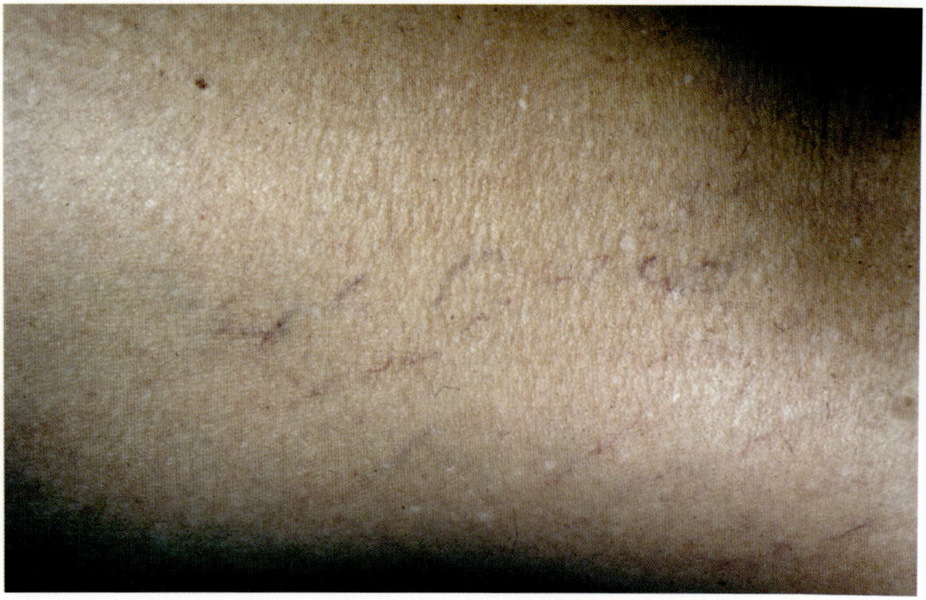

Figure 5.41. Spider veins before treatment with an intense pulsed light source

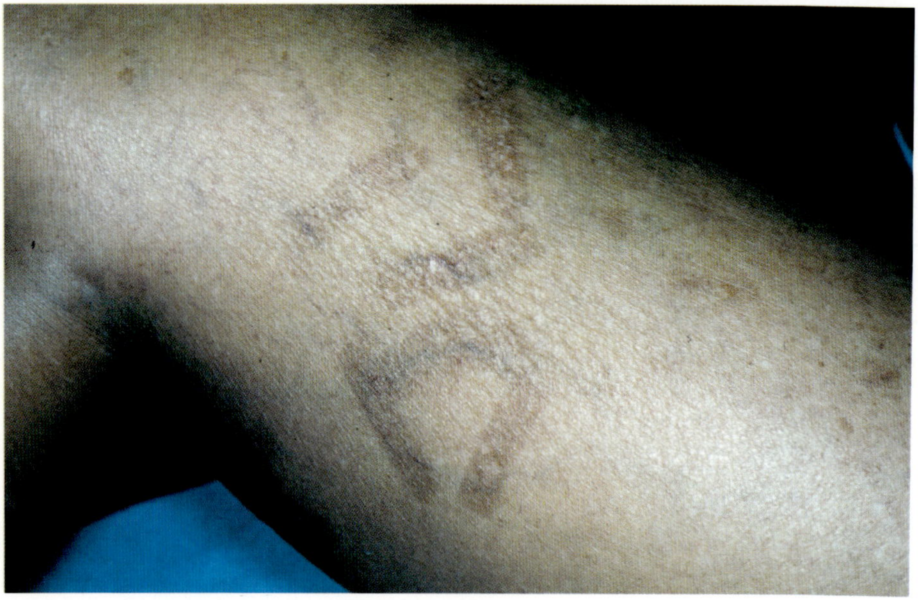

Figure 5.42. Post-inflammatory hyperpigmentation after treatment of spider veins with an intense pulsed light source

Hypopigmentation

Hypopigmentation is a relatively uncommon complication after laser treatment of vascular lesions. It is slightly more common in females than males. Females with fair complexions are more likely to experience hypopigmentation. Hypopigmentation is seen more commonly after treatment of red PSW as compared to pink or purple PSW. Hypopigmentation is most commonly seen in patients between the third and sixth decades. Hypopigmentation can also occur in 3.2% of dark-skinned patients.[62] Persistent hypopigmentation is more common on the neck, legs, and chest (Figures 5.43–5.46).

INFLAMMATORY REACTIONS

FLPDL-induced swelling and erythema are commonly seen features immediately after treatment. These findings generally resolve within 24 hours.[57] Scaling, crusting,[34,49,56] and even vesiculation,[56] have been seen, but are considered uncommon after FLPDL treatment.

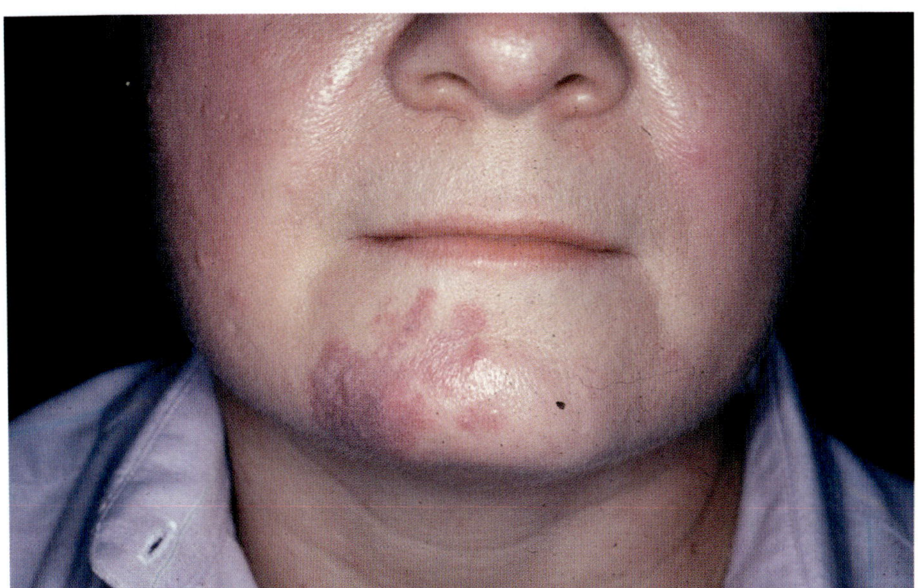

Figure 5.43. Port wine stain before treatment with the argon laser

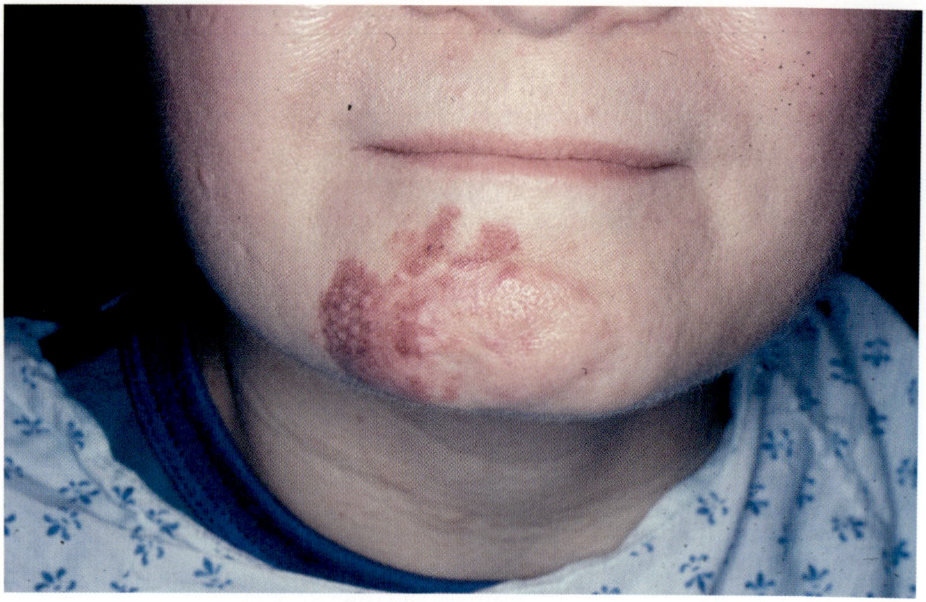

Figure 5.44. Scarring and hypopigmentation after treatment with the argon laser

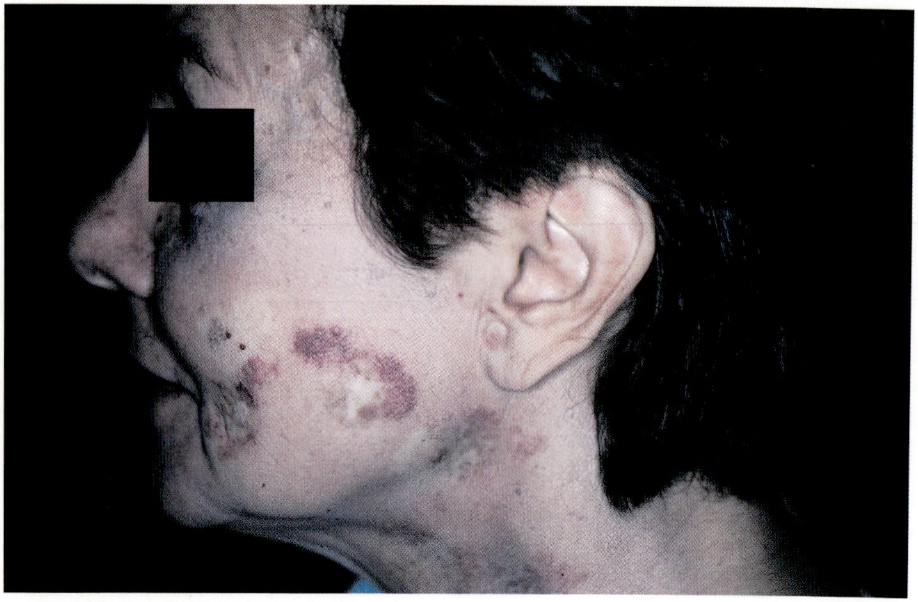

Figure 5.45. Hypopigmentation after treatment with the argon laser

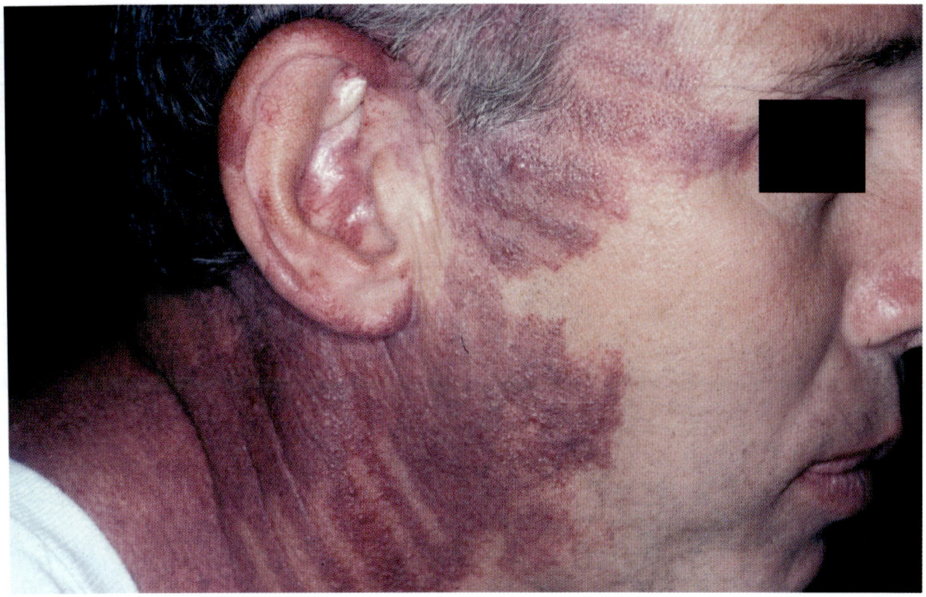

Figure 5.46. Linear streaks of hypopigmentation induced by intense pulsed light treatment of port wine stain

DERMATITIS

In some port wine stain (PWS) patients, a pruritic scaly patch may develop after FLPDL treatment. In one report, 64% of affected patients were 13 years of age or younger. All had a personal or family history of atopy. Histologic examination revealed a spongiotic dermatitis.[63]

PYOGENIC GRANULOMA

Post laser-induced pyogenic granuloma has been reported in 0.23% of laser-treated cases. It has been reported to develop in the area of laser therapy, generally seen 6 weeks after port wine stain (PWS) treatment.[49,64]

Of note, pyogenic granuloma, de novo, may occur as part of the natural history of an untreated PWS (Figure 5.47).

PAIN AND DISCOMFORT

Laser irradiation of the skin generally leads to a certain degree of discomfort. The degree of discomfort is generally laser energy-dependent, increasing with higher

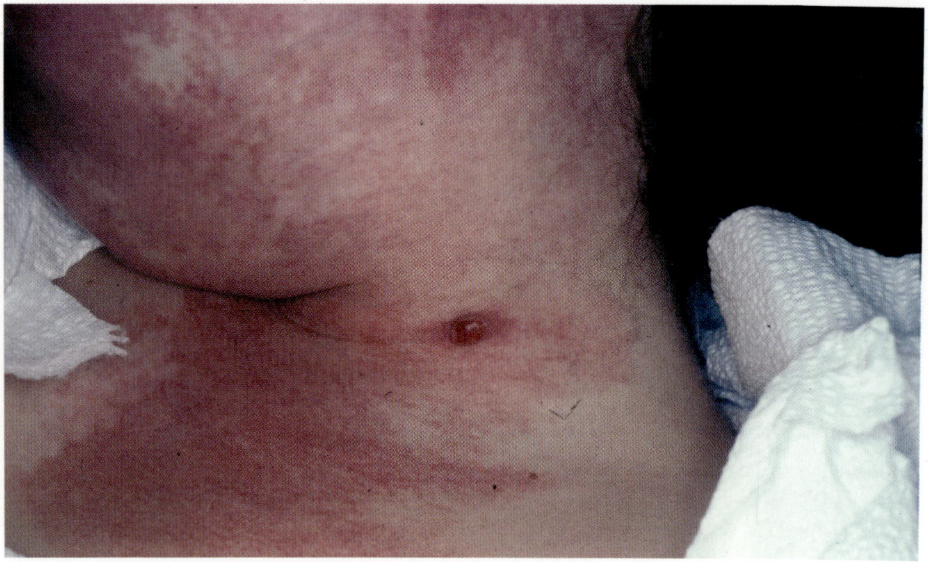

Figure 5.47. Pyogenic granuloma arising in port wine stain after FLPDL treatment

energies. It also varies with the sensitivity of the treated anatomic site. Areas, such as the central face, temple, periorbital, digital, anogenital, and plantar regions, are more sensitive to pain. Post-treatment pain is generally short-lived. However, it can last for 3 days to 3 weeks with its intensity reported as mild to severe.

CHANGE IN LIFESTYLE

A total of 45% of patients report a change in lifestyle after laser treatment of vascular lesions. They may not go out of the house for a mean of 5.6 days (range 2–14 days) after treatment. Some patients avoid social events and personal interactions. Restriction of activity in most cases occurs until post-FLPDL purpura has resolved. Swelling was also recorded as a cause of reduced activity.[49]

CONCLUSION

Flashlamp pulsed dye laser (FLPDL)-induced complications are rare and generally short-lived. A greater incidence of scarring and post-treatment pigmentary changes can be expected with the newer intense pulsed light sources and near infrared vascular lesion lasers.

REFERENCES

1 Owens N, Stephenson KL. Hemangioma: An evaluation of treatment by injection and surgery. Plast Reconstr Surg 1948;3:109–123.

2 McElfresh AE, Robbins RR. Radiation therapy of hemangiomas. J Pediatr 1961;59:311–312.

3 Brown SH Jr, Neerhont RC, Fonkalsrud EW. Prednisone therapy in the management of large hemangiomas in infants and children. Surgery 1972;71:168–173.

4 Zarem HA, Edgerton MT. Induced resolution of cavernous hemangiomas following prednisone therapy. Plast Reconstr Surg 1967;39:76–83.

5 Goldman L, Blaney DJ, Kindel DJ, et al. Pathology of the effect of the laser beam on the skin. Nature 1963;197:912–914.

6 Arndt KA. Treatment technics in argon laser therapy. J Am Acad Dermatol 1984;11:90–97.

7 Noe JM, Barsky SH, Geer DE, Rosen S. Port-wine stains and the response to argon laser therapy: Successful treatment and the predictive role of color, age, and biopsy. Plast Reconstr Surg 1980;65: 130–136.

8 Dixon JA, Huether S, Rotering R. Hypertrophic scarring in argon laser treatment of port-wine stains. Plast Recontr Surg 1984;73:771–779.

9 Tan OT, Carney JM, Margolis R, et al. Histologic responses of port-wine stains treated by argon, carbon dioxide, and tunable dye lasers: A preliminary report. Arch Dermatol 1986;122:1016–1022.

10 Cosman B. Experience in the argon laser therapy of port-wine stains. Plast Reconstr Surg 1980;65:119–129.

11 Apfelberg DB, Maser MR, Lash H. Extended clinical use of the argon laser for cutaneous lesions. Arch Dermatol 1979;115:719–721.

12 Apfelberg DB Maser MR, Lash H, Rivers JL. Progress report on extended clinical use of the argon laser for cutaneous lesions. Lasers Surg Med 1980;1:71–83.

13 Apfelberg DB, Maser MR, Lash H. Argon laser treatment of cutaneous vascular abnormalities: Progess report. Ann Plast Surg 1981;1:14–18.

14 Cosman B. Role of retreatment in minimal-power argon laser therapy for port-wine stains. Lasers Surg Med 1982;2:43–57.

15 Alster TS, Kurban AK, Grove GL, Grove MJ, Tan OT. Alteration of argon laser induced scars by the pulsed dye laser. Lasers Surg Med 1993;13:368–373.

16 Van Gemert MJC, Hulsbergen-Henning JP. A model approach to laser coagulation of dermal vascular lesions. Arch Dermatol Res 1981;270:429–439.

17 A new ray of hope for port-wine stains. Lancet 1981;1:480 [editorial].

18 Apfelberg DB, Flores JT, Maser MR, Lash H. Analysis of complications of argon laser treatment for port-wine hemangiomas with reference to striped technique. Lasers Surg Med 1983;2:357–371.

19 Gilchrest BA, Rosen S, Noe JM. Chilling port wine stains improves the response to argon lasers therapy. Plast Reconstr Surg 1982;69:278–283.

20 Barsky SH, Rosen S, Geer DE, Noe JM. The nature and evolution of port-wine stains: A computer-assisted study. J Invest Dermatol 1980;74:154–157.

21 Finley JL, Barsky SH, Geer DE, Karrat BR, Noe JM, Roen S. Healing of port-wine stains after argon laser therapy. Arch Dermatol 1981;117:486–489.

22 Fitzpatrick RE, Feinberg JA. Low dose argon laser therapy of port-wine stains. International Congress of Applied Lasers and Electric Optics '83 Proc 6:47, 1981.

23 Ohmori S, Huang CK, Takada H. Experiences upon the utilization of argon laser for treatment of port-wine stains. Transactions of the Seventh International Congress: Plastic and Reconstructive Surgery, Rio de Janeiro, 1979.

24 Scheibner A, Wheeland RG. Argon-pumped tunable dye laser therapy for facial port-wine stain hemangiomas in adults: A new technique using small spot size and minimal power. J Dermatol Surg Oncol 1989;15:277–282.

25 Dixon JA, Rotering RH, Huether SE. Patient's evaluation of argon laser therapy of port-wine stains, decorative tattoo, and essential telangiectasia. Lasers Surg Med 1984;4:181–190.

26 Rottenleur G, Mordon S, Buys B, et al. Robotized scanning laser handpiece for the treatment of port wine stains and other angiodysplasias. Lasers Surg Med 1988;8:283–287.

27 Carruth JAS. The establishment of precise physical parameters for the treatment of port-wine stains with the argon laser. Lasers Surg Med 1982;2:37–42.

28 West TB, Alster TS. Comparison of the long pulse dye (590–595 nm) and KTP (532 nm) lasers in the treatment of facial and leg telangiectasias. Dermatol Surg 1998;24:221–226.

29 Arndt KA. Treatment techniques in argon laser therapy: Comparison of pulsed and continuous exposures. J Am Acad Dermatol 1984;11:90–97.

30 Apfelberg DB, Maser MR, Lash H. Argon laser management of cutaneous vascular deformities. West J Med 1976;124:99–101.

31 Anderson RR, Parish JA. The optics of human skin. J Invest Dermatol 1981;77:13–19.

32 Tonge AKF, Tan OT, Boll J, Parrish JA, Murphy GF. Ultrastructure: effects of melanin pigment on target specificity using a pulsed dye laser (577 nm). J Invest Dermatol 1987;88:747–752.

33 Patterson MS, Wilson BC, Wyman DR. The propagation of optical properties of tissue and resulting fluence distributions. Lasers Med Sci 1991;6:379–390.

34 Swinehart JM. Hypertrophic scarring resulting from flashlamp-pumped pulsed dye laser surgery. J Am Acad Dermatol 1991;25:845–846.

35 Bailin PL. Treatment of port-wine stains with the CO_2 laser: Early results. In: Arndt KA, Noe JM, Rosen S, eds. Cutaneous Laser Therapy: Principles and Methods. New York: Wiley; 1983:129–136.

36 Anderson RR, Parrish JA. Microvasculature can be selectively damaged using lasers: A basic theory and experimental evidence in human skin. Lasers Surg Med 1981;1:263–276.

37 Greenwald J, Rosen S, Anderson RR, et al. Comparative histological studies of the tunable dye (at 577 nm) laser and argon laser: Specific vascular effects of the dye laser. J Invest Dermatol 1981;77:305–310.

38 Garden JM, Tan OT, Kerschmann R, et al. Normal human skin response to varying parameters of pulsed dye laser irradiation. J Invest Dermatol 1982; 78: 172–175.

39 Nakagama H, Tan OT, Parrish JA. Ultrastructural changes after pulsed laser radiation. J Invest Dermatol 1985;84:396–400.

40 Tan OT, Kerschmann R, Parrish JA. The effects of epidermal pigmentation on selective vascular effects of pulsed laser. Lasers Surg Med 1984;4:365–374.

41 Anderson RR, Parrish JA. Selective photothermolysis: Precise microsurgery by selective absorption of pulsed radiation. Science 1983;220:524–527.

42 Tan OT, Kerschmann R, Parrish JA. Effects of skin temperature on selective vascular injury caused by pulsed laser irradiation. J Invest Dermatol 1985;85:441–444.

43 Goldman MP, Fitzpatrick RE. Treatment of cutaneous vascular lesions. In: Goldman MP, Fitzpatrick RE, eds. Cutaneous Laser Surgery: The Art and Science of Selective Thermolysis. St. Louis, MO: Mosby; 1994:91–105.

44 Ashinoff R, Geronemus RG. Treatment of a port-wine stain in a black patient with the pulsed dye laser. J Dermatol Surg Oncol 1992;18:147–148.

45 Tan OT, Stafford TJ. Treatment of port-wine stains at 577 nm: Clinical results. Med Instrum 1987;21:218–221.

46 Polla LL, Tan OT, Garden JM, Parrish JA. Tunable pulsed dye laser for treatment of benign cutaneous vascular ectasia. Dermatologica 1987;174:11–17.

47 Garden JM, Tan OT, Parrish JA. The pulsed dye laser: Its use at 577 nm wave length. J Dermatol Surg Oncol 1987;13:134–138.

48 Tan OT, Sherwood K, Gilchrest BA. Successful treatment of children with port wine stains using the flashlamp-pulsed tunable dye laser. N Engl J Med 1989;320:416–421.

49 Lanigan SW. Patient-reported morbidity following flashlamp-pumped pulsed tunable dye laser treatment of port-wine stains. Br J Dermatol 1995;133:423–425.

50 Garden JM, Polla LL, Tan OT. The treatment of port-wine stains by pulsed dye laser. Arch Dermatol 1988;124:889–896.
51 Bernstein LJ, Geronemus RG. Keloid formation with the 585 nm pulsed dye laser during isotretinoin treatment. Arch Dermatol 1997;133:111–112.
52 Zachariea H. Delayed wound healing and keloid formation following argon laser treatment or dermabrasion during isotretinoin treatment. Br J Dermatol 1988;118:703–706.
53 Rubenstein R, Roenigk HH, Stegman S, Hanke CW. Atypical keloids after dermabrasion of patients taking isotretinoin. J Am Acad Dermatol 1986;15:280–285.
54 Bauer EA, Seltzer JL, Eisen AZ. Inhibition of collagen degradative enzymes by retinoic acid in vitro. J Am Acad Dermatol 1982;6:603–607.
55 Olbricht SM, Stern RS, Tang SV, Noe JM, Arndt KA. Complications of cutaneous laser surgery: A survey. Arch Dermatol 1987;123:345–349.
56 Garden JM, Bakus AD. Clinical efficacy of the pulsed dye laser in the treatment of vascular lesions. J Dermatol Surg Oncol 1993;19:321–326.
57 Reyes BA, Geronemus RG. Treatment of port-wine stains during childhood with the flashlamp-pumped pulsed dye laser. J Am Acad Dermatol 1990;23:1142–1148.
58 Glassberg E, Lask GP, Tan EML, Uitto J. The flashlamp-pumped 577 nm pulsed tunable dye laser: Clinical efficacy and in vitro studies. J Dermatol Surg Oncol 1988;14:1200–1208.
59 Renfro L, Geronemus RG. Anatomical differences of port-wine stains in response to treatment with the pulsed dye laser. Arch Dermatol 1993;129:182–188.
60 Tomita Y, Maeda K, Tegami H. Mechanisms for hyperpigmentation in post inflammatory pigmentation, urticaria pigmentosa and sunburn. Dermatologica 1989;179 (Suppl 1):49–53.
61 Goldman MP, Fitzpatrick RE. Pulsed dye laser treatment of leg telangiectasia: with and without simultaneous sclerotherapy. J Dermatol Surg Oncol 1990;16:338–344.
62 Archauer BM, Vander Kam VM, Padilla III JF. Clinical experience with the tunable pulsed dye laser (585 nm) in the treatment of capillary vascular malformations. Plast Reconstr Surg 1993;92:1233.
63 Lavine VJ, Geronemus RG. Adverse effects associated with the 577 and 585 nm pulsed dye laser in the treatment of cutaneous vascular lesions: A study of 500 patients. J Am Acad Dermatol 1988;124:889–896.
64 Abd-Al-Raheem TA, Hohenleutner U, Landthaler M. Granuloma pyogenicum as a complication of flashlamp-pumped pulsed dye laser. Dermatology 1994;189:283–285.

INDEX